HPV, Colposcopy, and Prevention of Squamous Anogenital Tract Malignancy

Editors

ALAN G. WAXMAN
MARIA LINA DIAZ

OBSTETRICS AND GYNECOLOGY CLINICS OF NORTH AMERICA

www.obgyn.theclinics.com

Consulting Editor
WILLIAM F. RAYBURN

June 2013 • Volume 40 • Number 2

ELSEVIER

1600 John F. Kennedy Boulevard • Suite 1800 • Philadelphia, Pennsylvania, 19103-2899

http://www.theclinics.com

OBSTETRICS AND GYNECOLOGY CLINICS OF NORTH AMERICA Volume 40, Number 2
June 2013 ISSN 0889-8545, ISBN-13: 978-1-4557-7128-8

Editor: Stephanie Donley

Obstetrics and Gynecology Clinics (ISSN 0889-8545) is published quarterly by Elsevier Inc., 360 Park Avenue South, New York, NY 10010-1710. Months of issue are March, June, September, and December. Periodicals postage paid at New York, NY, and additional mailing offices. Subscription price per year is $293.00 (US individuals), $518.00 (US institutions), $146.00 (US students), $353.00 (Canadian individuals), $652.00 (Canadian institutions), $214.00 (Canadian students), $428.00 (foreign individuals), $652.00 (foreign institutions), and $214.00 (foreign students). To receive student/resident rate, orders must be accompanied by name of affiliated institution, date of term, and the signature of program/residency coordinator on institution letterhead. Orders will be billed at individual rate until proof of status is received. Foreign air speed delivery is included in all *Clinics* subscription prices. All prices are subject to change without notice. POSTMASTER: Send address changes to *Obstetrics and Gynecology Clinics*, Elsevier Health Sciences Division, Subscription Customer Service, 3251 Riverport Lane, Maryland Heights, MO 63043. **Customer Service: Telephone: 1-800-654-2452 (U.S. and Canada); 314-447-8871 (outside U.S. and Canada). Fax: 314-447-8029. E-mail: journalscustomerservice-usa@elsevier.com (for print support); journalsonlinesupport-usa@elsevier.com (for online support).**

Reprints. For copies of 100 or more of articles in this publication, please contact the Commercial Reprints Department, Elsevier Inc., 360 Park Avenue South, New York, New York 10010-1710. Tel.: 212-633-3818; Fax: 212-462-1935; E-mail: reprints@elsevier.com.

Obstetrics and Gynecology Clinics of North America is also published in Spanish by McGraw-Hill Interamericana Editores S.A., P.O. Box 5-237, 06500, Mexico; in Portuguese by Reichmann and Affonso Editores, Rio de Janeiro, Brazil; and in Greek by Paschalidis Medical Publications, Athens, Greece.

Obstetrics and Gynecology Clinics of North America is covered In MEDLINE/PubMed (Index Medicus), Excerpta Medica, Current Concepts/Clinical Medicine, Science Citation Index, BIOSIS, CINAHL, and ISI/BIOMED.

Printed and bound by CPI Group (UK) Ltd, Croydon, CR0 4YY

Transferred to digital print 2012

Contributors

CONSULTING EDITOR

WILLIAM F. RAYBURN, MD, MBA
Department of Obstetrics and Gynecology, University of New Mexico School of Medicine, Albuquerque, New Mexico

EDITORS

ALAN G. WAXMAN, MD, MPH
Professor, Department of Obstetrics and Gynecology, University of New Mexico School of Medicine, Albuquerque, New Mexico

MARIA LINA DIAZ, MD, FACOG
Head, Section of Ambulatory Gynecology, Department of Gynecology, Cleveland Clinic Florida, Weston, Florida

AUTHORS

KEVIN AULT, MD
Department of Gynecology and Obstetrics, Emory University School of Medicine, Atlanta, Georgia

LORI A. BOARDMAN, MD, ScM
Assistant Dean of Medical Education and Professor of Obstetrics and Gynecology, Departments of Clinical Sciences and Medical Education, Health Sciences Campus at Lake Nona, University of Central Florida College of Medicine, Orlando, Florida

JACOB BORNSTEIN, MD, MPA
Professor and Chairman, Department of Obstetrics and Gynecology, Western Galilee Hospital, Nahariya, Israel

PHILIP E. CASTLE, PhD, MPH
Global Cancer Initiative, Chestertown, Maryland

DAVID CHELMOW, MD
Professor, Department of Obstetrics and Gynecology, Virginia Commonwealth University School of Medicine, Richmond, Virginia

MIRIAM CREMER, MD, MPH
Assistant Professor, Department of Obstetrics and Gynecology, University of Pittsburgh, Pittsburgh, Pennsylvania; The Mount Sinai Medical Center, Basic Health International, New York, New York

MARIA LINA DIAZ, MD, FACOG
Head, Section of Ambulatory Gynecology, Department of Gynecology, Cleveland Clinic Florida, Weston, Florida

iv   Contributors

LISA FLOWERS, MD
Associate Professor, Division of Gynecologic Oncology, Department of Gynecology and Obstetrics, Emory University School of Medicine, Atlanta, Georgia

FRANCISCO GARCÍA, MD, MPH, FACOG
Center of Excellence in Women's Health, University of Arizona, Tucson, Arizona

LEDA GATTOC, MD
Department of Gynecology and Obstetrics, Emory University School of Medicine, Atlanta, Georgia

JULIE GOBER-WILCOX, MD
Department of Pathology, University of New Mexico Health Sciences Center, Albuquerque, New Mexico

NANCY JOSTE, MD
Professor of Pathology, Director, Division of Anatomic Pathology, Department of Pathology, University of New Mexico Health Sciences Center, Albuquerque, New Mexico

NICOLE KARJANE, MD
Associate Professor, Department of Obstetrics and Gynecology, Virginia Commonwealth University School of Medicine, Richmond, Virginia

MICHELLE J. KHAN, MD, MPH
Clinical Instructor, Department of Obstetrics, Gynecology, and Reproductive Sciences, University of California, San Francisco, San Francisco, California

LAWRENCE LEEMAN, MD, MPH
Professor, Departments of Family and Community Medicine and Obstetrics and Gynecology, University of New Mexico, Albuquerque, New Mexico

STEPHANIE LONG, MD
Maternal Child Health Fellow, Department of Family and Community Medicine, University of New Mexico, Albuquerque, New Mexico

E.J. MAYEAUX Jr, MD
Professor of Family Medicine, Professor of Obstetrics and Gynecology, Departments of Family Medicine and Obstetrics and Gynecology, Family Medicine Program Director and Vice-Chair, Louisiana State University Health Sciences Center, Shreveport, Louisiana

NAVYA NAIR, MD, MPH
Department of Gynecology and Obstetrics, Emory University School of Medicine, Atlanta, Georgia

ERIN L. NELSON, MD
Assistant Professor, Department of Obstetrics and Gynecology, University of Texas, San Antonio, Texas

MINH LY NGUYEN, MD, MPH
Assistant Professor, Division of Infectious Disease, Department of Internal Medicine, Emory University School of Medicine, Atlanta, Georgia

TOMAS NUÑO, PhD
The Clinical Outcomes and Comparative Effectiveness Research Fellowship Program, The Arizona Cancer Center, Center of Excellence in Women's Health, University of Arizona, Tucson, Arizona

WALTER PRENDIVILLE, FRCOG
The Gynae Clinic, Mount Carmel Hospital, Churchtown, Dublin, Ireland

KATINA ROBISON, MD
The Program in Women's Oncology, Women and Infants' Hospital of Rhode Island,
Assistant Professor of Obstetrics and Gynecology, The Warren Alpert Medical School of
Brown University; Providence, Rhode Island

COLLEEN K. STOCKDALE, MD, MS
Associate Clinical Professor, Department of Obstetrics and Gynecology, University of
Iowa, Iowa City, Iowa

JODY STONEHOCKER, MD
Assistant Professor, Division of Gynecology, Department of Obstetrics and Gynecology,
University of New Mexico, Albuquerque, New Mexico

SILVIO TATTI, MD, MSc, PhD
Buenos Aires University Hospital de Clinicas, Austria, Caba, Argentina

ALAN G. WAXMAN, MD, MPH
Professor, Department of Obstetrics and Gynecology, University of New Mexico School
of Medicine, Albuquerque, New Mexico

COSETTE MARIE WHEELER, PhD
Regents Professor, Departments of Pathology and Obstetrics and Gynecology,
University of New Mexico Health Sciences Center, Albuquerque, New Mexico

MEGGAN ZSEMLYE, MD
Associate Professor, Department of Obstetrics and Gynecology, University of
New Mexico School of Medicine, Albuquerque, New Mexico

Contents

> Genital human papillomavirus (HPV) infection is the most common sexually
> transmitted infection. Most HPV infections are benign and resolve on their
> own, but some women develop persistent HPV infections. Persistent HPV
> infection with certain high-risk HPV genotypes is the necessary cause of
> most epithelial lesions of the uterine cervix. The importance of latent or
> quiescent HPV, waning immunity, hormonal milieu, microbiota, and other
> factors modifying the natural history of HPV infections across a woman's
> lifetime deserves further study. Promising biomarkers are emerging that
> may aid in defining which HPV-infected women are at risk of developing
> invasive cervical cancer.

> Human papillomavirus (HPV) is one of the most common sexually trans-
> mitted infections affecting both men and women worldwide. The develop-
> ment of the prophylactic HPV vaccines is a significant pharmaceutical
> innovation with potential to reduce HPV-related morbidity. However,
> barriers to the universal use and acceptability of the HPV vaccines
> continue to exist in both economically privileged and disadvantaged
> countries. It may be decades before the impact of preventive vaccines
> on HPV-related diseases caused by the considerable burden of HPV
> infections will be seen. Collaborative efforts must continue to promote
> vaccine implementation.

> New recommendations for screening intervals across different age groups
> is leading to a diminished role for the cytology laboratory and an increased
> role for the human papillomavirus (HPV) testing laboratory. With the intro-
> duction of the liquid-based Papanicolaou test, high-risk HPV testing, and
> computer-assisted screening, the cytology laboratory is at the forefront
> of efforts to improve screening for the provision of better patient care.
> Cytology laboratories are ideally positioned to facilitate important basic
> and applied research involving cervical cancer.

Guidelines for cervical cancer screening have continued to evolve as we have accumulated new information about the pathogenesis of cervical cancer and the role of the human papilloma virus. Most recently, the American Cancer Society, the American Society for Colposcopy and Cervical Pathology, and the American Society for Clinical Pathology issued revised joint recommendations for the prevention and early detection of cervical cancer. In addition, the US Preventative Services Task Force revised its guidelines, and the American College of Obstetricians and Gynecologists updated its practice bulletin.

Based on a growing need for unified terminology to describe the pathologic and clinical spectrum of lesions, the American Society for Colposcopy and Cervical Pathology and the College of American Pathologists Pathology and Laboratory Quality Center convened the Lower Anogenital Squamous Terminology (LAST) Project to reassess and harmonize the terminology used to describe human papillomavirus-associated squamous lesions of the lower anogenital tract as manifested in a variety of end organs. The distinction between cancer precursors and those without malignant potential leads to consistency in the interpretation of management guidelines and the therapeutic options.

This article describes the current nomenclature of colposcopic findings in the lower genital tract as defined by the International Federation for Cervical Pathology and Colposcopy (IFCPC) and agreed at their Triennial General Meeting in July 2012 in Rio de Janeiro. It builds on previous nomenclature published by the IFCPC over the last two decades and introduces for the first time the concept of transformation zone excision types. Vulval and vaginal colposcopic terminology is described.

Developments from late 2011 to early 2013, including consensus conferences and the introduction of low-cost, rapid-turnaround testing of human papillomavirus, will change prevention strategies for cervical cancer in the United States and in low- and middle-income countries.

Recent guidelines from multiple organizations stress screening initiation no earlier than the age of 21 years and increased screening intervals for women aged 21 to 29 years. Primary prevention with human papillomavirus vaccination has the potential to significantly affect the development of high-grade cervical lesions, including cancer, and will likely affect screening guidelines in the future.

Cervical cancer is the most commonly diagnosed malignancy during pregnancy with an incidence of 1.5 to 12 per 100,000 pregnancies. In the United States between 2% and 7% of all pregnant women will have an abnormal Pap test. The management of these abnormal results during pregnancy can present a challenge to the practitioner. This article reviews recently published guidelines and current evidence for evaluation and management of abnormal cervical cytology and cervical cancer in pregnancy.

The management of low-grade squamous intraepithelial lesions (LSIL) has changed greatly over the past 2 decades. The most recent recommendations propose avoiding treatment while continuing to monitor patients for clearance of disease or a change to a more severe diagnosis. Knowledge of the correct way to manage LSIL is important because LSIL is a relatively common diagnosis found on cervical cytology. Especially since the introduction of liquid-based cytology, the diagnosis of LSIL has become more frequent. The College of American Pathologists estimated in 2003 that the reporting rate for LSIL was 2.9%.

The introduction of testing for high-risk HPV types and P16 Immunostaining of CIN2 histologic specimens allows for determination of the risk of progression versus regression for a woman with a particular cytologic or histologic specimen. Observation with serial cytological or colposcopic examinations is now appropriate for women with low-grade histologic lesions as well as pregnant and young women with certain high-grade histologic lesions. Current recommendations for management of high-grade lesions, the efficacy of treatment options (cryotherapy and LEEP), and the immediate (bleeding, infection) and longer term complications (cervical incompetence, preterm delivery) of cervical dysplasia treatment are presented.

Human papillomavirus (HPV) is the most common viral cause of cancer, and is responsible for 5% of cancers worldwide. Following demonstration of the causative link between HPV and cervical cancer, HPV has been shown to be associated with several anogenital malignancies and with oral pharyngeal cancers. HPV-related anal and oral pharyngeal disease is rising in incidence and includes anal warts and neoplasia, recurrent

clinician can build counseling strategies. It is paramount to relay accurate, timely, and clear information in a reassuring manner. Emphasis is placed on encouraging patients to adopt healthy and protective measures, such as lifestyle changes, testing for other sexually transmitted diseases, compliance with surveillance and screening visits, and vaccination against HPV in age-appropriate individuals.

OBSTETRICS AND GYNECOLOGY CLINICS

DOWNLOAD
Free App!

Review Articles
THE CLINICS

NOW AVAILABLE FOR YOUR iPhone and iPad

Foreword

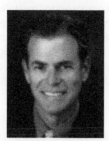

William F. Rayburn, MD, MBA
Consulting Editor

This issue, guest edited by Dr Alan Waxman and Dr Maria Diaz, provides a comprehensive review on the prevention of and screening for cervical cancer. Keeping updated can be challenging, and understanding guidelines for screening for cervical cancer and its precursors requires periodic clarification. As Dr Waxman and Dr Diaz mention in their preface, this field has undergone numerous changes since our last issue on this subject published five years ago.

Screening for cervical cancer represents a true success story, since most cases now occur among women who were either never screened or inadequately screened. As a result, the incidence of cervical cancer in the United States has decreased by more than 50% in the past 30 years. Despite this, women who are immigrants to the United States, those lacking a regular source of health care, and the uninsured are especially at risk. Cervical cancer is much more common worldwide, especially in countries without screening programs.

This issue highlights risk-benefit considerations for women at different ages. Screening should begin at age 21 years. Women aged 21 to 29 years should be tested with cervical cytology alone, and screening should be performed every 3 years. For those aged 30 to 65 years, cotesting with cytology and HPV testing every 5 years is preferred. Women with negative cytology and positive HPV cotesting results who are aged 30 years and older should be evaluated by either repeat cotesting in 12 months or immediate HPV genotype-specific testing for HPV-16 and HPV-18. Women who received the HPV vaccine should be screened according to the same guidelines as those who have not been vaccinated.

Both liquid-based and conventional methods of cervical cytology collection remain acceptable for screening. As highlighted in this issue, new technologies and novel tools for cervical cancer screening continue to evolve as do recommendations for managing the results. Evidence-based information from national consensus conferences and reports offer major redefinitions and nomenclature changes for the histopathology of squamous intraepithelial lesions across the lower anogenital tract. Another major change in terminology for findings seen on colposcopy is mentioned in this issue.

Obstet Gynecol Clin N Am 40 (2013) xiii–xiv
http://dx.doi.org/10.1016/j.ogc.2013.03.010
0889-8545/13/$ – see front matter © 2013 Published by Elsevier Inc.

obgyn.theclinics.com

Also noteworthy are clinically relevant articles pertaining to screening adolescents and young women, colposcopy in pregnancy, nongenital HPV disease, special considerations for immunocompromised patients, and current advice in counseling the patient with HPV disease. It is my desire that this comprehensive issue activates the reader's attention to topics of cutting-edge interest in cervical cancer prevention and screening. On behalf of Dr Waxman, Dr Diaz, and their excellent group of knowledgeable contributors, I hope that the practical information provided herein will aid in the implementation of well-planned approaches in evaluating and recommending treatment for our patients of all ages.

William F. Rayburn, MD, MBA
Department of Obstetrics and Gynecology
University of New Mexico School of Medicine
MSC10 5580; 1 University of New Mexico
Albuquerque, NM 87131-0001, USA

E-mail address:
wrayburn@salud.unm.edu

Preface

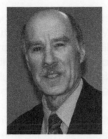 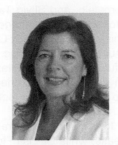

Alan G. Waxman, MD, MPH   Maria Lina Diaz, MD, FACOG
Editors

In the 5 years since *Obstetrics and Gynecology Clinics of North America* last published an issue devoted to colposcopy and the prevention of cervical cancer, there have been significant developments in the field. While our understanding of the natural history of squamous lesions caused by infections with the human papillomavirus (HPV) has undergone incremental changes, the regimens for prevention of HPV-related cancers have changed more dramatically. In this issue we highlight some of those changes.

Between November 2011 and September 2012, the American Society for Colposcopy and Cervical Pathology (ASCCP) cosponsored 3 major consensus conferences devoted to different aspects of preventing cancers of the cervix and other organs of the anogenital tract. The first, in collaboration with the American Cancer Society (ACS) and American Society for Clinical Pathology (ASCP), resulted in new guidelines for screening for cervical cancer and its precursors.[1] The timing of the release of these recommendations was coordinated to coincide with very similar guidelines from the US Preventive Services Task Force.[2] Subsequently, the American College of Obstetricians and Gynecologists (ACOG) endorsed the recommendations in its practice bulletin no. 131.[3] In this issue, Dr David Chelmow, a participant in both the ACS/ASCCP/ASCP and the ACOG processes along with Dr Nicole Karjane, explains these recommendations from onset of screening to when to stop and the various permutations of cytology and HPV testing in between. A consensus conference, held in September 2012 by ASCCP, with results published in March 2013,[4] used new data to refine the 2006 ASCCP Consensus Guidelines for management of abnormal screening and biopsy results. Because these recommendations cross a number of clinical situations, we have chosen to include them within several articles that examine specific clinical situations. These are ably written by Drs Meggan Zsemlye, Larry Leeman with Stephanie Long, Jody Stonehocker, and Lori Boardman with Katina Robison.

Drs Tomas Nuño and Francisco Garcia discuss the recommendations of the LAST project conference—cosponsored by ASCCP and the College of American Pathologists.[5] This evidence-based consensus conference recommended a major redefinition and nomenclature change for the histopathology of squamous intraepithelial lesions across the lower anogenital tract. Another major change in terminology has been proposed for findings seen on colposcopy. This nomenclature proposed

Obstet Gynecol Clin N Am 40 (2013) xv–xvi
http://dx.doi.org/10.1016/j.ogc.2013.03.009
0889-8545/13/$ – see front matter © 2013 Published by Elsevier Inc.

by the International Federation for Cervical Pathology and Colposcopy is presented in this monograph along with an international perspective of colposcopy by Drs Walter Prendiville, Jacob Bornstein, and Silvio Tatti.

In addition to new guidelines for screening, management, and terminology, we've included updates on the natural history of HPV by Dr Cosette Wheeler and the status of HPV vaccines by Drs Kevin Ault and Leda Gattoc. Drs Philip Castle and Miriam Cremer discuss the current and future uses of HPV testing, focusing on its potential for cervical cancer prevention in developing countries. Drs Nancy Joste and Julie Gober-Wilcox give us a close-up look at cytology screening and HPV testing from the laboratorian's viewpoint.

In their respective articles, Dr Maria Diaz gives practical guidance for counseling the patient with HPV-related disease, while Dr Lisa Flowers discusses management of the immunocompromised patient. Dr EJ Mayeaux and Drs Erin Nelson and Colleen Stockdale discuss HPV-related lesions beyond the cervix.

In sum, we've tried in this small monograph to provide the clinician with a comprehensive update on the clinical, basic science, and public health aspects of HPV-related lower anogenital tract disease. We hope you find it useful for your practice.

Alan G. Waxman, MD, MPH
University of New Mexico School of Medicine
Department of Obstetrics and Gynecology
MSC 10 5580
1 University of New Mexico
Albuquerque, NM 87131-0001, USA

Maria Lina Diaz, MD, FACOG
Department of Gynecology
Cleveland Clinic Florida
2950 Cleveland Clinic Boulevard
Weston, FL 33331, USA

E-mail addresses:
awaxman@salud.unm.edu (A.G. Waxman)
marialinadiaz@gmail.com (M.L. Diaz)

REFERENCES

1. Saslow D, Solomon D, Lawson HW, et al. American Cancer Society, American Society for Colposcopy and Cervical Pathology, and American Society for Clinical Pathology Screening Guidelines for the Prevention and Early Detection of Cervical Cancer. J Low Genit Tract Dis 2012;16(3):175–204.
2. Moyer VA. U.S. Preventive Services Task Force. Screening for cervical cancer: U.S. Preventive Services Task Force recommendation statement. Ann Intern Med 2012;156:880–91.
3. ACOG practice bulletin 131. Screening for cervical cancer. Obstet Gynecol 2012; 120(5):1222–38.
4. Massad LS, et al. Updating guidelines for the management of abnormal cervical cancer screening tests and cancer precursors. J Lower Genital Tract Dis, in press.
5. Darragh TM, Colgan T, Cox JT, et al. The Lower Anogenital Squamous Terminology Standardization Project for HPV-associated lesions: background and consensus recommendations from the College of American Pathologists and the American Society for Colposcopy and Cervical Pathology. J Low Genit Tract Dis 2012;16:205–42.

The Natural History of Cervical Human Papillomavirus Infections and Cervical Cancer

Gaps in Knowledge and Future Horizons

Cosette Marie Wheeler, PhD[a,b],*

KEYWORDS

- Human papillomavirus (HPV) infection • Human papillomavirus natural history
- Age-specific HPV prevalence • HPV immunity • HPV persistence • HPV genotypes
- Cervical intraepithelial neoplasia • Global cervical cancer burden

KEY POINTS

- Human papillomavirus (HPV) infections are the most common sexually transmitted agents known. Compared with the low transmission probabilities of other sexually transmitted infections such as human immunodeficiency virus (HIV) and herpes simplex virus type 2 (HSV-2), the transmission rate from male to female per coital act has been estimated for genital HPVs to be between 0.4 and 0.8.
- Although most genital HPV infections clear on their own, a small proportion of women develop persistent infection. HPV genotype is the best predictor of risk of persistence, with HPV16 being uniquely persistent and carcinogenic. HPV genotyping for HPV16/HPV18 has been recommended for triage in clinical practice.
- Regional differences in age-specific HPV prevalence are not well understood. Differences in sexual behaviors, waning immunity, changing hormonal milieu, coinfections with other organisms including parasitic and viral infections and the overall microbiota, as well as potential contributions from quiescent or latent HPV infections require further study to shed light on the natural history of HPV infections across a woman's lifetime.

Continued

Disclosures: CMW has received funding for research through the University of New Mexico from the US National Institute of Allergy and Infectious Diseases (Program Director U19AI084081), the US National Cancer Institute (Program Director U54CA164336), Merck & Co, Inc, GlaxoSmith Kline (for HPV vaccine studies), and Roche Molecular Systems (equipment and reagents for HPV genotyping).

[a] Department of Pathology, University of New Mexico Health Sciences Center, Albuquerque, NM, USA; [b] Department of Obstetrics and Gynecology, University of New Mexico Health Sciences Center, Albuquerque, NM, USA
* House of Prevention Epidemiology (HOPE), Department of Pathology, 1 University of New Mexico, MSC 02-1670, 1816 Sigma Chi Road Northeast, Albuquerque, NM 87131.
E-mail address: cwheeler@salud.unm.edu

Obstet Gynecol Clin N Am 40 (2013) 165–176
http://dx.doi.org/10.1016/j.ogc.2013.02.004
0889-8545/13/$ – see front matter © 2013 Elsevier Inc. All rights reserved.

obgyn.theclinics.com

Continued

- Most knowledge of HPV natural history has been derived from cohort studies of young women when HPV is first acquired at sexual initiation and in the subsequent 2 decades. Future studies of HPV natural history must turn to understanding HPV infections in women aged 40 years and older. Given that primary (vaccination) and secondary (screening) cervical cancer prevention strategies are being implemented using age-specific approaches, current gaps in knowledge must be filled.
- Beyond HPV genotype, other biomarkers (HPV variants, protein markers of cell proliferation, and epigenetic markers including both host-specific and HPV-specific gene methylation) seem promising for potential improved risk stratification and clinical implementation.
- Most women are at risk for high-risk HPV (HR-HPV) infections. In spite of the advent of highly efficacious HPV vaccines, these women will remain a significant public health challenge for decades to come. Gaps in knowledge of the natural history of HPVs offer opportunities for scientific breakthroughs to improve the management of HR-HPV infections and to prevent invasive cervical cancers.

Genital human papillomavirus infections (HPVs) are the most common of all sexually transmissible agents.[1] The rate of HPV transmission probability is higher than that of human immunodeficiency virus (HIV) or herpes simplex virus, type 2 (HSV-2), with the median transmissibility of HPV (as estimated by computer simulation studies of university students) being 40% per coital act.[2] Computer simulation models and HPV16 seroprevalence data have found a per-partner male to female transmission probability of 60% to 80% for HPV type 16 (HPV16).[3,4] Any variable linked to sexual activity, including young age, number of sexual partners, recent sexual partners, and having sex with partners who have other partners including both men and women is a risk factor for genital HPV infection.[5]

Although the best data come from a murine animal model,[6] it was generally accepted long before this model that microabrasion or wounding was necessary for HPV to access and infect the basal cells of the stratified genital epithelium. The stratified squamous epithelium of the ectocervix meets the columnar epithelium of the endocervix in the transformation zone (T-zone) where there are stem cells to support the continuous turnover of both cell types. It remains unclear whether HPVs can infect and transform nonstem cells of the columnar epithelium or the basal and parabasal layers of the stratified epithelium.

Studies of prevalent and incident infections detected during longitudinal follow-up of young women show that most cervical HPV infections are benign and resolve on their own.[7–9] HPV infections are generally thought to include a productive life cycle in which infectious virions are produced and HPV DNA becomes readily detectable. Once HPV infection is acquired and productive, autoinoculation seems common at the anus and vagina, and conversely from the vagina to the anus, but whether there is a long-term HPV reservoir within the genital tract remains unknown.[10] The average duration of cervical HPV infection has been reported to vary by HPV genotype but reasons for these differences are not understood and results are inconsistent.[11–15] Most cervical HPV infections likely clear within in a few months and more than 90% of infections become undetectable in less than 2 years. It is unknown whether some individuals might be highly resistant to HPV infections. Cohort studies fail to identify individuals who resolve infection in a few days to a few weeks because infrequent (4–6 months) sampling intervals are typically used. It is also unknown why some women develop persistent cervical HPV infections, but it is these women who are at greatest risk for the development of invasive cervical cancer. Cervical HPV persistence irrespective of age is necessary for the development of cervical cancer worldwide. However, data suggest that, in some instances, long-term persistence of high-risk HPVs (HR-HPV) may not always result in high-grade cervical intraepithelial neoplasia (CIN).[16] In the search for improved risk stratification of HPV-infected women who will ultimately develop cervical disease, it is worth considering whether identifying and characterizing any subset of super-responders would shed light on HPV persistence.

Cervical HPV prevalence peaks at young ages on sexual initiation and in the United States, population-based prevalence remains low across the lifespan after about the age of 30 years.[17,18] Age-specific regional differences in cervical HPV prevalence are not well understood.[19] Given that HPV testing and vaccination have been incorporated into cervical cancer prevention programs on an age-specific basis, it is becoming increasingly important to clarify outstanding issues in the natural history of HPV infection and any potential relationship to precancer and cancer outcomes.

So-called U-shaped HPV prevalence curves characterized by high cervical HPV prevalence at young ages followed by a significant decline and subsequent increase in prevalence beginning at different later ages have been observed in a variety of settings. In other instances, HPV increases in prevalence at young ages and then remains constant with age. Obvious potential factors contributing to these age-specific regional HPV prevalence differences at older ages could include (1) continuing new sexual exposures; (2) reappearance of quiescent/latent HPV; (3) changes in immune status, such as decline in immune function and hormonal milieu at older ages or immunosuppression caused by coinfection with other viral or parasitic agents; and (4) cofactors including the cervicovaginal microbiota and pH or factors yet to be determined. In the first 2 instances, region-specific and age-specific patterns of sexual behavior would be expected to contribute to differences in HPV prevalence. In the third and fourth instances, changes in immune responsiveness and the local microenvironment could modify the risk of acquisition of new HPV infection, activation of previously acquired but quiescent or latent HPV infections, or persistence of both.

Data supporting quiescent or latent HPV infections being common come from studies of immunosuppressed women with HIV infections[20,21] and clinical observations of increased HPV-associated lesions following organ transplantation.[22] A role for immune regulation of HPV infections has thus been assumed. In a large cohort study of midadult women,[23] risk estimates suggested that new sexual partners could account for 21% of HPV incidence, whereas 21% was attributed to increasing lifetime number of sexual partners and 12% was explained by decreasing immune function. The proportion of HPV infections that stem from sexual acquisition versus reactivation related to lifetime number of sexual partners (a surrogate for likely prior HPV exposures) is difficult to estimate but could be similar based on these data. Assuming that some portion of HPV prevalence arises through a quiescent reservoir related to prior HPV exposures, it is not clear how often HPV reappears and whether reappearances occur consistently across the lifespan versus with an increasing frequency at older ages. A recent model of HPV infection natural history that includes redetection/reactivation of quiescent or latent HPV and that considers sexual initiation, sexual behavior at younger ages, and ongoing sexual behaviors within time-period cohorts deserves attention as greater understanding is achieved of population variability in the natural history of genital HPV infections across the lifespan.[24]

In concert with, or in the absence of, a productive viral infection, HPV entry into nondividing or minimally dividing cervical basal epithelial cells could allow HPV genomes to become residents in quiescent or latent states until a triggered replication, division, or differentiation event of the host stem cell. It seems reasonable that total numbers of lifetime sexual partners and viral load at sexual exposures might be related to the numbers of basal cells harboring resident HPV genomes under some probability that would then, subject to a variety of potential cofactors, reappear as programmed cell division ensues to replenish the epithelial strata.

Although efforts have been expended to distinguish and understand HPV reappearance, latency, and/or reactivation from a basic biologic perspective[25,26] and in population studies,[23,27–31] establishing a definition of HPV latency or identification of a latent state by analogy to other viruses such as herpes[32] will likely be difficult to establish. Sensitive tools to measure HPV genomes and characteristic transcripts within single cells may prove helpful in this regard but quiescent or latent HPV genomes in the reservoir of stem cells may be few among many, therefore the challenge in identifying these potential reservoir cells may remain. Understanding quiescence or latency has implications when considering age-related patterns of HPV prevalence, but some argue that this is important to extending HPV vaccination beyond current young age targets. Support for vaccination of women to prevent subsequent new infection, reinfection, or reappearance has been suggested,[33,34] but presently there is no evidence that newly acquired or reappearing HPV infections are more prone to subsequent persistence or risk for cervical cancer.

To better understand the natural history of HPV infection and correlates of disease outcomes, it would be useful to identify markers of declining HPV immunity, but acquired and innate immunity are, in general, poorly understood for HPVs. Human leukocyte antigen (HLA) and HLA-related genes, alleles, haplotypes, and single nucleotide polymorphisms (SNPs) have been identified as risks or protective factors, although study designs and results have varied in different populations.[35–38] Although it is thought that cell-mediated immunity plays a critical role in the clearance of HPV infections, measures of HPV-specific cell-mediated immunity remain elusive, with responses being largely undetectable or less than the detection limits of existing assays. More is known about HPV-specific humoral immunity than cell-mediated immunity, although, in general, humoral responses are also low, with variability in the development of antibodies by HPV genotype and among women.[39] A significant proportion of HPV-infected women fail to develop detectable HPV-specific antibodies. Why some women develop antibodies and others do not is not well understood. From a practical perspective, this observation makes it unlikely that a simple blood test for HPV infection will ever become available. Low-level or lack of detectable immune responses in HPV-infected women is likely caused by HPVs having coevolved with their hosts over millennia[40,41] and having mechanisms of immune evasion including their tropism for epithelium in an immune-privileged environment.

Irrespective of being able to measure HPV-specific immune responses, it is generally thought that acquired HPV type-specific immunity modifies, at least to some degree, the risk of subsequent reinfection with the same HPV genotype. In women with detectable HPV-specific antibodies during or following cervical infection, studies have assessed whether serum antibodies coincident with natural HPV infections show type-specific protection against reinfection.[42,43] The emerging body of evidence suggests that high levels of serum antibodies provide some protection against subsequent risk of infection, although high levels of antibodies could serve as markers of some broader or extended immune responsiveness. With the implementation of HPV vaccination and the desire to better understand immune function in HPV natural history across the lifespan, efforts to understand the usefulness of general immune measurements will remain important and development of HPV-specific measures of immunity will need to continue. Furthermore, the relationship of inflammation and the local microenvironment to HPV infections[44,45] and their potential role in the development of HPV-related disease is continuing as another area of interest.

In the future, there will be a need to implement more complex measures in population studies to fill the gaps in knowledge. If seen as a priority, long-term cohort studies, especially in women 35 to 40 years of age and older, will be needed to better understand disease risks associated with general waning immunity, waning HPV type-specific immunity, latent/reappearing HPV infections, and the lack of decline or increases in HPV prevalence observed in some populations at older ages.

As noted previously, HPV persistence is the known necessary exposure for the development of cervical cancer. Several cofactors with moderate risks for cervical cancer outcomes have been well established (ie, smoking, long-term oral contraceptive use, multiparity, and HIV infection)[46–51] but HPV genotype remains the best predictor of risk for disease progression. If a woman is negative for HR-HPV at any age, risk of precancer and cancer for the next 5 years is small.[52] Infection with HPV16 has been determined to be the most important HPV genotype predicting likelihood of progression.[53] It remains unclear why HPV16 is the most successful or apparently the most fit HPV type based on population prevalence and why HPV16 is uniquely carcinogenic.[54] HPV genotyping of cervical samples during cervical screening has recently been incorporated into clinical practice recommendations.[55] The most recent US cervical screening guidelines acknowledge that the presence of cervical HPV16 and HPV18 supports an increased risk of detecting a high-grade cervical lesion. A role for viral load measurements for any HPV genotype has not proved clinically useful thus far.

Beyond HPV type, intratypic HPV variants are associated with differing risk of developing high-grade cervical lesions[56,57] but little to no information is available to assess risk for invasive cervical cancer outcomes. The largest body of work on HPV intratypic variant disease risk is available for HPV16. Non-European HPV16 variants have been associated with greater disease risk than variants belonging to the European lineage, which includes the original HPV prototypic HPV16 genome. Polymorphism in the HPV16 long control region (LCR), which has also been referred to as the upstream regulatory region (URR) or the noncoding region (NCR), and E6 genes of HR-HPVs may be useful in distinguishing which lesions may progress or regress but currently no standardized assay are available to enable further progress in this area.

The search for biomarkers continues as researchers look for improved risk stratifiers of women who are positive for HR-HPV genotypes. To date, immunostaining for the overexpression of cyclin-dependent kinase inhibitor p16INK4a in HPV-infected cells has been the most widely applied biomarker. p16INK4a staining has been used for many years to augment cytology and histology diagnosis, and recently it was formally recommended to clarify histologic interpretation and enhance diagnostic accuracy.[58–61] It remains to be seen whether p16INK4a can be used to predict HPV-related risks of precancer and cancer outcomes. Other markers of cell proliferation such as Ki-67, a cellular marker for proliferation that is expressed at all stages during the cell cycle except G0; minichromosome maintenance protein [MCM2], a member of the DNA licensing protein family; and topoisomerase IIa [TOP2A], a nuclear enzyme involved in DNA replication have also shown potential clinical usefulness but further studies are needed.[62]

One of the most promising areas of research in defining HPV disease risk lies in epigenetics related to gene expression silencing via methylation. Data support a role for methylation in HPV-related cervical carcinogenesis and suggest a potential prognostic usefulness beyond HPV testing or cytology. Death-associated protein kinase 1 (DAPK1), cell adhesion molecule 1 (CADM1), and retinoic acid receptor beta (RARB) are host genes that have shown consistently increased methylation levels in studies of cervical cancers and these and other targets deserve further study.[63] HPV-specific gene methylation shows the greatest promise as a modifier or marker of risk for disease progression. HPV16 genome methylation at CpG sites in L1 and L2 capsid genes, and the E2/E4 genes have been shown to be predictors for detecting high-grade cervical lesions.[64–66] Reasons for methylation are unclear but different methylation patterns may be useful in predicting which HPV infections will persist or clear and which could facilitate improvement in risk stratification and clinical management.

Having noted some of the gaps in knowledge and highlighted promises of future biomarkers, it is appropriate to review the basic stepwise model of cervical carcinogenesis previously proposed.[67,68] In this model, HPV infections are easily acquired by sexual exposure and, at any age, most HPV infections resolve within a few months to a few years. After approximately 2 years of HPV persistence, there is an increasing risk of a precancer diagnosis. The major abnormal cervical cytology and histology diagnostic categories and their relationship to HPV infections leading to precancer is described earlier.[69] CIN1 or low-grade cervical intraepithelial neoplasia is pathognomonic for HPV infection. Cervical intraepithelial neoplasia grade 2 (CIN2) is a controversial high-grade diagnosis that is the least reproducible of all cervical diagnoses,[70] and some consider it more of an equivocal histologic entity. The biologic behavior of CIN2 is not well understood and, although a large proportion of CIN2 regress,[71] it is nonetheless maintained as the conservative threshold for excisional therapy.[72] Cervical intraepithelial neoplasia grade 3 (CIN3) or lesions defined as the immediate cervical cancer precursors also can regress, but those that persist can lead, typically over decades, to invasive cancer. Invasive cervical cancers most often arise from HPV infections of the metaplastic epithelium at the squamocolumnar junction or T-zone but little is known about the final steps of carcinogenesis leading to invasion. It is unknown whether viral persistence precedes the development of a clonal transformation event or whether having CIN3 leads to HPV persistence. Estimates of the time from infection with a high-risk HPV genotype to the development of CIN3 depend on the frequency of screening and are hindered by the uncertainties of colposcopic biopsy.[73,74] The time from infection with a high-risk HPV to CIN3 is estimated to be much shorter than the typical decades needed from first development of a detectable CIN3 lesion to invasion, although there is considerable individual heterogeneity. Invasive cervical cancers, albeit uncommonly, are therefore observed in some women at young ages.

Recent cervical screening recommendations in the United States support lengthening of intervals between screens in women aged 30 to 65 years.[55] Screening at 3-year intervals with cytology alone or intervals of up to 5 years when cotesting for HR-HPV genotypes has been recommended when the cytology and HPV tests are negative and a negative history is reported. Based on current understanding of the natural history of HPV infection and the estimated transit time between HPV infection to the development of precancer and cancer, as well as cohort studies and randomized clinical trial data, the recommended intervals have been selected as safe and effective. In the absence of national organized screening, it remains important to ensure that women return for screening within the recommended screening intervals of 3 to 5 years, which may prove difficult in the absence of adequate surveillance for patient recall.

In conclusion, there is unequivocal evidence that evolutionarily related carcinogenic HPV genotypes cause cervical cancer and other cancers worldwide. In 2008, about 500,000 incident cases and 275,000 deaths per year were attributed to cervical cancer worldwide.[75] On a global basis, cervical cancer is the third most common cancer in women and it is a leading cause of cancer death among women in low-income countries where these deaths occur at young age while women are still raising their families. Although there are some differences in HPV genotype distribution in cancers regionally, the evidence is overwhelming that, of the more than 40 HPV genotypes infecting the human anogenital tract, about 8 HPV types (namely HPV16, HPV18, HPV31, HPV33, HPV35, HPV45, HPV52, and HPV58) are responsible for at least 90% of the global burden of cervical cancer.[76] HPV16 followed by HPV18 are the most frequently detected HPV genotypes in squamous cell carcinomas of the cervix, whereas HPV18 is more strongly associated with adenocarcinoma of the cervix.

Most women in the world today are at risk for HR-HPV infections. In spite of the advent of highly efficacious HPV vaccines, these women will remain a significant public health challenge for decades to come. In the future, gaps in knowledge will offer ongoing opportunities for scientific breakthroughs to improve the management of HR-HPV infections and to prevent invasive cervical cancers.

REFERENCES

1. Ebrahim SH, McKenna MT, Marks JS. Sexual behaviour: related adverse health burden in the United States. Sex Transm Infect 2005;81:38–40.
2. Burchell A, Richardson H, Mahmud SM, et al. Modelling the sexual transmissibility of human papillomavirus infection using stochastic computer simulation and empirical data from a cohort study of young women in Montréal, Canada. Am J Epidemiol 2006;163:534–43.
3. Barnabas RV, Laukkanen P, Koskela P, et al. Epidemiology of HPV 16 and cervical cancer in Finland and the potential impact of vaccination: mathematical modelling analyses. PLoS Med 2006;3:e138.
4. Hughes JP, Garnett GP, Koutsky LA. The theoretical population level impact of a prophylactic human papilloma virus vaccine. Epidemiology 2006;13:631–9.
5. Veldhuijzen NJ, Snijders PJ, Reiss P, et al. Factors affecting transmission of mucosal human papillomavirus. Lancet Infect Dis 2010;10:862–74.
6. Kines RC, Thompson CD, Lowy DR, et al. The initial steps leading to papillomavirus infection occur on the basement membrane prior to cell surface binding. Proc Natl Acad Sci U S A 2009;106(48):20458–63. http://dx.doi.org/10.1073/pnas.0908502106.
7. Rodriguez AC, Schiffman M, Herrero R, et al. Longitudinal study of human papillomavirus persistence and cervical intraepithelial neoplasia grade 2/3: critical role of duration of infection. J Natl Cancer Inst 2010;102(5):315–24.
8. Winer RL, Hughes JP, Feng Q, et al. Early natural history of incident, type-specific human papillomavirus infections in newly sexually active young women. Cancer Epidemiol Biomarkers Prev 2011;20(4):699–707.
9. Molano M, Van den Brule A, Plummer M, et al. Determinants of clearance of human papillomavirus infections in Colombian women with normal cytology: a population-based, 5-year follow-up study. Am J Epidemiol 2003;158:486–94.
10. Moscicki AB, Schiffman M, Burchell A, et al. Updating the natural history of human papillomavirus and anogenital cancers. Vaccine 2012;30(Suppl 5):F24–33. http://dx.doi.org/10.1016/j.vaccine.2012.05.089.
11. Moscicki AB. Impact of HPV infection in adolescent populations. J Adolesc Health 2005;37:S3–9.
12. Ho GY, Burk RD, Klein S, et al. Persistent genital human papillomavirus infection as a risk factor for persistent cervical dysplasia. J Natl Cancer Inst 1995;87:1365–71.
13. Rositch AF, Koshiol J, Hudgens MG, et al. Patterns of persistent genital human papillomavirus infection among women worldwide: a literature review and meta-analysis. Int J Cancer 2012. http://dx.doi.org/10.1002/ijc.27828.

14. Muñoz N, Hernandez-Suarez G, Méndez F, et al, Instituto Nacional de Cancerología HPV Study Group. Persistence of HPV infection and risk of high-grade cervical intraepithelial neoplasia in a cohort of Colombian women. Br J Cancer 2009; 100(7):1184–90. http://dx.doi.org/10.1038/sj.bjc.6604972.

15. Koshiol J, Lindsay L, Pimenta JM, et al. Persistent human papillomavirus infection and cervical neoplasia: a systematic review and meta-analysis [review]. Am J Epidemiol 2008;168(2):123–37. http://dx.doi.org/10.1093/aje/kwn036.

16. Castle PE, Rodriguez AC, Burk RD, et al. Long-term persistence of prevalently detected human papillomavirus infections in the absence of detectable cervical precancer and cancer. J Infect Dis 2011;203(6):814–22.

17. Hariri S, Unger ER, Sternberg M, et al. Prevalence of genital human papillomavirus among females in the United States, the national health and nutrition examination survey, 2003–2006. J Infect Dis 2011;204:566–73.

18. Wheeler CM, Hunt WC, Cuzick J, et al. A population-based study of human papillomavirus genotype prevalence in the United States: baseline measures prior to mass human papillomavirus vaccination. Int J Cancer 2013;132(1):198–207. http://dx.doi.org/10.1002/ijc.27608.

19. Franceschi S, Herrero R, Clifford GM, et al. Variations in the age-specific curves of human papillomavirus prevalence in women worldwide. Int J Cancer 2006;119: 2677–84.

20. Theiler RN, Farr SL, Karon JM, et al. High-risk human papillomavirus reactivation in human immunodeficiency virus-infected women: risk factors for cervical viral shedding. Obstet Gynecol 2010;115(6):1150–8. http://dx.doi.org/10.1097/AOG.0b013e3181e00927.

21. Strickler HD, Burk RD, Fazzari M, et al. Natural history and possible reactivation of human papillomavirus in human immunodeficiency virus-positive women. J Natl Cancer Inst 2005;97(8):577–86.

22. Grulich AE, van Leeuwen MT, Falster MO, et al. Incidence of cancers in people with HIV/AIDS compared with immunosuppressed transplant recipients: a meta-analysis [review]. Lancet 2007;370(9581):59–67.

23. González P, Hildesheim A, Rodríguez AC, et al. Behavioral/lifestyle and immunologic factors associated with HPV infection among women older than 45 years. Cancer Epidemiol Biomarkers Prev 2010;19(12):3044–54. http://dx.doi.org/10.1158/1055-9965.EPI-10-0645.

24. Gravitt PE. The known unknowns of HPV natural history [review]. J Clin Invest 2011;121(12):4593–9. http://dx.doi.org/10.1172/JCI57149.

25. Zhang P, Nouri M, Brandsma JL, et al. Induction of E6/E7 expression in cottontail rabbit papillomavirus latency following UV activation. Virology 1999;263(2): 388–94.

26. Maglennon GA, McIntosh P, Doorbar J. Persistence of viral DNA in the epithelial basal layer suggests a model for papillomavirus latency following immune regression. Virology 2011;414(2):153–63.

27. Insinga RP, Perez G, Wheeler CM, et al, FUTURE I Investigators. Incidence, duration, and reappearance of type-specific cervical human papillomavirus infections in young women. Cancer Epidemiol Biomarkers Prev 2010;6:1585–94. http://dx.doi.org/10.1158/1055-9965.EPI-09-1235.

28. Trottier H, Ferreira S, Thomann P, et al. Human papillomavirus infection and reinfection in adult women: the role of sexual activity and natural immunity. Cancer Res 2010;70(21):8569–77.

29. Rositch AF, Burke AE, Viscidi RP, et al. Contributions of recent and past sexual partnerships on incident human papillomavirus detection: acquisition and

reactivation in older women. Cancer Res 2012;72(23):6183–90. http://dx.doi. org/10.1158/0008-5472.CAN-12-2635.

30. Gravitt PE, Rositch AF, Silver MI, et al. A cohort effect of the sexual revolution may be masking an increase in human papillomavirus detection at menopause in the United States. J Infect Dis 2013;207(2):272–80. http://dx.doi.org/10.1093/ infdis/jis660.

31. Winer RL, Hughes JP, Feng Q, et al. Prevalence and risk factors for oncogenic human papillomavirus infections in high-risk mid-adult women. Sex Transm Dis 2012;39(11):848–56. http://dx.doi.org/10.1097/OLQ.0b013e3182641f1c.

32. Preston CM, Efstathiou S. Chapter 33. Molecular basis of HSV latency and reactivation. In: Arvin A, Campadelli-Fiume G, Mocarski E, et al, editors. Human herpesviruses: biology, therapy, and immunoprophylaxis. Cambridge University Press; 2007.

33. Olsson SE, Kjaer S, Sigurdsson K, et al. Evaluation of quadrivalent HPV 6/11/16/ 18 vaccine efficacy against cervical and anogenital disease in subjects with serological evidence of prior vaccine type HPV infection. Hum Vaccin 2009;5: 696–704.

34. Szarewski A, Poppe WA, Skinner SR, et al, HPV PATRICIA Study Group. Efficacy of the human papillomavirus (HPV)-16/18 AS04-adjuvanted vaccine in women aged 15-25 years with and without serological evidence of previous exposure to HPV-16/18. Int J Cancer 2012;131(1):106–16. http://dx.doi.org/10.1002/ijc.26362.

35. Apple RJ, Becker TM, Wheeler CM, et al. Comparison of human leukocyte antigen DR-DQ disease associations found with cervical dysplasia and invasive cervical carcinoma. J Natl Cancer Inst 1995;87(6):427–36.

36. Wang SS, Wheeler CM, Hildesheim A, et al. Human leukocyte antigen class I and II alleles and risk of cervical neoplasia: results from a population-based study in Costa Rica. J Infect Dis 2001;184(10):1310–4.

37. Madeleine MM, Johnson LG, Smith AG, et al. Comprehensive analysis of HLA-A, HLA-B, HLA-C, HLA-DRB1, and HLA-DQB1 loci and squamous cell cervical cancer risk. Cancer Res 2008;68(9):3532–9. http://dx.doi.org/10.1158/0008-5472. CAN-07-6471.

38. Wang SS, Hildesheim A, Gao X, et al. Comprehensive analysis of human leukocyte antigen class I alleles and cervical neoplasia in 3 epidemiologic studies. J Infect Dis 2002;186(5):598–605.

39. Carter JJ, Koutsky LA, Wipf GC, et al. The natural history of human papillomavirus type 16 capsid antibodies among a cohort of university women. J Infect Dis 1996; 174:927–36.

40. Bernard HU, Burk RD, Chen Z, et al. Classification of papillomaviruses (PVs) based on 189 PV types and proposal of taxonomic amendments. Virology 2010;401:70–9.

41. Schiffman M, Herrero R, Desalle R, et al. The carcinogenicity of human papillomavirus types reflects viral evolution. Virology 2005;337:76–84.

42. Safaeian M, Porras C, Schiffman M, et al, Costa Rican Vaccine Trial Group. Epidemiological study of anti-HPV16/18 seropositivity and subsequent risk of HPV16 and -18 infections. J Natl Cancer Inst 2010;102:1653–62.

43. Viscidi RP, Snyder B, Cu-Uvin S, et al. Human papillomavirus capsid antibody response to natural infection and risk of subsequent HPV infection in HIV-positive and HIV-negative women. Cancer Epidemiol Biomarkers Prev 2005;14:283–8.

44. Smith BC, McAndrew T, Chen Z, et al. The cervical microbiome over 7 years and a comparison of methodologies for its characterization. PLoS One 2012;7(7): e40425. http://dx.doi.org/10.1371/journal.pone.0040425.

45. Clarke MA, Rodriguez AC, Gage JC, et al. A large, population-based study of age-related associations between vaginal pH and human papillomavirus infection. BMC Infect Dis 2012;12:33. http://dx.doi.org/10.1186/1471-2334-12-33.
46. Castellsague X, Munoz N. Chapter 3: Cofactors in human papillomavirus carcinogenesis-role of parity, oral contraceptives, and tobacco smoking. J Natl Cancer Inst Monogr 2003;20–8.
47. Plummer M, Herrero R, Franceschi S, et al. Smoking and cervical cancer: pooled analysis of the IARC multi-centric case-control study. Cancer Causes Control 2003;14:805–14.
48. Moreno V, Bosch FX, Munoz N, et al. Effect of oral contraceptives on risk of cervical cancer in women with human papillomavirus infection: the IARC multicentric case-control study. Lancet 2002;359:1085–92.
49. Munoz N, Franceschi S, Bosetti C, et al. Role of parity and human papillomavirus in cervical cancer: The IARC multicentric case-control study. Lancet 2002;359: 1093–101.
50. Serraino D, Carrieri P, Pradier C, et al. Risk of invasive cervical cancer among women with, or at risk for, HIV infection. Int J Cancer 1999;82:334–7.
51. Frisch M, Biggar RJ, Goedert JJ. Human papillomavirus-associated cancers in patients with human immunodeficiency virus infection and acquired immunodeficiency syndrome. J Natl Cancer Inst 2000;92:1500–10.
52. Katki HA, Kinney WK, Fetterman B, et al. Cervical cancer risk for women undergoing concurrent testing for human papillomavirus and cervical cytology: a population-based study in routine clinical practice. Lancet Oncol 2011;12(7): 663–72. http://dx.doi.org/10.1016/S1470-2045(11)70145-0.
53. Khan MJ, Castle PE, Lorincz AT, et al. The elevated 10-year risk of cervical precancer and cancer in women with human papillomavirus (HPV) type 16 or 18 and the possible utility of type-specific HPV testing in clinical practice. J Natl Cancer Inst 2005;97:1072–9.
54. Munoz N, Bosch FX, de Sanjose S, et al. Epidemiologic classification of human papillomavirus types associated with cervical cancer. N Engl J Med 2003;348: 518–27.
55. Saslow D, Solomon D, Lawson HW, et al, ACS-ASCCP-ASCP Cervical Cancer Guideline Committee. American Cancer Society, American Society for Colposcopy and Cervical Pathology, and American Society for Clinical Pathology screening guidelines for the prevention and early detection of cervical cancer. CA Cancer J Clin 2012;62(3):147–72. http://dx.doi.org/10.3322/caac.21139.
56. Xi LF, Koutsky LA, Hildesheim A, et al. Risk for high-grade cervical intraepithelial neoplasia associated with variants of human papillomavirus types 16 and 18. Cancer Epidemiol Biomarkers Prev 2007;16(1):4–10.
57. Schiffman M, Rodriguez AC, Chen Z, et al. A population-based prospective study of carcinogenic human papillomavirus variant lineages, viral persistence, and cervical neoplasia. Cancer Res 2010;70(8):3159–69. http://dx.doi.org/10. 1158/0008-5472.CAN-09-4179.
58. Tsoumpou I, Arbyn M, Kyrgiou M, et al. p16(INK4a) immunostaining in cytological and histological specimens from the uterine cervix: a systematic review and meta-analysis [review 50]. Cancer Treat Rev 2009;35(3):210–20. http://dx.doi. org/10.1016/j.ctrv.2008.10.005.
59. Cuschieri K, Wentzensen N. Human papillomavirus mRNA and p16 detection as biomarkers for the improved diagnosis of cervical neoplasia [review]. Cancer Epidemiol Biomarkers Prev 2008;17(10):2536–45. http://dx.doi.org/10.1158/ 1055-9965.EPI-08-0306.

60. Darragh TM, Colgan TJ, Cox JT, et al, Members of LAST Project Work Groups. The Lower Anogenital Squamous Terminology Standardization Project for HPV-Associated Lesions: background and consensus recommendations from the College of American Pathologists and the American Society for Colposcopy and Cervical Pathology [review]. J Low Genit Tract Dis 2012;16(3):205–42.

61. Waxman AG, Chelmow D, Darragh TM, et al. Revised terminology for cervical histopathology and its implications for management of high-grade squamous intraepithelial lesions of the cervix. Obstet Gynecol 2012;120(6):1465–71. http://dx.doi.org/10.1097/AOG.0b013e31827001d5.

62. Martin CM, O'Leary JJ. Histology of cervical intraepithelial neoplasia and the role of biomarkers [review]. Best Pract Res Clin Obstet Gynaecol 2011;25(5):605–15. http://dx.doi.org/10.1016/j.bpobgyn.2011.04.005.

63. Wentzensen N, Sherman ME, Schiffman M, et al. Utility of methylation markers in cervical cancer early detection: appraisal of the state-of-the-science. Gynecol Oncol 2009;112(2):293–9.

64. Wentzensen N, Sun C, Ghosh A, et al. Methylation of HPV18, HPV31, and HPV45 genomes and cervical intraepithelial neoplasia grade 3. J Natl Cancer Inst 2012; 104(22):1738–49. http://dx.doi.org/10.1093/jnci/djs425.

65. Mirabello L, Schiffman M, Ghosh A, et al. Elevated methylation of HPV16 DNA is associated with the development of high grade cervical intraepithelial neoplasia. Int J Cancer 2013;132(6):1412–22. http://dx.doi.org/10.1002/ijc.27750.

66. Lorincz AT, Brentnall AR, Vasiljević N, et al. HPV16 L1 and L2 DNA methylation predicts high grade cervical intraepithelial neoplasia in women with mildly abnormal cervical cytology. Int J Cancer 2013. http://dx.doi.org/10.1002/ijc.28050.

67. Schiffman M, Castle PE, Jeronimo J, et al. Human papillomavirus and cervical cancer [review]. Lancet 2007;370(9590):890–907.

68. Wright TC Jr, Schiffman M. Adding a test for human papillomavirus DNA to cervical-cancer screening. N Engl J Med 2003;348:489–90.

69. Wheeler CM. Natural history of human papillomavirus infections, cytologic and histologic abnormalities, and cancer [review]. Obstet Gynecol Clin North Am 2008;35(4):519–36. http://dx.doi.org/10.1016/j.ogc.2008.09.006, vii.

70. Stoler MH, Schiffman M, Atypical Squamous Cells of Undetermined Significance-Low-grade Squamous Intraepithelial Lesion Triage Study (ALTS) Group. Interobserver reproducibility of cervical cytologic and histologic interpretations: realistic estimates from the ASCUS-LSIL Triage Study. JAMA 2001; 285(11):1500–5.

71. Castle PE, Schiff man M, Wheeler CM, et al. Evidence for frequent regression of cervical intraepithelial neoplasia-grade 2. Obstet Gynecol 2009;113:18–25.

72. Wright TC Jr, Massad LS, Dunton CJ, 2006 American Society for Colposcopy and Cervical Pathology-sponsored Consensus Conference. 2006 consensus guidelines for the management of women with cervical intraepithelial neoplasia or adenocarcinoma in situ [Erratum appears in J Low Genit Tract Dis 2008;12:63]. J Low Genit Tract Dis 2007;11:223–39.

73. Gage JC, Hanson VW, Abbey K, et al, ASCUS LSIL Triage Study (ALTS) Group. Number of cervical biopsies and sensitivity of colposcopy. Obstet Gynecol 2006;108(2):264–72.

74. Stoler MH, Vichnin MD, Ferenczy A, et al, FUTURE I, II and III Investigators. The accuracy of colposcopic biopsy: analyses from the placebo arm of the Gardasil clinical trials. Int J Cancer 2011;128(6):1354–62. http://dx.doi.org/10.1002/ijc.25470.

75. Ferlay J, Shin HR, Bray F, et al. Estimates of worldwide burden of cancer in 2008: GLOBOCAN 2008. Int J Cancer 2011;127:2893–917.

76. de Sanjose S, Quint WG, Alemany L, et al, Retrospective International Survey and HPV Time Trends Study Group. Human papillomavirus genotype attribution in invasive cervical cancer: a retrospective cross-sectional worldwide study. Lancet Oncol 2010;11(11):1048–56. http://dx.doi.org/10.1016/S1470-2045(10)70230-8.

Human Papillomavirus Vaccination
Current Indications and Future Directions

Leda Gattoc, MD, Navya Nair, MD, MPH, Kevin Ault, MD*

KEYWORDS

- Vaccination • HPV cervical cancer • Cervical dysplasia • Vulvar dysplasia
- Genital warts

KEY POINTS

- Human papillomavirus (HPV) infection is the underlying cause of cervical, vulvar, vaginal, anal and orapharyngeal cancers.
- Multiple randomized prospective clinical trials have demonstrated that HPV vaccination prevents HPV-related diseases such as cervical and anal cancer.
- Clinical guidelines concerning HPV vaccination have evolved since its introduction in 2006. Current guidelines recommend the vaccination of adolescent and adult males and females aged 9 to 26 years.
- New HPV vaccines are currently being developed to protect against more HPV types. Investigators are also developing therapeutic vaccines that can potentially treat HPV-related diseases.

INTRODUCTION

Human papillomavirus (HPV) is one of the most common sexually transmitted infections in the United States with an estimated 20 million currently infected, and 6.2 million becoming newly infected annually.[1] A large national study that looked at more than 4000 women found that the overall prevalence of HPV infection among females aged 14 to 59 years was 42.5%. It also demonstrated that HPV infection significantly increased after age 14 to 19 years and peaked at age 20 to 24 years, consistent with the hypothesis that HPV is acquired shortly after onset of sexual activity (**Fig. 1**).[2]

Supported by the National Center for Advancing Translational Sciences of the National Institutes of Health under Award Number UL1TR000454. The content is solely the responsibility of the authors and does not necessarily represent the official views of the National Institutes of Health.

Department of Gynecology and Obstetrics, Emory University School of Medicine, 1365 Clifton Road, Atlanta, GA 30322, USA

* Corresponding author. Department of Gynecology and Obstetrics, Emory University School of Medicine, 69 Jesse Hill Jr Drive, Atlanta, GA 30303.

E-mail address: kevin.ault@emory.edu

Obstet Gynecol Clin N Am 40 (2013) 177–197

http://dx.doi.org/10.1016/j.ogc.2013.03.007

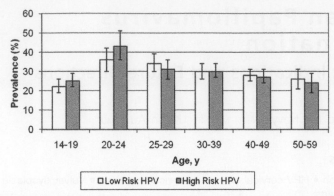

Fig. 1. Prevalence of low-risk and high-risk HPV among female respondents 14 to 59 years of age. (*Data from* Hariri S, Unger ER, Sternberg M, et al. Prevalence of genital human papillomavirus among females in the United States, the National Health And Nutrition Examination Survey, 2003–2006. J Infect Dis 2011;204(4):566–73.)

HPV has been linked to various benign and malignant lesions occurring in mucosal and skin epithelia. Currently, there are 148 recognized HPV types, classified into 33 species.[3] Forty HPV types infect the mucosal epithelium with a subset of approximately 12 high-risk subtypes that are etiologically linked to cervical cancer and its immediate premalignant precursors.[4] Two of the most important high-risk subtypes, HPV 16 and 18, account for 70% of cervical cancer cases.[5] Low-risk subtypes cause low-grade cervical dysplasia, genital warts, respiratory papillomas, and nasopharyngeal papillomas.[6] HPV 6 and 11 account for 90% of genital warts found in males and females. In the United States, an analysis of cancer registry data estimated that the total burden of all other HPV-related cancers (excluding cervical cancer) equals that of the cervical cancer burden. According to the National Program of Cancer Registries (NPCR) and Surveillance, Epidemiology, and End Results (SEER) databases, HPV-associated cancers accounted for 3.3% of all cancer cases among women and 2.0% of the total cancer cases among men diagnosed in 2009.[7] Jemal and colleagues[7] reported an increase in incidence rates of HPV-associated cancer of the oropharynx among white men and women, anal cancer among white and black men and women, and vulvar cancer among white and black women from 2000 to 2009. The increases in incidence rates for these cancers were more notable among persons aged 55 to 64 years compared with the younger age groups.[7] Sexually active men and women have more than a 50% lifetime risk of becoming infected with HPV, and it is estimated that 80% of women will contract an HPV-related disease by age 50 years.[8] Women aged 25 years and younger are at greatest risk of HPV infection, with a second peak of infection occurring after age 55 years.[9]

Cervical cancer is the second most commonly occurring cancer in women worldwide.[10] Most of the global burden (>85%) of cervical cancer occurs in developing countries.[11] In 1942, George Papanicolaou published a report on the use of cytology to screen for cervical cancer.[12] Since then, cytologic screening has dramatically reduced the prevalence of cervical cancer in developed countries with well-established screening programs. However, millions of women worldwide harbor chronic persistent HPV infections that increase their risk of developing cervical cancer. In 2008, 530,000 women were newly diagnosed with cervical cancer and 280,000 died of the disease.[11] It is projected that by 2030, 10 to 14 million women will be newly diagnosed with cervical cancer and 5 to 8 million will die of the disease unless preventive efforts are improved, particularly in developing countries where there is still significant disease burden.[13]

Cancer of the cervix is the end result of a long process that begins with infection with HPV.[14] Once a cell is infected with an oncogenic HPV strain, there are typically 4 steps that lead to cervical cancer: HPV transmission, viral persistence, progression of a clone of persistently infected cells to a precancerous lesion, and finally invasion. Forward progression in this process is not always the case. Clearance of HPV infection and regression of precancerous lesions can also occur.[15] With a competent immune system, most cervical HPV infections are cleared by cell-mediated immunity within 1 to 2 years of exposure (**Fig. 2**).[16]

The human papillomavirus consists of 8000-basepair long circular DNA molecules wrapped in a protein shell. This protein shell contains 2 molecules, L1 and L2. The HPV genome is composed of 6 early genes, 2 late genes, and a noncoding region. Once the virus infects a cell, the early proteins (E1, E2, E4, E5, E6, E7) are transcribed first, followed by the late proteins (L1 and L2), each of which are necessary for viral replication and assembly of newly formed virus particles in infected cells.[17] Both of the currently available vaccines target the L1 protein on different HPV types, but investigators are currently developing new vaccines against the L2 protein.

CURRENT HPV VACCINES

Given the well-established etiologic relationship between HPV infection and cervical cancer, a vaccine to immunize against HPV may reduce the burden of cervical caner and other HPV-related diseases.[18] In 2006, the US Food and Drug Administration (FDA) approved the first vaccine against HPV by Merck & Co, Inc. Gardasil or HPV4 is a quadrivalent vaccine consisting of 4 different types of virallike particles from the 4 serotypes of HPV (types 6, 11, 16, and 18). In 2009, a second bivalent HPV vaccine (HPV2; Cervarix by GlaxoSmithKline) targeting HPV types 16 and 18 was also approved by the FDA. These were the first vaccines developed specifically to prevent a sexually transmitted infection and the second (after the hepatitis B vaccine) designed to prevent cancer.[19] Gardasil is adjuvated with simple aluminum salt and is produced in yeast.[19] Cervarix contains the adjuvant ASO4, which includes monophosphoryl lipid A and an aluminum salt, and it is produced in insect cells.[19] Both vaccines are delivered via intramuscular injection in 3 doses over 6 months.

The Gardasil vaccine was initially licensed for use in females aged 9 to 26 years of age. In March 2007, the Centers for Disease Control Advisory Committee on Immunization Practices (ACIP) recommended routine vaccination with HPV4 for all girls aged

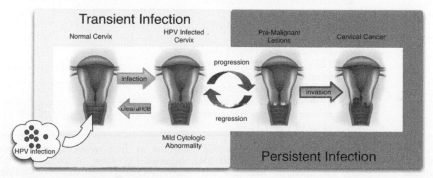

Fig. 2. Pathogenesis of HPV infection.

11 to 12 years old. The vaccine can be administered as early as 9 years of age and catch-up vaccination is recommended for those aged 13 to 26 years old who have not been vaccinated previously.[20,21] Cervarix was initially approved for use in females from 10 to 25 years of age in October 2009. The ACIP also approved its routine use in girls aged 11 to 12 years, starting as early as 10 years of age and catch-up vaccination from 13 to 25 years of age (**Table 1**).[22]

NEW INDICATIONS

HPV vaccination efforts have focused heavily on women and young adolescent girls. However, more than 25% of all HPV-related cancers occur in men and an estimated 250,000 cases of genital warts that occur each year in the United States affect sexually active men.[23] HPV-related malignancies affecting men include anal, penile, and oropharyngeal cancers, which are caused primarily by HPV 16.[24–26] There has been an increased incidence of oropharyngeal and anal cancer in men.[24,26] In October

Table 1
FDA-approved HPV vaccines

	Gardasil	Cervarix
Proper name	HPV quadrivalent (types 6, 11, 16, 18) vaccine, recombinant	HPV bivalent (types 16 and 18) vaccine, recombinant
Manufacturer	Merck & Co.	GlaxoSmithKline Biologicals
VLP types	6, 11, 16, 18	16, 18
Adjuvant	225 µg aluminum hydroxyphosphate sulfate	500 µg aluminum hydroxide, 50 µg 3-O-deacylated-4'-monophosphoryl lipid A
Schedule	0, 2, 6 mo	0, 1, 6 mo
Indications	Vaccination in females between 9 and 26 y of age for prevention of diseases caused by HPV 6/11/16/18: Cervical cancer Genital warts Cervical adenocarcinoma in situ (AIS) Cervical intraepithelial neoplasia (CIN) grades 1, 2, and 3 Vulvar intraepithelial neoplasia (VIN) grade 2 and grade 3 Vaginal intraepithelial neoplasia (VaIN) grade 2 and grade 3 Prevention of vulvar and vaginal cancer Vaccination in boys and men between 9 and 26 y of age for the prevention of genital warts caused by HPV 6/11 Vaccination in people aged 9 to 26 y for the prevention of anal cancer and associated precancerous lesions caused by HPV 6/11/16/18	Vaccination in females between 9 and 25 y of age for the prevention of disease caused by HPV 16/18: Cervical cancer CIN grades 1, 2, and 3 AIS

Data from FDA-approved indications for Gardasil. Available at: http://www.fda.gov/Biologics BloodVaccines/Vaccines/ApprovedProducts/UCM094042. Accessed December 10, 2012; and FDA-approved indications for Cervarix. Available at: http://www.fda.gov/BiologicsBloodVaccines/ Vaccines/ApprovedProducts/UCM094042. Accessed December 10, 2012.

2009, the FDA approved the use of Gardasil in males aged 9 to 26 years of age.[27] The ACIP subsequently approved permissive guidance to vaccinate males aged 9 to 26 years of age to decrease their risk of acquiring genital warts, although it was not recommended for routine use in males at that time.[28]

Infection with HPV 16 and 18 accounts for 90% of anal cancers and the incidence of anal cancers has been steadily increasing for the past 3 decades. Anal carcinoma is still relatively rare when compared with cervical cancer, with 5820 estimated new cases and 770 deaths in the United States in 2011. According to a population-based review of the SEER cancer registry, there has been a 2.8-fold increase in the incidence of anal cancer from 1973 to 1998,[29] and there has been a similar increased trend in mortality over the past few years.[30] Anal cancer is more prevalent in individuals infected with human immunodeficiency virus (HIV) and men who have sex with men, even those without HIV infection.[29,31] However, there is a higher disease burden in women. In 2003, the Centers for Disease Control and Prevention (CDC) reported that anal cancer was more common in women (1.6 per 100,000 women) than in men (1.3 per 100,000 men).[32] They estimate 1600 new cases of HPV-related anal cancers in women compared with only 900 new cases in men in the United States.[32] In 2010, the FDA included prevention of anal cancer in men and women as an additional indication for use of the HPV4 vaccine.[33]

Guiliano and colleagues[34] demonstrated that the quadrivalent vaccine was effective in preventing the development of anal intraepithelial neoplasia in men. In this study, the vaccine had an 89.3% efficacy in the prevention of HPV 6/11/16/18–related genital warts in the per protocol population. A substudy of the phase III efficacy trial was performed and included 598 men who have sex with men aged 16 to 26 years.[35] The subanalysis demonstrated an 88.1% per protocol efficacy in preventing HPV 6/11/16/18–related genital warts. The per protocol efficacy for prevention of HPV 6/11/16/18–related anal intraepithelial neoplasia (AIN) grades 1 to 3 was 77.5% and AIN lesions grades 2 to 3 was 74.9%. In October 2011, the ACIP extended their recommendations to include routine vaccination for all boys aged 11 to 12 years. It can be administered as early as 9 years and catch-up vaccination is recommended for boys aged 13 to 21 years. Men aged 22 to 26 years may be vaccinated. For special populations such as immunocompromised men and men who have sex with men, vaccination is recommended up to 26 years of age (**Fig. 3**).[35]

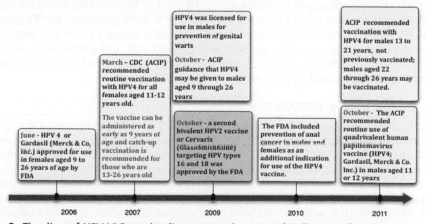

Fig. 3. Timeline of HPV VLP vaccine licensure and approved indications for use.

In 2011, the Costa Rica Vaccine Trial, 1 of the phase III efficacy studies performed on the HPV 2 vaccine, reported that the vaccine may be as effective in preventing anal HPV infection.[36] The bivalent vaccine demonstrated 62% efficacy against prevalent HPV 16/18 infection in the anus. In the HPV-naive cohort, vaccine efficacy against anal HPV 16/18 infection was 83.6%, which was similar to its efficacy in preventing cervical HPV 16/18 infection (87.9%). However, the bivalent vaccine has not yet been approved for use for the prevention of anal HPV infection.

HPV VACCINE EFFICACY TRIALS
Quadrivalent HPV Vaccine: FUTURE I and II Trials

There have been several randomized clinical trials conducted to investigate the efficacy of the quadrivalent vaccine. A phase II randomized placebo-controlled trial enrolled 1158 female participants, aged 16 to 23 years who were randomized to receive placebo or the quadrivalent vaccine. In this study, there was a 90% reduction in the incidence of HPV 6/11/16/18–related cervical or genital diseases in the vaccinated group.[37] The interim analyses performed in this study helped establish the dose of the vaccine used in phase III studies.

The phase III efficacy trials for the HPV4 vaccine were primarily designed to demonstrate its efficacy in preventing new-onset vaccine-related HPV infection as well as precancerous lesions that result from persistent infection. The FUTURE I trial also evaluated its participants for the development of HPV 6/11/16/18–associated cervical intraepithelial neoplasia grade 1 and higher (CIN 1+) and external genital lesions, including genital warts and vulvar/vaginal intraepithelial neoplasia.[38] The primary end points for the FUTURE II study included premalignant precursors such as high-grade dysplasia (CIN 2 or 3), adenocarcinoma in situ (AIS), and cervical cancer associated with HPV 16 and 18.[39] Both trials collectively enrolled and randomized 17,622 women and were designed to have at least 4 years of follow-up (**Table 2**).

The end-of-study analyses for both trials showed promising results in the prevention of vaccine-related HPV genital and cervical disease. There was 100% efficacy in the prevention of HPV 6/11/16/18–related CIN 3 in the cohort of women with no baseline cervical cytologic abnormality or prevalent infection of any HPV types (14 types were tested) and serologic evidence of previous exposure to the vaccine-related HPV types. Women in the intention-to-treat group (ITT) had lower efficacy, 45.1%, because this group included women with previous exposure to HPV at enrollment.[39,40] There was greater than 95% efficacy in the prevention of HPV 6/11/16/18–related vulvar intraepithelial neoplasia grade 2 and 3 (VIN 2/3) in both the HPV-naive group and the ITT group. The HPV4 vaccine also demonstrated greater than 75% efficacy in the prevention of vaginal intraepithelial neoplasia grade 2 and 3 (VaIN 2/3) and genital warts in the same cohort.[40] In addition, there was high efficacy in prevention of VIN 2/3, VaIN 2/3, and genital warts caused by non–vaccine-related HPV types.[41]

Bivalent HPV Vaccine: PATRICIA Trial

The Papilloma Trial against Cancer In young Adults (PATRICIA) study was a randomized double-blind study conducted in 14 countries to study the efficacy of the bivalent HPV vaccine against HPV types 16 and 18. Women were randomized to receive either the bivalent HPV vaccine or a control hepatitis A vaccine. More than 18,000 women were enrolled and a total of 17,106 women completed the vaccine series. The primary end point was to evaluate vaccine efficacy against CIN 2+ that was associated with HPV 16 or HPV 18 in women who were seronegative at baseline, and DNA negative at baseline and at month 6.[42] The average duration of follow-up was 35 months after

Table 2
Phase III efficacy trials on HPV vaccines

Trial	FUTURE I Trial	FUTURE II Trial	PApilloma TRial Against Cancer In Young Adults (PATRICIA)
Vaccine	Quadrivalent vaccine against HPV 6/11/16/18	Quadrivalent vaccine against HPV 6/11/16/18	Bivalent vaccine against HPV 16/18
Study type	Phase III double-blinded randomized controlled trial	Phase III double-blinded randomized controlled trial	Phase III double-blinded randomized controlled trial
Length of follow-up (y)	4	4	4
Age of participants (y)	16–24	15–26	15–25
Lifetime no. of sexual partners	≤4	≤4	≤6
Exclusion criteria	Pregnancy, history of abnormal Pap smear or genital warts History of severe allergic reaction; known immune disorders; receipt of attenuated or live vaccines within 14–21 d of enrollment		Pregnancy, breastfeeding, history of colposcopy, autoimmume disease, or immunodeficiency
Primary end points	Incident HPV 6/11/16/18-associated genital warts, CIN 1–3, VIN 1–3, ValN 1–3, AIS and cervical, vaginal, or vulvar cancer	Incident HPV 16/18/18-associated CIN 2–3, AIS, or cervical cancer	Incident HPV 16/18-associated CIN 2+
Outcome	96% efficacy against CIN 1 in unexposed Protection from high-grade cervical dysplasia: 86.3% in placebo vs 20.1% in vaccinated 98% efficacy in high-grade disease related to HPV 16/18 in unexposed 44% efficacy in high-grade disease related to HPV 16/18 in exposed Protection from noncervical low-grade disease: 81.5% in placebo vs 21.7% in vaccinated 100% efficacy against VIN 1 and ValN 1 in unexposed 99% efficacy against condyloma in unexposed		92% efficacy against ≥CIN 2 related to HPV 16/18 54% efficacy against ≥CIN 2 related to nonvaccine HPV types 100% efficacy against ≥CIN 3 related to HPV 16/18 90% efficacy against ≥CIN 3 overall 100% efficacy against adenocarcinoma in situ in those negative for HPV 77% efficacy against AIS in all Reduction in high-grade disease caused by other nonvaccine HPV types

Data from Refs.[39,42,43,45,95–99]

completion of the vaccine series. The analysis was done according to the protocol cohort, the total vaccinated cohort (TVC, which included all women receiving at least 1 vaccine dose, regardless of baseline HPV status and including those who were sexually active), and TVC-naive (women with no evidence of oncogenic HPV infection at baseline.)

The PATRICIA trial demonstrated 100% efficacy in the prevention of CIN 3+ caused by HPV 16/18 in the TVC-naive group. As expected, the efficacy in the TVC group was lower at 45.7%. There was a 93.2% efficacy in the prevention of CIN 3 in the TVC-naive group irrespective of HPV type.[43,44] In addition, there was also 100% efficacy in the prevention of AIS in the TVC-naive group and 76.9% in the TVC group. The vaccine had a 90% efficacy in preventing all CIN 3+ lesions in all age groups in the TVC-naive cohort. Among the TVC group, there was a progressive decline in vaccine efficacy against all HPV 16/18–associated CIN 3+ among different age groups. The highest efficacy (65.5%) was seen in women aged 15 to 17 years of age; 33.1% efficacy was seen in the group aged 18 to 20 years and 19.5% in those aged 21 to 25 years. The investigators attributed this decline in efficacy among the older age group to the higher exposure to HPV at baseline among older women (see **Table 2**).

The bivalent vaccine has also been shown to reduce the risk of high-grade cervical disease caused by nonvaccine HPV types, including HPV 31, 33, 35, 39, 45, 51, 52, 56, 58, 59, 66, and 68.[45]

Comparison of Quadrivalent and Bivalent HPV Vaccines

The cross-protective effects of both available vaccines have become a focus of interest, particularly among public health figures in countries that are in the midst of deciding which vaccine to use in their national programs. However, because of differences in participant characteristics and the prevalence of HPV infections among trial participants, comparisons between the 2 vaccines have been difficult. Malagon and colleagues[46] performed a systematic review and meta-analysis comparing the cross-protective effects of the quadrivalent vaccine versus the bivalent vaccine. To minimize differences in study design and participants, they focused the analysis on HPV-naive populations. In this comparison, it was demonstrated that both the quadrivalent and bivalent vaccines offer cross-protection against disease caused by nonvaccine HPV types. Pooled data from PATRICIA and FUTURE I/II showed that cross-protective efficacy was greater with the bivalent vaccine compared with the quadrivalent vaccine. The quadrivalent vaccine was noted to be efficacious against HPV 31 whereas the bivalent vaccine showed greater efficacy against HPV 31, 33, and 45 for persistent infection and CIN 2+ disease. Both vaccines showed little evidence of cross-protection against HPV 52 and 58. Prolonged follow-up in the bivalent trials showed decreasing efficacy against HPV 31 and 45 suggesting waning of cross-protection over time.[46]

IMMUNOGENICITY TRIALS

The 2 currently available HPV viruslike particle (VLP) vaccines have been developed using innovative recombinant molecular technology and consist only of the major viral capsid protein L1. VLP vaccines confer their protective effect by inducing high concentrations of type-specific virion neutralizing antibodies and they have demonstrated remarkable efficacy against genital diseases caused by the vaccine HPV types.[47] Clinical trials have shown that both vaccines are highly immunogenic demonstrating 100% seroconversion, and showing peak geometric antibody titers (GMTs) to be 10-fold to 100-fold higher compared with GMTs after natural infection.[48,49] Studies measuring the antibody responses of both vaccines used different assays, which make it impossible to make quantitative comparisons based on published studies; Gardasil was evaluated with a Luminex-based assay whereas Cervarix was evaluated with a VLP-based enzyme-linked assay (ELISA).[50] Nevertheless, titers for both vaccines peaked 1 month after the third dose and declined over the next year but remained relatively stable for the duration of follow-up (4 years for Cervarix and 4.5 years for Gardasil).[51,52] Women vaccinated with Cervarix showed titers greater than the GMT observed after natural infection during the plateau stage. However, almost one-third of those vaccinated with Gardasil experienced a drop in HPV 18 titers to less than the level of detection. This may be due to the intrinsic immunogenicity of HPV 18 VLPs or merely confounded by the monoclonal antibody assay used to detect the HPV 18 antibodies.

Immunogenic studies on adolescent boys and girls not only demonstrated vaccine safety in this age group but also exhibited a noninferior antibody response to the vaccine by boys compared with girls.[53,54] In addition, the GMT of VLP-specific antibodies in boys and girls were 2-fold higher than that found in young women.[55,56]

A phase III randomized study was conducted to compare the immunogenicity and safety of the bivalent vaccine and the quadrivalent vaccine in 1106 healthy women aged 18 to 45 years (they were stratified by age groups: 18–26 years, 27–35 years, and 36–45 years).[57] At month 7 after first vaccination, all women in the according-to-protocol cohort who were seronegative/DNA negative before vaccination had seroconverted for HPV 16 and HPV 18 serum neutralizing antibodies except for 2 women aged 27 to 35 years in the Gardasil group who did not seroconvert for HPV 18 (98%). However, geometric mean titers of serum neutralizing antibodies ranged from 2.3-fold to 4.8-fold higher for HPV 16 and 6.8-fold to 9.1-fold higher for HPV 18 after vaccination with Cervarix compared with Gardasil, across all age groups. At month 24, 100% of the women who received the HPV 16/18 vaccine and 97.5% to 100% of those who received the HPV 6/11/16/18 vaccine remained seropositive for HPV 16; 99% to 100% of the women who received the bivalent vaccine and 72.3% to 84.4% of the women who received the quadrivalent vaccine remained seropositive for HPV 18.[58] Higher antibody levels among the HPV 16/18 group compared with the HPV 6/11/16/18 group were similarly noted at month 24. In accordance with other immunogenicity studies, the geometric mean titer ratios of anti-HPV 16 and 18 antibodies between the 2 vaccine groups were greater in the younger age group (18–26 years and 27–36 years) compared with the older age group (35–45 years) from month 7 to month 24.

Other immunobridging studies have been implemented to generate data that can support the use and efficacy of the vaccine outside the recommended guidelines. Romanowski and colleagues[59] conducted a partially blinded randomized controlled trial evaluating a 2-dose vaccine schedule versus a 3-dose schedule of the HPV 16/18 vaccine in healthy young females aged 9 to 25 years. The study participants were stratified into age groups (9–14 years, 15–19 years, and 20–25 years) and randomized to receive 2 or 3 doses of 20 μg of HPV 16 and 18 L1 VLP or 2 higher doses of 40 μg of HPV 16 and 18 L1 VLP. Results showed that the 2-dose schedule of HPV 16/18 in the age group 9 to 14 years was noninferior to the 3-dose schedule in women aged 15 to 25 years at 1 month after the last dose and this was maintained at month 24 after completion of the vaccine series. The safety profiles were similar in all 3 groups and this study supports that a 2-dose schedule may infer adequate immunogenic response in younger females.

In a subanalysis of the Costa Rica Vaccine Trial, the investigators also aimed to analyze the efficacy of less than 3 vaccine doses of the bivalent vaccine.[60] Excluding women who had no follow-up or who were HPV 16 or 18 DNA positive at enrollment, they compared 5967 women who received all 3 vaccines, 802 women who received 2 doses, and 384 women who only received 1 dose. The efficacy of the vaccine against incident HPV 16 or 18 infection that persisted at least 1 year was 80.9% for those who received 3 doses, 84.1% for those who received 2 doses, and 100% for those who received 1 dose only. This subanalysis, although obtained from a nonrandomized sample, contributes further evidence that less than 3 doses of the vaccines may confer adequate immunoprotection.

Currently, ongoing studies are also investigating the safety and immunogenic effect of the HPV vaccine in individuals infected with HIV. Women infected with HIV have been shown to have a higher prevalence of HPV coinfection and HPV-related diseases.[61] Linkage studies also demonstrate a 2-fold to 22-fold increase in cervical cancer in HIV-positive women compared with the general population.[62] In addition to safety and efficacy studies, investigators are also looking to determine if there is any difference in antibody titers between HIV-negative and HIV-infected individuals and to determine the difference in antibody titers among HIV-infected individuals on antiretroviral therapy versus those who are not.[63] Preliminary results of a phase II trial of the bivalent vaccine performed in South Africa showed that both HIV-negative and HIV-infected women seroconverted to HPV 16 and 18 regardless of baseline HPV status.[51] However, women with HIV had significantly lower geometric mean titers compared with their HIV-negative counterparts. There are many other studies looking at adolescents, young women, and men infected with HIV. Several of these studies are being conducted in countries where both HIV and HPV pose a significant public health problem.[52,64] Administering the HPV vaccine to this population, who are at a higher risk for HPV-related morbidity, provides reasonable rationale for disease prevention and infection control.

HPV VACCINE UPTAKE

Given the positive results from multiple efficacy studies on the 2 currently available HPV vaccines, widespread uptake and administration before sexual debut can potentially reduce the public health burdens brought about by HPV-related infections. However, there are impediments to widespread vaccine acceptability and barriers in achieving high vaccination rates among the preferred target age group. In adolescents, disparities in HPV vaccination use have been demonstrated by age, race, insurance, and poverty level.[65] Several studies among women, adolescents, and parents have documented concerns regarding vaccine safety, efficacy, and cost.[56,66,67] Among parents, there is concern regarding the potential influence of early vaccination on adolescent sexual behavior.[68–70]

The CDC tracks vaccination coverage among adolescents aged 13 to 17 years through the National Immunization Survey–Teen (NIS-Teen).[65] An analysis of the NIS-Teen data for 2010 was performed to provide updated vaccination coverage estimates (Fig. 4). The 2010 data demonstrated that (among females in this age group) those receiving 1 or more dose of HPV increased from 44.3% to 48.7%, and 26.7% to 32.0% received 3 more doses of HPV compared with 2009 estimates. Among females who initiated the HPV series, 94.3% met the minimum period needed to complete the series and 69.6% received 3 or more doses. Among adolescent males, 1.4% (confidence interval 1.1–1.8) received 1 or more doses of HPV.

HPV vaccine initiation was observed to be lower among the white population than among Hispanic and American Indian/Alaskan Native populations. However, the racial disparities in vaccine completion showed that completion of the 3 doses was lower among the black and Hispanic populations than among the white population. There

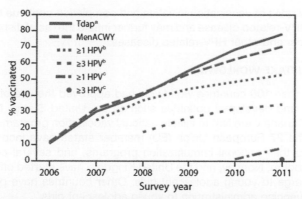

Fig. 4. National immunization survey-Teen, United States, 2006–2011. Estimated vaccination coverage with selected vaccines and doses among adolescents aged 13 to 17 years, by survey year. [a] On or after age 10 years. [b] Among females. [c] Among males. Adolescent vaccination coverage increased from 2006 to 2011, although the rate of increase differed by vaccine. MenACWY, meningococcal conjugate vaccine; Tdap, tetanus toxoid, diphtheria toxoid, acellular pertussis vaccine. (*Data from* Morbidity and Mortality Weekly Report (MMWR). National and state vaccination coverage among adolescents aged 13–17 years — United States, 2011. Available at: http://www.cdc.gov/mmwr/preview/mmwrhtml/mm6134a3.htm?s_cid=mm6134a3_e%0d%0a#fig. Accessed February 28, 2013.)

was no difference observed by poverty status for initiation of the vaccine. However, completion of the series among adolescents living below the poverty line was lower compared with those living at or above the poverty line. The price for the complete 3-dose series of Gardasil is about $399 and $386 for the Cervarix vaccine.[71] Most insurance covers the cost of the ACIP recommended vaccines, and the federally funded Vaccine for Children program has also helped to alleviate the financial barrier to children who may not otherwise have access because of lack of insurance coverage. Having insurance coverage has been associated with higher rates of vaccination (both initiation and completion) among adolescent females. Completion of the vaccine series has also varied by type of insurance coverage; higher rates of completion were observed within the private insurance sector.[72]

There is also a paucity of information on the use of the HPV vaccine among young adult women.[64] Women aged 19 to 26 years of age, perhaps, have the highest rates of HPV infection and HPV-related diseases.[73,74] Seventy-four percent of the new HPV infections annually occur among women aged 15 to 24 years.[75] However, reports by the CDC 2 to 5 months after HPV vaccination approval showed that only 10% of women aged 18 to 26 years had initiated the vaccine series.[76] Another study by Dempsey and colleagues[64] showed that the rates of HPV vaccination between 2007 and 2009 among women aged 19 to 26 years continued to be low with only 18% initiating the series and only 10% completing all 3 vaccine doses within a period of 30 months. National Health Interview Survey (NHIS) data in 2010 showed that 20.7% of women aged 19 to 26 years received at least 1 dose of HPV vaccine, which was a significant increase from 17.1% in 2009 and 10.5% in 2008. Less than 1% of men aged 19 to 26 years received at least 1 dose of the vaccine.[77]

Disparities in vaccine series initiation by race and insurance type were also found to worsen over time. African Americans in this study, as in other studies of younger age groups,[78] were shown to have decreased rates of completing the vaccine series. Minority women are at increased risk of HPV-related disease and mortality. The persistently low rates of vaccination initiation and completion continue to be a barrier in eradicating HPV-related disease and may further inflate the racial disparities in rates of cervical cancer and other HPV-related diseases.

HPV VACCINE UPTAKE WORLDWIDE

By 2008, more than 100 countries worldwide had approved the use of either one or both vaccines, and developed countries such as the United States, New Zealand, Australia, and Canada were first to initiate national vaccination programs.[34,79] In addition, most of the 27 European Union (EU) member states have incorporated HPV vaccination into their national immunization programs, and several countries such as Italy, Luxembourg, Norway, and the United Kingdom have started offering the vaccine free of charge to young adolescent girls. Other countries have provided reimbursement for vaccine administration to young adolescent girls.

In low-income and middle-income countries, uptake of HPV vaccine into national vaccination programs has not been implemented as easily because of financial constraints, lack of infrastructure, and competing health priorities.[80] However, in 2008, the Global Alliance for Vaccines and Immunization (GAVI), an organization that subsidizes vaccines for poor countries, pledged to secure funds to make the HPV vaccine available in underdeveloped countries. Recently, the GAVI Alliance announced a price of US$5 per dose for HPV vaccine, which makes the vaccine more affordable for low-resource countries that are eligible for subsidized vaccine purchase and increases the likelihood of introducing the vaccine.[81] The GAVI hopes to make funds available to eligible countries interested in HPV vaccine implementation between 2010 and 2020. Panama and Mexico were the first middle-income countries to introduce HPV vaccination; Rwanda and Bhutan have also started national vaccination campaigns after receiving adequate donations to fund their programs.[82] From 2006 to 2010, PATH, a global nongovernmental health organization, collaborated with the governments of India, Peru, Uganda, and Vietnam to gather evidence to support decisions on whether and how to introduce HPV vaccines.[83] The objective was to determine what level of complete HPV vaccination coverage in the target population could be achieved for each country with a specific strategy for vaccine distribution. High HPV vaccination coverage was achieved where school-based delivery strategies were used. The coverage achieved through school-based programs was 82.6% in Peru and 88.9% in 2009 in Uganda. In Vietnam, there was an improvement in coverage in the second year of the program with rates increasing from 83.0% to 96.1%. A combination of school-based and health center–based delivery was used in India. The coverage achieved by the program ranged from 77.2% to 87.8%.

The positive impact of widespread HPV vaccination has been recently demonstrated in Australia. A significant decline in the incidence of genital warts as well as histologically confirmed high-grade cervical lesions has been observed since the implementation of free universal HPV vaccination in 2007.[84–86] Australia's vaccination program has resulted in complete vaccination of 70.8% of females aged 12 to 26 years. As a result, they observed a 39% reduction in the incidence of genital warts in nonvaccinated heterosexual men of the same age range, which is probable evidence of the herd immunity effect of the HPV vaccine.[84]

NEW VACCINES

The results of vaccine trials worldwide will provide important information that can be used in implementing national policies on vaccine administration and perhaps extend coverage to include secondary populations such as older women and

Table 3
HPV vaccines in development

Vaccine Type	Immunogen	Target	Sponsor
Prophylactic Vaccines			
Octavalent vaccine	L1 virus like particle of HPV types 6, 11, 16,18, 31, 45, 52, 58	Cervical, Anal, Vaginal, Vulvar dysplasia and cancer	Merck
V504 (administered with Gardasil)	L1 virus like particles of HPV types 31, 33, 45, 52, 58	Cervical, Anal, Vaginal, Vulvar dysplasia and cancer	Merck
MEDI-517	Virus like particles of HPV types 16, 18	Cervical dysplasia and cancer	Glaxo Smith Kline
9-valent vaccine (V503)	L1 virus like particles of HPV types 6, 11, 16, 18, 31, 33, 45, 52, 58	Cervical, Anal, Vaginal, Vulvar dysplasia and cancer Genital Warts	Merck
VGX-3100	Plasmids targeting E6 and E7 proteins of HPV types 16, 18	Cervical dysplasia and cancer	Inovio Pharmaceuticals
Therapeutic Vaccines			
pNGVL-4a-CRT/E7 (detox) DNA vaccine	E7 DNA of HPV 16	Cervical dysplasia Head and neck cancers	Sidney Kimmel Comprehensive Cancer Center
HPV-16 vaccine	4 HPV 16 E6 proteins	Cervical dysplasia	University of Arkansas
TA-HPV	E6 and E7 proteins of HPV 16/18	Cervical cancer	European Organization for Research and Treatment of Cancer
VGX-3100	Plasmids targeting E6 and E7 proteins of HPV 16/18	Cervical dysplasia and cancer	Inovio Pharmaceuticals
HPV 16 E6 and E7 vaccine	E6 and E7 proteins HPV 16	Cervical cancer, anal cancer, esophageal cancer, head and neck cancer, penile cancer, vulvar cancer	National Cancer Institute
MAGE-A3-HPV 16	Trojan peptide complexes containing MAGE-A3 and HPV 16	Head and neck cancer	University of Maryland
ADXS11-001	E7 protein of HPV 16	Cervical dysplasia and cancer, anal cancer, oropharyngeal cancer	Advaxis
Hsp-E7	Recombinant DNA fusion of heat shock protein 65 and E7 protein of HPV type 16	Cervical dysplasia	National Cancer Institute, Dana-Farber/Brigham and Women's Cancer Center

(continued on next page)

Table 3 *(continued)*			
Vaccine Type	Immunogen	Target	Sponsor
Alternating E7 vaccine and dendritic cells presenting E7	E7 protein of HPV 16 vaccine and dendritic cells presenting E7 protein	Recurrent or persistent cervical cancer	Steward St. Elizabeth's Medical Center of Boston, National Cancer Institute
Gp100: 209–217 and HPV 16 E7: 12–20 peptide	Amino acids 209–217 of glycoprotein 100 melanoma antigen and amino acids 12–20 of E7 protein of HPV 16	Melanoma	Providence Cancer Center, Earle A. Chiles Research Institute, National Cancer Institute

Data from Search term "HPV vaccine." Available at: www.clinicaltrials.gov. Accessed February 28, 2013.

individuals infected with HIV. However, the 2 currently available vaccines have a limited efficacy on other high-risk HPV types and the cost of the vaccine limits widespread access, especially in low-income countries. In addition, storage requires refrigeration, and administration requires multiple doses and intramuscular injection. Second-generation vaccines are currently being developed to address these shortcomings. The objectives in developing second-generation vaccines will be to (1) broaden coverage to include protection against other genital oncogenic HPV types; (2) induce long-term protection; (3) make the vaccines more affordable and easily stored; (4) allow vaccines to be administered easily via noninjectable methods; and (5) potentially provide therapeutic efficacy. Multiple companies are investigating new vaccines targeting various immunogens in the HPV virus. The nonavalent vaccine being investigated by Merck is the closest to approval for use (**Table 3**).[87]

L2-Based Vaccine

The amino terminus of the L2 capsid protein of HPV contains a major cross-neutralizing epitope. This has been the basis of investigations into L2-based vaccines.[88] Research done using mouse monoclonal antibodies shows that there are at least 2 cross-neutralization episodes in the amino acid 56 to 75 region that show neutralization against oncogenic HPV strains.[89] Studies on mice and rabbits show that immunization with VLPs expressing the L2 protein of HPV 16 and 31 induced robust antibody titers against various HPV types.[90] Mouse studies show that oral administration of a vaccine targeted at the L2 capsid protein induced significant neutralizing activities against genital infection by HPV 16/18/45/58.[91]

Nonavalent Vaccine

Studies have shown that both HPV vaccines have moderate cross-protection against other high-risk HPV types.[27,28] In addition to HPV 16 and 18, other high-risk subtypes that have been associated with 90% of cervical cancer cases worldwide include types 31, 33, 45, 52, and 58.[92] Merck has been studying the efficacy of a nonavalent vaccine containing VLPs of 9 high-risk HPV types (6, 11, 16, 18, 31, 33, 45, 52, and 58).[19] They are currently in phase III clinical trials and they anticipate presenting their results to the FDA shortly.[87] The nonavalent vaccine has potential to significantly reduce cervical precancerous and cancerous lesions.[93]

Therapeutic Vaccines

The development of a vaccine with both a therapeutic and prophylactic component should prove to be beneficial for individuals who have already been exposed to HPV. Therapeutic vaccines can prevent reinfection and control reactivation of already acquired HPV types. The goal for therapeutic vaccines is to eliminate preexisting lesions and even malignant tumors by generating cell-mediated immunity against HPV-infected cells.[94] Current approaches include live vector–based, peptide-based, protein-based, nucleic acid-based, and cell-based vaccines. The antigens targeted in therapeutic vaccines include the HPV early proteins that are expressed throughout the life cycle of the infected cells and cancer cells. In particular, the HPV-encoded proteins E6 and E7 represent ideal targets for the development of these vaccines. Investigators have primarily focused on stimulating the production and activation of T cells by targeting E6 and/or E7 proteins.

SUMMARY

HPV is one of the most common sexually transmitted infections affecting both men and women worldwide. The development of prophylactic HPV vaccines is a significant pharmaceutical innovation with the potential to reduce HPV-related morbidity as shown by the positive results of several efficacy trials. However, barriers to the universal use and acceptability of the HPV vaccines continue to exist in both economically privileged and disadvantaged countries. It may be decades before the impact of preventive vaccines on HPV-related diseases will be seen because of the considerable burden of HPV infections. However, collaborative efforts should continue to promote vaccine administration and extension of coverage to other vulnerable populations that may benefit from the vaccines' prophylactic properties.

REFERENCES

1. Weinstock H, Berman S, Cates W Jr. Sexually transmitted diseases among American youth: incidence and prevalence estimates, 2000. Perspect Sex Reprod Health 2004;36(1):6–10.
2. Hariri S, Unger ER, Sternberg M, et al. Prevalence of genital human papillomavirus among females in the United States, the National Health And Nutrition Examination Survey, 2003-2006. J Infect Dis 2011;204(4):566–73.
3. Bernard HU, Burk RD, Chen Z, et al. Classification of papillomaviruses (PVs) based on 189 PV types and proposal of taxonomic amendments. Virology 2010;401:70–9.
4. Bouvard V, Baan R, Straif K, et al. A review of human carcinogens—Part B: biological agents. Lancet Oncol 2009;10:321–2.
5. Bosch FX, de Sanjose S. Chapter 1: human papillomavirus and cervical cancer–burden and assessment of causality. J Natl Cancer Inst Monogr 2003;(31):3 13.
6. Markowitz LE, Dunne EF, Saraiya M, et al. Quadrivalent human papillomavirus vaccine. Recommendations of the Advisory Committee on Immunization Practices (ACIP). MMWR Recomm Rep 2007. Available at: http://www.cdc.gov/mmwr/preview/mmwrhtml/rr5602a1.htm?s_cid=rr5602a1_e. Accessed May 25, 2011.
7. Jemal A, Simard EP, Dorel C, et al. Annual report to the nation on the status of cancer, 1975–2009, featuring the burden and trends in human papillomavirus

(HPV)–associated cancers and HPV vaccination coverage levels. J Natl Cancer Inst 2013;105(3):175–201.

8. Myers ER, McCrory DC, Nanda K, et al. Mathematical model for the natural history of human papillomavirus infection and cervical carcinogenesis. Am J Epidemiol 2000;151(12):1158–71.

9. Herrero R, Hildesheim A, Bratti C, et al. Population-based study of human papillomavirus infection and cervical neoplasia in rural Costa Rica. J Natl Cancer Inst 2000;92(6):464–74.

10. Castellsague X, de Sanjose S, Aguado T, et al. WHO/ICO Information Centre on HPV and Cervical Cancer (HPV Information Centre). HPV and cervical cancer in the world [Report]. Geneva (Switzerland), Barcelona (Spain): WHO, ICO; 2007. Available at: http://www.who.int/hpvcentre/en/. Accessed February 7, 2013.

11. Ferlay J, Shin HR, Bray F, et al. Estimates of worldwide burden of cancer in 2008: GLOBOCAN 2008. Int J Cancer 2010;127(12):2893–917.

12. Papanicolaou GN. A new procedure for staining vaginal smears. Science 1942; 95(2469):438–9.

13. Sahasrabuddhe V, Sherman ME. Human papillomavirus vaccines for cervical cancer prevention: translating possibility into reality. J Natl Cancer Inst 2012; 104(22):1698–701.

14. Schiffman M, Wentzensen N, Wacholder S, et al. Human papillomavirus testing in the prevention of cervical cancer. J Natl Cancer Inst 2011;103(5):368–83.

15. Schiffman M, Castle PE, Jeronimo J, et al. Human papillomavirus and cervical cancer. Lancet 2007;370(9590):890–907.

16. Stanley M. Immune responses to human papillomavirus. Vaccine 2006;24(Suppl 1): S16–22.

17. Muñoz N, Castellsagué X, de González AB, et al. Chapter 1: HPV in the etiology of human cancer. Vaccine 2006;24(Suppl 3):S3/1–10.

18. Schiffman M, Castle PE. The promise of global cervical-cancer prevention. N Engl J Med 2005;353(20):2101–4.

19. Schiller JT, Lowy DR. Immunogenicity testing in human papillomavirus virus-like-particle vaccine trials. J Infect Dis 2009;200:166–71.

20. CDC. Quadrivalent human papillomavirus vaccine: recommendations of the Advisory Committee on Immunization Practices (ACIP). MMWR Recomm Rep 2007;56:RR-2.

21. Centers for Disease Control and Prevention (CDC). FDA licensure of bivalent human papillomavirus vaccine (HPV2 Cervarix) for use in females and updated HPV vaccination recommendations from the Advisory Committee on Immunization Practices (ACIP). MMWR Recomm Rep 2010;59(20):626–9.

22. GlaxoSmithKline. CDC Advisory Committee recommends Cervarix to prevent cervical cancer in girls and young women. Available at: http://us.gsk.com/html/media-news/pressreleases/2009/2009_us_pressrelease_10075.htm. Accessed November 10, 2009.

23. Hu D, Goldie S. The economic burden of noncervical human papillomavirus disease in the United States. Am J Obstet Gynecol 2008;198:500–7.

24. Joseph DA, Miller JW, Wu X, et al. Understanding the burden of human papillomavirus-associated anal cancers in the US. Cancer 2008;113(Suppl 10): 2892–900.

25. Chaturvedi AK, Engels EA, Pfeiffer RM, et al. Human papillomavirus and rising oropharyngeal cancer incidence in the United States. J Clin Oncol 2011;29: 4294–301.

26. Saraiya M. Burden of HPV-associated cancers in the United States. Presentation before the Advisory Committee on Immunization Practices (ACIP), February 24, 2011. Atlanta (GA): US Department of Health and Human Services, CDC; 2011. Available at: http://www.cdc.gov/vaccines/recs/acip/downloads/mtg-slides-feb11/11-2-hpv-rela-cancer.pdf. Accessed March 2, 2013.

27. Food and Drug Administration Center for Biologics Evaluation and Research. Briefing document for the Vaccines and Related Biological Products Advisory Committee. Subject: Male indication for Gardasil. Available at: http://www.fda. gov/downloads/AdvisoryCommittees/CommitteesMeetingMaterials/Blood VaccinesandOtherBiologics/VaccinesandRelatedBiologicalProductsAdvisory Committee/UCM181361.pdf. Accessed September 24, 2009.

28. FDA. FDA approves new indication for Gardasil to prevent genital warts in men and boys. 2009 10/16/2009. Available at: http://www.fda.gov/NewsEvents/ Newsroom/PressAnnouncements/ucm187003.htm. Accessed October 20, 2009.

29. Maggard MA, Beanes SR, Ko CY. Anal canal cancer: a population-based reappraisal. Dis Colon Rectum 2003;46(11):1517–23.

30. Howlader N, Noone AM, Krapcho M, et al. SEER cancer statistics review, 1975-2008. Bethesda (MD): National Cancer Institute [based on November 2010 SEER data submission, posted to the SEER web site, 2011]. Available at: http://seer.cancer.gov/csr/1975_2008/. Accessed December 7, 2012.

31. Johnson LG, Madeleine MM, Newcomer LM, et al. Anal cancer incidence and survival: the surveillance, epidemiology, and end results experience, 1973–2000. Cancer 2004;101:281–8.

32. Centers for Disease Control and Prevention. Human papilloma virus (HPV) associated cancers. Available at: http://www.cdc.gov/cancer/hpv/statistics/anal.htm. Accessed March 1, 2013.

33. Food and Drug Administration. Highlights of prescribing information. Gardasil (human papillomavirus quadrivalent [types 6, 11, 16 and 18]). Silver Spring (MD): Food and Drug Administration; 2011. Available at: http://www.fda.gov/ downloads/biologicsbloodvaccines/vaccines/approvedproducts/ucm111263. pdf. Accessed December 13, 2012.

34. Giuliano AR, Palefsky JM, Goldstone S, et al. Efficacy of quadrivalent HPV vaccine against HPV infection and disease in males. N Engl J Med 2011;364(5):401–11.

35. Centers for Disease Control and Prevention (CDC). Recommendations for the quadrivalent human papillomavirus vaccine in males – Advisory Committee on Immunization Practices (ACIP). MMWR Recomm Rep 2011;60(50):1705–8.

36. Kreimer AR, González P, Katki HA, et al. Efficacy of a bivalent HPV 16/18 vaccine against anal HPV 16/18 infection among young women: a nested analysis within the Costa Rica Vaccine Trial. Lancet Oncol 2011;12(9):862–70.

37. Villa LL, Costa RL, Petta CA, et al. Prophylactic quadrivalent human papillomavirus (types 6, 11, 16, and 18) L1 virus-like particle vaccine in young women: a randomised double-blind placebo-controlled multicentre phase II efficacy trial. Lancet 2005;6(5):271–8.

38. Garland SM, Hernandez-Avila M, Wheeler CM, et al. Quadrivalent vaccine against the human papillomavirus to prevent anogenital diseases. N Engl J Med 2007;356(19):1928–43.

39. FUTURE II Study Group. Quadrivalent vaccine against human papillomavirus to prevent high-grade cervical lesions. N Engl J Med 2007;356(19):1915–27.

40. Kjaer SK, Sigurdsson K, Iversen OE, et al. A pooled analysis of continued prophylactic efficacy of quadrivalent human papillomavirus (types 6/11/16/18)

vaccine against high-grade cervical and external genital lesions. Cancer Prev Res (Phila) 2009;2(10):868–78.

41. Munoz N, Kjaer SK, Sigurdsson K, et al. Impact of human papillomavirus (HPV)-6/11/16/18 vaccine on all HPV-associated genital diseases in young women. J Natl Cancer Inst 2010;102(5):325–39.

42. Paavonen J, Jenkins D, HPV PATRICIA Study Group, et al. Efficacy of a prophylactic adjuvanted bivalent L1 virus-like-particle vaccine against infection with human papillomavirus types 16 and 18 in young women: an interim analysis of a phase III double-blind, randomised controlled trial. Lancet 2007; 369(9580):2161–70.

43. Lehtinen M, Paavonen J, Wheeler CM, et al. Overall efficacy of HPV-16/18 AS04-adjuvanted vaccine against grade 3 or greater cervical intraepithelial neoplasia: 4-year end-of-study analysis of the randomised, double-blind PATRICIA trial. Lancet Oncol 2012;13(1):89–99.

44. Schiller JT, Castellsagué X, Garland SM. A review of clinical trials of human papillomavirus prophylactic vaccines. Vaccine 2012;30S:F123–38.

45. Wheeler CM, Castellsagué X, HPV PATRICIA Study Group, et al. Cross-protective efficacy of HPV-16/18 AS04-adjuvanted vaccine against cervical infection and precancer caused by non-vaccine oncogenic HPV types: 4-year end-of-study analysis of the randomised, double-blind PATRICIA trial. Lancet Oncol 2012;13(1):100–10.

46. Malagón T, Drolet M, Boily MC, et al. Cross-protective efficacy of two human papillomavirus vaccines: a systematic review and meta-analysis. Lancet Infect Dis 2012;12(10):781–9.

47. Stanley M, Gissman L, Nardelli-Haeflinger D. Immunobiology of human papillomavirus infection and vaccination–implications for second generation vaccines. Vaccine 2008;26(Suppl 10):K62–7.

48. Harper DM, Franco EL, Wheeler C, et al. Efficacy of a bivalent L1 virus-like particle vaccine in prevention of infection with human papillomavirus types 16 and 18 in young women: a randomised controlled trial. Lancet 2004;364(9447): 1757–65.

49. Villa LL, Ault KA, Giuliano AR, et al. Immunologic responses following administration of a vaccine targeting human papillomavirus types 6, 11, 16, and 18. Vaccine 2006;24(27–28):5571–83.

50. Schiller JT, Castellsague X, Villa L, et al. An update of prophylactic human papillomavirus L1 virus-like particle vaccine clinical trials. Vaccine 2008;26(Suppl 10):K53–61.

51. Denny L, Hendricks B, Gordon C, et al. Safety and immunogenicity of the HPV-16/18 ASO4-adjuvanted vaccine in HIV positive women in South Africa. Abstract no. 599. Presented at AORTIC 7th International Conference. 2011.

52. Available at: http://www.clinicaltrials.gov/ct2/results?term=HPV+and+HIV&pg=1. Accessed January 26, 2013.

53. Reisinger KS, Block SL, Lazcano-Ponce E, et al. Safety and persistent immunogenicity of a quadrivalent human papillomavirus types 6, 11, 16, 18 L1 virus-like particle vaccine in preadolescents and adolescents: a randomized controlled trial. Pediatr Infect Dis J 2007;26(3):201–9.

54. Block SL, Nolan T, Sattler C, et al. Comparison of the immunogenicity and reactogenicity of a prophylactic quadrivalent human papillomavirus (types 6, 11, 16, and 18) L1 virus-like particle vaccine in male and female adolescents and young adult women. Pediatrics 2006;118(5):2135–45.

55. Pedersen C, Petaja T, Strauss G, et al. Immunization of early adolescent females with human papillomavirus type 16 and 18 L1 virus-like particle vaccine containing AS04 adjuvant. J Adolesc Health 2007;40(6):564–71.
56. Boehner CW, Howe SR, Bernstein DI, et al. Viral sexually transmitted disease vaccine acceptability among college students. Sex Transm Dis 2003;30(10): 774–8.
57. Einstein MH, Baron M, Levin MJ, et al. Comparison of the immunogenicity and safety of Cervarix and Gardasil human papillomavirus (HPV) cervical cancer vaccines in healthy women aged 18-45 years. Hum Vaccin 2009;5(10):705–19.
58. Einstein MH, Baron M, Levin MJ, et al. Comparison of the immunogenicity and safety of Cervarix and Gardasil human papillomavirus (HPV) cervical cancer vaccines in healthy women aged 18-45 years – Follow up from months 12-24 in a phase III randomized study of healthy women aged 18-45 years. Hum Vaccin 2011;7(12):1343–58.
59. Romanowski B, Schwarz TF, Ferguson LM, et al. Immunogenicity and safety of the HPV-16/18 AS04-adjuvanted vaccine administered as a 2-dose schedule compared with the licensed 3-dose schedule: results from a randomized study. Hum Vaccin 2011;7(12):1374–86.
60. Kreimer AR, Rodriguez AC, Hildesheim A, et al. Proof-of-principle evaluation of the efficacy of fewer than three doses of a bivalent HPV16/18 vaccine. J Natl Cancer Inst 2011;103(19):1444–51.
61. De Vuyst H, Lillo F, Broutet N, et al. HIV, human papillomavirus, and cervical neoplasia and cancer in the era of highly active antiretroviral therapy. Eur J Cancer Prev 2008;17:545–54.
62. Harris TG, Burk RB, Palefsky JM, et al. Incidence of cervical squamous intraepithelial lesions associated with HIV serostatus, CD4 cell counts, and human papillomavirus test results. JAMA 2005;293:1471–6.
63. Denny LA, Franceschi S, de Sanjosé S, et al. Human papillomavirus, human immunodeficiency virus and immunosuppression. Vaccine 2012;30(Suppl 5): F168–74.
64. Dempsey A, Cohn L, Dalton V, et al. Worsening disparities in HPV vaccine utilization among 19-26 year old women. Vaccine 2009;29:528–34.
65. CDC. National, state, and local area vaccination coverage among adolescents aged 13–17 years--United States, 2009. MMWR Recomm Rep 2010;59:1018–23. Available at: http://www.cdc.gov/mmwr/preview/mmwrhtml/mm6033a1.htm#Tab1. Accessed February 23, 2013.
66. Dempsey AF, Zimet GD, Davis RL, et al. Factors that are associated with parental acceptance of human papillomavirus vaccines: a randomized intervention study of written information about HPV. Pediatrics 2006;117(5):1486–93.
67. Wong LP. Young multiethnic women's attitudes toward the HPV vaccine and HPV vaccination. Int J Gynaecol Obstet 2008;103(2):131–5.
68. Davis K, Dickman ED, Ferris D, et al. Human papillomavirus vaccine acceptability among parents of 10- to 15-year-old adolescents. J Low Genit Tract Dis 2004;8(3):188–94.
69. Zimet GD, Perkins SM, Sturm LA, et al. Predictors of STI vaccine acceptability among parents and their adolescent children. J Adolesc Health 2005;37(3): 179–86.
70. Kahn JA, Ding L, Huang B, et al. Mothers' intention for their daughters and themselves to receive the human papillomavirus vaccine: a national study of nurses. Pediatrics 2009;123(6):1439–45.

71. Stobbe M. Panel recommends a 2nd cervical cancer vaccine as alternative for girls and young women. New York: New York Times; 2009.
72. Etter DJ, Zimet GD, Vaughn RI. Human papillomavirus vaccine in adolescent women: a 2012 update. Curr Opin Obstet Gynecol 2012;24:305–10.
73. Dunne EF, Unger ER, Sternberg M, et al. Prevalence of HPV infection among females in the United States. JAMA 2007;297(8):813–9.
74. Ault KA. Epidemiology and natural history of human papillomavirus infections in the female genital tract. Infect Dis Obstet Gynecol 2006;2006:40470.
75. Huang CM. Human papillomavirus and vaccination. Mayo Clin Proc 2008;83(6): 701–7.
76. Jain N, Euler GL, Shefer A, et al. Human papillomavirus (HPV) awareness and vaccination initiation among women in the United States, national immunization survey-adult 2007. Prev Med 2009;48(5):426–31.
77. Williams WW, Lu PJ, Singleton JA, et al. Adult vaccination coverage — United States, 2010. MMWR Recomm Rep 2012;61(4):66–70.
78. Dempsey A, Cohn L, Dalton VA, et al. Patient and clinic factors associated with adolescent human papillomavirus vaccine utilization within a university based health system. Vaccine 2010;28(4):989–95.
79. Barr E, Sings HL. Prophylactic HPV vaccines: new interventions for cancer control. Vaccine 2008;26:6244–57.
80. Graham J, Mishra A. Global challenges of implementing human papillomavirus vaccines. Int J Equity Health 2011;10:27.
81. GAVI welcomes lower prices for life-saving vaccines. Geneva (Switzerland): GAVI Alliance; 2011. Available at: http://www.gavialliance.org/library/news/press-releases/2011/gavi-welcomes-lower-prices-for-life-saving-vaccines/. Accessed August 8, 2011.
82. Poljak M. Prophylactic human papillomavirus vaccination and primary prevention of cervical cancer: issues and challenges. Clin Microbiol Infect 2012; 18(Suppl 5):64–9.
83. LaMontagne DS, Barge S, Thi Le N, et al. Human papillomavirus vaccine delivery strategies that achieved high coverage in low- and middle-income countries. Bull World Health Organ 2011;89:821–30.
84. Donovan B, Franklin N, Guy R, et al. Quadrivalent human papillomavirus vaccination and trends in genital warts in Australia: analysis of national sentinel surveillance data. Lancet Infect Dis 2011;11:39–44.
85. Read TR, Hocking JS, Chen MY, et al. The near disappearance of genital warts in young women 4 years after commencing a national human papillomavirus (HPV) vaccination programme. Sex Transm Infect 2011;87:544–7.
86. Brotherton JM, Fridman M, May C, et al. Early impact of the HPV vaccination program on cervical abnormalities in Victoria, Australia: an ecological study. Lancet 2011;377:2085–92.
87. Peres J. For cancers caused by HPV, two vaccines were just the beginning. J Natl Cancer Inst 2011;103(5):360–2.
88. Seitz H, Schmitt M, Böhmer G, et al. Natural variants in the major neutralizing epitope of human papillomavirus minor capsid protein L2. Int J Cancer 2013; 132(3):E139–48.
89. Nakao S, Mori S, Kondo K, et al. Monoclonal antibodies recognizing cross-neutralization epitopes in human papillomavirus 16 minor capsid protein L2. Virology 2012;434(1):110–7.
90. Nieto K, Weghofer M, Sehr P, et al. Development of AAVLP(HPV16/31L2) particles as broadly protective HPV vaccine candidate. PLoS One 2012;7(6):e39741.

91. Yoon SW, Lee TY, Kim SJ, et al. Oral administration of HPV-16 L2 displayed on *Lactobacillus casei* induces systematic and mucosal cross-neutralizing effects in Balb/c mice. Vaccine 2012;30(22):3286–94.
92. Franceschi S, Cuzick J, Herrero R, et al. EUROGIN 2008 roadmap on cervical cancer prevention. Int J Cancer 2009;125(10):2246–55.
93. Van de Velde N, Boily MC, Drolet M, et al. Population-level impact of the bivalent, quadrivalent, and nonavalent human papillomavirus vaccines: a model-based analysis. J Natl Cancer Inst 2012;104(22):1712–23.
94. Hung CF, Ma B, Monie A, et al. Therapeutic human papillomavirus vaccines: current clinical trials and future directions. Expert Opin Biol Ther 2008;8(4):421–39.
95. Joura EA, Garland SM, Paavonen J, et al, FUTURE I and II Study Group. Effect of the human papillomavirus (HPV) quadrivalent vaccine in a subgroup of women with cervical and vulvar disease: retrospective pooled analysis of trial data. BMJ 2012;344:e1401.
96. FUTURE I/II Study Group, Dillner J, Kjaer SK, et al. Four year efficacy of prophylactic human papillomavirus quadrivalent vaccine against low grade cervical, vulvar, and vaginal intraepithelial neoplasia and anogenital warts: randomised controlled trial. BMJ 2010;341:c3493.
97. Ault KA, Future II Study Group. Effect of prophylactic human papillomavirus L1 virus-like-particle vaccine on risk of cervical intraepithelial neoplasia grade 2, grade 3, and adenocarcinoma in situ: a combined analysis of four randomised clinical trials. Lancet 2007;369(9576):1861–8.
98. Brown DR, Kjaer SK, Sigurdsson K, et al. The impact of quadrivalent human papillomavirus (HPV; types 6, 11, 16, and 18) L1 virus-like particle vaccine on infection and disease due to oncogenic nonvaccine HPV types in generally HPV-naive women aged 16-26 years. J Infect Dis 2009;199(7):926–35.
99. Paavonen J, Naud P, HPV PATRICIA Study Group, et al. Efficacy of human papillomavirus (HPV)-16/18 AS04-adjuvanted vaccine against cervical infection and precancer caused by oncogenic HPV types (PATRICIA): final analysis of a double-blind, randomised study in young women. Lancet 2009;374(9686):301–14.

The Modern Cytology Laboratory
Moving Beyond the Pap Test

Nancy Joste, MD*, Julie Gober-Wilcox, MD

KEYWORDS

- Cytology laboratory • Papanicolaou test • Squamous dysplasia • Cervical cancer
- Human papillomavirus test • Primary HPV screening • Biomarkers • p16

KEY POINTS

- New recommendations for screening intervals across different age groups is leading to a changing role for the cytology laboratory with an increased role for the human papillomavirus (HPV) testing laboratory.
- With the introduction of the liquid-based Pap test, high-risk HPV (hrHPV) testing, and computer-assisted screening, the cytology laboratory is at the forefront of efforts to improve screening for the provision of better patient care.
- Cytology laboratories are ideally positioned to facilitate important basic and applied research involving cervical cancer.

The cytology laboratory of today has come a great distance from the days of cervical cancer screening relying solely on searching for abnormal cells on a smeared slide. With the introduction of the liquid-based Papanicolaou (Pap) test, high-risk (hr) human papillomavirus (HPV) testing, and computer-assisted screening, the cytology laboratory is at the forefront of efforts to improve screening for the provision of better patient care. The Pap test is known for its excellent specificity, but a single test is associated with a sensitivity of approximately 50% to 70%.[1] Some laboratory efforts have primarily focused on the goals of improving the sensitivity of the Pap test and reducing false-negative cytology diagnoses, whereas efforts such as hrHPV testing work to increase specificity of those Pap tests with atypical results, such as atypical squamous cells of undetermined significance (ASC-US).

This article reviews some of the more recent efforts along these lines, keeping in mind that some of such efforts lead to a diminished role of the conventional cytology laboratory as we know it while also creating a greater role for the laboratory in other testing modalities. Topics covered include the current generation of hrHPV tests, current status of computer-assisted screening, use of biomarkers in improving the sensitivity of Pap tests, the possible role of HPV testing in primary screening, the

---

Division of Anatomic Pathology, Department of Pathology, University of New Mexico Health Sciences Center, MSC04 4640, 1 University of New Mexico, Albuquerque, NM 87131-0001, USA
* Corresponding author.
E-mail address: njoste@salud.unm.edu

Obstet Gynecol Clin N Am 40 (2013) 199–210
http://dx.doi.org/10.1016/j.ogc.2013.02.001
0889-8545/13/$ – see front matter © 2013 Elsevier Inc. All rights reserved.

use of hrHPV in triaging diagnoses beyond ASC-US and cotesting, the cytology laboratory as a biorepository, and, finally, changes that will occur the laboratory following efforts to increase patients' access to their medical information and implementation of electronic medical records. The goal of this article is to provide clinicians with a good working understanding of what their cytology laboratory can currently offer in our joint efforts to provide high-quality cervical cancer screening.

HUMAN PAPILLOMAVIRUS TESTING

Since the initial introduction of HPV testing in 1999, the field has been dominated by hybrid capture technology, specifically the Hybrid Capture 2 (HC2) HPV DNA test (Qiagen, Gaithersburg, MD). Worldwide, this test remains the most frequently used HPV test and the test standard with which other tests are compared. The past few years have witnessed approval of several other tests with varying methodology, and soon laboratories may be offering hrHPV testing different from the familiar HC2 test. This section provides an overview of the current commercially available HPV tests and discusses their advantages and limitations (**Table 1**).

All of the Food and Drug Administration (FDA)-approved and commercially available hrHPV tests are designed for detection of multiple HPV nucleic acids in cervical and/or vaginal samples.[2] All are approved for use in reflex testing with ASC-US cytology and in cotesting in women 30 years of age and older. The tests can be grouped into the following 4 categories:

1. hrHPV DNA-based screening assays
2. hrHPV DNA-based screening assays with reflex or concurrent HPV 16, 18 genotype detection
3. hrHPV DNA-based genotyping assays
4. hrHPV E6/E7 mRNA screening assays

High-Risk HPV DNA-Based Screening Assays

These tests include the Qiagen HC2 test and the Cervista HPV HR test (Hologic Gen-Probe, Inc, Bedford, MA). Results from both HC2 and Cervista simply indicate

Table 1
Current hrHPV testing platforms

Test Type	Test Name	Methodology	Results Format	Test Medium
hrHPV DNA screening assays	HC2 Cervista	Hybrid capture Invader chemistry	Pooled hrHPV	PreservCyt or STM PreservCyt
hrHPV DNA screening assays with HPV 16 and 18	Cervista HPV 16/18	Invader chemistry	HPV 16	PreservCyt or STM
hrHPV DNA genotyping assays	Cobas 4800	Real-time polymerase chain reaction (PCR)	Pooled hrHPV or HPV 16 and 18	Cobas PCR Cell Collection Media or PreservCyt
hrHPV E6/E7 mRNA screening assays using Tigris platform	Aptima	Transcription-mediated amplification of E6/E7 mRNA transcripts	Pooled hrHPV or HPV 16 and 18/45	Aptima Cervical Specimen Collection or PreservCyt

the presence or absence of high-risk HPV types with no information regarding specific HPV types. Both tests use multiplex probe sets including the most prevalent high-risk types (HPV 16, 18, 31, 33, 45, 51) as well as several HPV types (HPV 52, 58, 59, 68) noted to be uncommonly associated with cervical cancers. Cervista also includes HPV 66.

HC2 is an in vitro DNA hybridization assay using a specific hrHPV RNA probe cocktail with signal amplification and qualitative chemiluminescence for detection of 13 high-risk HPV nucleic acids using a luminometer. The test does not include an internal control to assess specimen adequacy or the presence of interfering substances.

The Cervista HPV HR test also uses a signal-amplification method using fluorescent detection of high-risk HPV nucleic acids. This test uses Invader chemistry with a series of binding and cleavage reactions to the DNA target sequence using the probe cocktail and a second invader probe. A final reaction produces a fluorescent signal. Internal negative and positive controls are present which are useful for quality control (QC) in this test.

Both HC2 and Cervista have the potential for cross-reactivity with untargeted HPV types yielding false-positive results. False-negative results may result from very low levels of infection. HC2 and Cervista tests are approved only for use with ThinPrep Pap tests and with specimens collected in Qiagen PreservCyt solution. HC2 can additionally be collected in Qiagen Specimen Transport Medium (STM).

High-Risk HPV DNA-Based Tests with Reflex or Concurrent HPV 16, 18 Detection

Cervista HPV HR test has a sister test, the Cervista HPV 16/18 test, which uses the same Invader technology as the HPV HR test. This test allows qualitative fluorescent detection of HPV types 16 and 18 DNA. The test is approved by the FDA for use adjunctively with the Cervista HPV HR test to determine presence or absence of HPV 16 and 18. According to the package insert, the Cervista HPV 16/18 test has problems with cross-reactivity with high levels of HPV 31 and false-negative results noted with low viral load. It is approved only for use with ThinPrep Pap tests and with specimens collected in Qiagen PreservCyt solution.

HPV DNA-Based Genotyping Assays

The FDA-approved test for HPV PCR-based DNA-based genotyping is the Cobas 4800 HPV test (Roche Molecular Diagnostics, Pleasanton, CA). This test uses real-time polymerase chain reaction (PCR) methodology to amplify sequences fluorescently labeled for detection. The results can be reported in 2 ways: (1) as a pooled result with 14 targeted hrHPV types or (2) results for HPV 16 and 18 separately and a pooled result for the other 12 high-risk types. Specimens can be collected in either ThinPrep PreservCyt solution or the Cobas PCR Cell Collection Media. The test has internal and positive and negative controls, and has clinical sensitivity and specificity comparable with that of HC2. The Cobas 4800 System is automated and has high-throughput capabilities.

High-Risk HPV E6/E7 mRNA Screening Assays

The Aptima HPV test (Hologic Gen-Probe, Inc, San Diego, CA) is an FDA-approved hrHPV E6/E7 mRNA-based screening assay. HPV E6 and E7 oncoproteins are known to be associated with the progression of HPV infection to cancer and may offer more specific information than testing for hrHPV DNA. The other testing modalities already discussed simply detect the presence of the virus without information on the integration of the virus into the host genome, a necessary step for a precancerous lesion. In this sense, those tests all suffer from a diminished specificity for true disease. E6/E7 transcripts are considered informative as indicators of actual disease and not just transient HPV infection. This transcription-mediated amplification-based assay allows detection of E6/E7 transcripts of 14 hrHPV types with no distinction between HPV types. An internal control is present for QC. Hologic recently received FDA approval for Aptima to report separate results for HPV 16 alone and HPV 18/45 combined.

Aptima testing requires specimen collection with the Aptima Cervical Specimen Collection and Transport Kit or ThinPrep PreservCyt solution. The testing platform is the Gen-Probe Tigris, a fully automated high-throughput testing system. Tigris also allows testing for other sexually transmitted diseases such as gonorrhea, *Chlamydia*, and *Trichomonas*. This testing method does not have problems with cross-reactivity and has sensitivity similar to that of HC2, with higher specificity.

None of the tests discussed thus far are approved for use for specimens collected for the SurePath Pap tests (BD Diagnostics, Durham, NC), the other major liquid-based Pap test in the United States. Despite multiple submissions to the FDA at the time of publication, BD has still not obtained FDA approval for HPV testing using HC2 or other HPV tests for their SurePath Pap test. The reason for this failure is not entirely clear, but there is the concern that the small amounts of formaldehyde in the BD SurePath collection medium could act to denature DNA to produce aberrant results. Many laboratories that offer SurePath Pap tests have addressed the lack of FDA approval by performing in-house validation of an HPV test, probably most commonly HC2. A validation study can be done by double collection of patient specimens in both SurePath and ThinPrep collection media and performing HC2 testing on both specimen sets to ensure concordance of results in HPV testing.

In June 2012 BD Diagnostics, the manufacturer of SurePath, issued a Technical Bulletin that was sent to clinical laboratories regarding performance of off-label HPV testing of SurePath samples with the Qiagen HC2 test. This bulletin stated the lack of FDA approval for this type of testing and the possibility of false-negative results, which could lead to inappropriate patient management and potentially compromise patient safety. The technical bulletin recommended cocollection of a cervical sample with Qiagen STM for HPV testing purposes.

ADVANCES IN COMPUTER-ASSISTED SCREENING OF PAP TESTS

Computer-assisted screening of Pap tests has been available since the early 2000s. Whereas the conventional Pap test has traditionally depended on human screening of the slide's cells by cytotechnologists, these computer advances have allowed an extra level of review based on computer-aided image analysis of features of dysplasia. This type of computerized review strives to reduce the false-negative rate that accompanies the Pap test whereby abnormal cells are present on the slide but escape detection by the human eye. If a computer can detect additional abnormal cells, this extra layer of computer review could serve to improve the sensitivity of the Pap test.

There are currently 2 such devices approved by the FDA and in use in the United States. One is the FocalPoint device (BD Diagnostics), which includes a primary screening instrument and a location-guided instrument. The other is the ThinPrep Imaging System (Cytyc Corp, Boxboro, MA), also a location-guided system. Both location-guided instruments are approved for use only on liquid-based SurePath or ThinPrep slides, respectively, and cannot be used to screen the Pap tests of the other manufacturers. Both systems use computerized image analyses for detection of nuclear abnormalities seen in dysplasias, such as nuclear hyperchromasia and increased nucleus to cytoplasm ratio.

The ThinPrep Imaging System with Dual Review functions in a single capacity. Dual Review implies that every slide is reviewed by both the computer and human. The Pap slide is first stained with a proprietary stain, then the instrument scans a slide and selects the 22 fields of view on the slide that are the most worrisome for a squamous intraepithelial lesion. These areas are noted by coordinates and are relayed by computer to a microscope, for the cytotechnologist to review these 22 areas and decide if abnormal cells are present. If abnormal cells are detected, the slide then goes to a pathologist for a final decision as to the diagnosis. There are no options for primary screening of samples or selection of cases by the system for QC purposes.

FocalPoint has 2 options for use. First, it can be used as a primary screening instrument, called the FocalPoint Slide Profiler, which can scans both SurePath and conventional slides for abnormalities. At the end of the computer scanning a given set of slides, up to 25% of the slides in the set, can be declared normal and need no further review by cytotechnologists or pathologists and can be "auto-archived" or filed away (no second review). The remaining 75% of Pap-test slides in a given set (considered the "most abnormal") are ranked into quintiles from 1 to 5 (quintile #1 being the most abnormal) and also receive a score related to the percent chance of having an abnormality compared with the other Pap slides in that set. This quintile and percentile information accompanies the slide to the cytotechnologist, who then completely screens the slide as usual. Because of the computer's prescreening and ranking capabilities, subsequent slide review by cytotechnologists and pathologists can give additional attention to slides considered at higher risk for abnormalities.

Although the FDA approval of the FocalPoint Slide Profiler allows for up to 25% of Pap tests to have no further human review (auto-archived), many laboratories do practice dual review and have these slides screened by cytotechnologists nonetheless. This approach allows the reassurance of all Pap tests being reviewed at least twice, by both a computer and 1 or 2 humans.

BD's location-guided screening system is called the FocalPoint GS Imaging System. It is somewhat similar to the ThinPrep Imaging System whereby it locates the 10 fields of view most likely to contain an abnormality based on the image analysis of the cells on the slide by the computer. This information is sent by the server to the computers and microscopes of cytotechnologists, and they are automatically directed to the 10 fields of view for review of possible abnormal cells. In practice, cytotechnologists frequently review more of the slide than just these 10 fields of view.

The manufacturers of both instruments claim that their computer-assisted screening can reduce the incidence of a laboratory's false-negative Pap tests. Laboratories using these instruments may not all see a huge reduction in false-negative rate, simply because their rate was initially low. Laboratories with problems with a higher rate of false-negative Pap smears may be the ones that benefit most from this technology.

The FocalPoint system also daily generates a certain percentage of random cases for QC review from the slides screened. After computer screening, these selected QC slides will be completely screened twice again by 2 different cytotechnologists. Laboratories have a federally mandated daily 10% slide second review QC, and the FocalPoint-generated QC slides can be added to this for an overall increase in daily QC, in some laboratories up to 25% of their daily slides. While the computer-assisted screening strives to reduce a laboratory's false-negative rate, the additional QC effort in itself may serve to do so.

BIOMARKERS FOR USE IN CERVICAL SPECIMENS

There is considerable interest in taking the microscopic examination of both Pap tests and cervical tissue samples beyond conventional morphologic review and diagnosis, again with the goal of improving diagnostic accuracy and increasing sensitivity.

Biomarkers informative for the presence of high-risk HPV are of use in several situations in the cytology and histology laboratories. First, biomarkers applied to Pap tests with ambiguous results such as ASC-US, atypical squamous cells that cannot exclude high-grade squamous intraepithelial lesion (HSIL) (ASC-H), and atypical glandular cells of undetermined significance (AGC), and negative cytology with positive hrHPV tests may allow more conclusive determination of risk of cervical cancer than hrHPV testing alone, with its specificity issues. Second, biomarkers are of use in cervical tissue samples, particularly cervical biopsies that are worrisome but not conclusively diagnostic for a high-grade dysplasia. The LAST project, discussed in an article by Garcia elsewhere in this issue, proposes specific recommendations for use of biomarkers in evaluating cervical tissue samples.[3]

Whether in cytologic or histologic specimens, the goal of any pathologic examination is to detect clinically significant lesions that may progress to cancer while not subjecting women with clinically insignificant lesions to unnecessary treatment interventions. The key is identifying transformed cells with HPV integration and a defined cancer risk, and excluding women with nonintegrated HPV in productive infections.

Informative biomarkers are ones that reflect transformed cells with HPV integration and increased proliferation. Here the ones most commonly used are discussed: p16[INK4a], Ki67 (mib-1), and ProEx C (BD Diagnostics). The use of these tests with Pap tests is examined here, comparing their sensitivity and specificity with those of hrHPV testing, mostly HC2.

p16 is a tumor-suppressor protein that serves as a biomarker for the presence of hrHPV, and as such is thought to serve as a surrogate marker for a transforming hrHPV infection. Its normal mechanism of action is deceleration of the cell cycle by inactivating cyclin-dependent kinases linked to the phosphorylation of the retinoblastoma protein. In the presence of hrHPV E7, oncogene cell cycling is increased and through a series of steps p16 transcription is induced, leading to p16 protein accumulation within the cell that is detectable by immunohistochemical or immunocytochemical analyses.

Ki67 is a cell-cycle proliferation marker which, in the presence of hrHPV in cervical specimens, can reflect an increase in dividing suprabasal cells. Normally only basal cells demonstrate proliferation, and HPV infection induces proliferation in upper levels of the squamous epithelium. Ki67 is also easily detected by immunostaining. Coexpression of both p16 and Ki67 is a powerful indicator of the presence of an HSIL. There is a commercially available product that provides dual immunostaining with both p16 and Ki67, called CINtec PLUS (Roche Molecular Diagnostics, Pleasanton, CA).

BIOMARKERS IN PAP TESTS

Several studies have investigated the use of biomarkers in Pap tests, which are ideally performed using immunocytochemistry assays on liquid-based cytologic preparations. Here the specific biomarkers (1) p16 alone, (2) p16 with Ki-67, and (3) ProEx C immunostain are discussed.

A recent review and meta-analysis of primarily p16 alone in Pap tests reviewed 17 studies comprising a combination of women with low-grade squamous intraepithelial lesion (LSIL), ASC-US, and both ASC-US and LSIL.[4] The results of these p16 studies were compared with the sensitivity and specificity of hrHPV testing by HC2 with the outcome of cervical intraepithelial neoplasia (CIN)2+ or CIN 3+ on subsequent tissue biopsy. In analyzing studies with ASC-US cytology, p16 and HC2 demonstrated equivalent sensitivities, but p16 showed an improved specificity compared with HC2. This trend for increased specificity of p16 compared with HC2 was also seen in the reviews with LSIL cytology. With LSIL cases, however, p16 showed diminished sensitivity for CIN2+ and CIN3+ compared with HC2.

Is there an advantage to combining p16 with other markers? Whereas individual staining with p16 and Ki67 is noted to stain benign squamous metaplastic cells and endocervical cells as sources of false-positive results, the 2 stains coexpressed in the same cell suggests a significant finding indicating a transformed HPV lesion. The commercial product with dual p16 and Ki67 staining, CINtec PLUS, has been investigated in several retrospective studies with ASC-US cytology[5] and in both ASC-US and LSIL cases.[6] These studies have shown that p16/Ki67 dual staining yields comparable sensitivity and an increase in specificity for CIN2+ compared with both p16 single staining and hrHPV testing. Another retrospective study used p16/Ki67 dual staining to triage Pap cytology–negative results with hrHPV-positive results, and found high sensitivity and specificity for the detection of CIN2+ and CIN3+ in these cases.[7]

Several recent studies have investigated dual p16/Ki67 immunostaining in the difficult problem of glandular atypia (AGC) in Pap tests. In this setting, one study demonstrated that dual staining using CINtec PLUS has a high positive predictive value for a subsequent tissue diagnosis of endocervical adenocarcinoma.[8] Another study showed that CINtec PLUS staining of Pap tests significantly improved the specificity and maintained the sensitivity for future tissue diagnoses of both CIN2/3 and glandular lesions, in comparison with testing for hrHPV by PCR.[9]

What remains to be determined is how these results with HC2 and HPV PCR compare in specificity with some of the newest generation of HPV tests such as the hrHPV E6/E7 mRNA screening assays (Aptima HPV assay). Large prospective studies looking at dual staining are under way, and their results will be critical in determining the role of dual staining in triaging abnormal cytology compared with HPV testing.

ProEx C Immunocytochemistry Test

ProEx C stain (BD Diagnostics) is another dual immunostain approved for use on tissue specimens, such as diagnostically difficult cervical biopsies, in efforts to improve detection of HSIL.[10] The company and researchers have also investigated the use of the stain as a marker to improve the sensitivity of the Pap test, specifically as an adjunct test for Pap tests diagnosed as either ASC-US or ASC-H. ProEx C is a dual stain containing 2 molecular markers found to be overexpressed in cervical squamous cell carcinoma, topoisomerase II, involved in cell-cycle progression and minichromosonal maintenance protein 2 a marker of cellular proliferation. Several studies have looked at the utility of the test in the detection of HSIL with ASC-US and ASC-H cytologies, and in both instances have found a higher sensitivity than with hrHPV testing.[11,12] The specificity was equivalent to hrHPV testing in ASC-US or in the case of ASC-H, ProEx C showed significantly higher specificity than HC2 in detecting CIN2+ lesions in subsequent tissue biopsy. The stain, however, does have problems with false-positive results owing to staining some types of normal cells.[13]

HPV TESTING AS PRIMARY SCREENING

With the inherent difficulty in improving the sensitivity of the Pap test, what are the other options for primary screening for cervical cancer? If using a screening test with increased sensitivity, would there be trade-offs with specificity and increased unnecessary treatment interventions?

The role of hrHPV testing in primary cervical cancer screening has been evaluated in several cross-sectional studies and randomized clinical trials in other countries. These studies have conclusively shown that hrHPV DNA testing is more sensitive in comparison with cytology alone in identifying CIN2 lesions or worse. Mayrand and colleagues[14] conducted the first large randomized clinical trial directly comparing hrHPV testing alone with conventional Pap testing in 10,154 Canadian women aged 30 to 69 years, and found that hrHPV testing was almost 40% more sensitive and only 2.7% less specific for detecting CIN2 or more. Recognizing the need to follow this primary screening with a test of high specificity, the investigators demonstrated that hrHPV screening followed by Pap triage led to fewer colposcopy referrals than either test alone (1.1% vs 2.9% with Pap testing alone or 6.1% with HPV testing alone).

A Swedish study evaluating hrHPV screening with Pap triage used data from a population-based randomized trial that compared 11 possible cervical screening strategies in women aged 32 to 38 years. In looking at different combinations of HPV testing and cytology, the investigators found that primary screening with hrHPV testing followed by cytology triage and repeat hrHPV testing was more efficacious than cotesting (concurrent hrHPV testing and cytology). Both strategies increased sensitivity of detecting CIN3+ by at least 30%, but cotesting required twice as many screening tests, whereas the triage strategy increased the number of screening tests by only 12%.[15]

At present in the United States, hrHPV as a primary screening test is recommended with concurrent cytology only in women aged 30 to 65 years. A prospective cohort study of approximately 332,000 women aged 30 years and older undergoing cotesting (hrHPV testing and cytology) found that the 3-year and 5-year cumulative incidence of CIN3 or worse in women who tested negative for both at baseline was 0.047% at 3 years and 0.16% at 5 years. Screening more frequently than every 3 years would not improve sensitivity, and potentially leads to increased cost and overtreatment.[16]

These findings are reflected in the new 2012 cervical cancer screening guidelines which recommend cotesting with hrHPV and cytology every 5 years or cytology alone every 3 years in women aged 30 to 65 years if results are negative.[17] Of note, it is estimated that only 30% of women aged 30 years or older are currently receiving hrHPV and Pap smear cotesting.[18] Adding more support for the use of hrHPV testing as primary screening is a United States population-based study that included more than 330,000 women. It found that the 5-year cumulative risk of developing cervical cancer in women who were hrHPV negative was 0.17%, which is almost equal to that of cotesting at 0.16%.[19] This finding suggests that testing with hrHPV without concurrent cytology may be sensitive enough for primary screening.

Although primary screening with HPV tests is an intriguing possibility, some researchers recommend caution. hrHPV testing is not a perfect test despite the often-cited figure of greater than 99.0% sensitivity. Several studies have noted an incidence of up to 10% negative hrHPV tests in the months preceding the finding of high-grade histology, including invasive squamous cell carcinoma.[20] A more cautious approach would be to adhere to the current recommendations of cytology and hrHPV cotesting as a way to circumvent the sensitivity issues of both cytology and HPV tests.

The role of hrHPV testing in low-resource settings is of interest in global efforts in cervical cancer prevention. Cervical cancer remains the second leading cause of death in women worldwide, with almost 500,000 new cases and 240,000 deaths every year attributable to ineffective screening programs, mostly in low-resource countries.[21] In these settings, infrastructure for effective cytology screening programs is often rudimentary at best, making other screening options attractive.

A prospective study by Sankaranarayanan and colleagues[22] showed that in low-resource settings a single round of hrHPV testing (HC2) was associated with a significant reduction in the number of deaths from cervical cancer compared with cytology, visual inspection with acetic acid (VIA), and counseling (control group). In their large randomized trial in rural India comprising 131,746 women aged 30 to 59 years, at 8 years of follow-up there was a significant reduction in the number of deaths from cervical cancer in the hrHPV testing group compared with the control, cytology, and VIA group. This study highlights the potential impact of hrHPV testing in developing nations for cervical cancer screening, but raises other issues such as the current prohibitively high expense of hrHPV testing and the difficulties in acquiring test samples from women in these settings. Some answers to these problems are being addressed in studies investigating hrHPV test self-sampling by women[23] and the use of alternative hrHPV tests such as careHPV (Qiagen), a low-cost and rapid HPV test that holds promise for use in cervical cancer screening efforts in low-resource settings.[24]

HPV TESTING IN LOW-GRADE SQUAMOUS INTRAEPITHELIAL LESIONS

The results from the landmark ALTS trial, published in 2003, demonstrated the utility of HPV testing and triage in women with ASC-US and LSIL Pap results.[25] A single HPV test appropriately triaged 93% of women with ASC-US cytology who were ultimately found to have CIN3, whereas a single repeat Pap test had a sensitivity of only 44.1%. In addition, the negative predictive value of HPV testing in women with ASC-US cytology was estimated at 99.5%. The trial also found high prevalence of HPV in women with LSIL in that 83% were found to be HPV positive, thereby negating the utility of HPV testing in this group.

A recent study by Cuzick and colleagues,[26] however, looked at the findings from the ATHENA HPV trial, an ongoing study sponsored by Roche Diagnostics that includes more than 47,000 women aged 21 and older undergoing routine cervical cancer screening. The investigators found that HPV testing is a cost-effective strategy in triaging women older than 40 years with LSIL. Of 925 cases of LSIL, more than 70% tested positive for hrHPV; however, the proportion was nearly 80% for women in their 20s but just 56% for women age 40 or older. In this older age group CIN2 was found in 19 women, and all but 1 tested positive for high- risk HPV. There were 10 cases of CIN3, all of which tested positive. Given the lower prevalence rate of hrHPV in women 40 years and older with LSIL and the high negative predictive value of HPV testing in detecting CIN2 or worse, it appears that HPV testing in this subset of women shows promise in avoiding unnecessary referrals for colposcopy.

CYTOLOGY LABORATORIES AS BIOREPOSITORIES FOR RESEARCH

Cytology laboratories are ideally positioned to facilitate important basic and applied research involving cervical cancer. In particular, molecular epidemiology studies can make use of residual fluid from liquid-based Pap tests (usually discarded) as an excellent source of cellular material for a variety of tests. Conventional Pap smears are also of value, as cells can be scraped off the slide surface or microdissected. Cytology laboratories can also provide linkage information to diagnoses and patient demographics.

DNA and RNA are extractable from the methanol-based fixative of liquid-based Pap tests, and can be used for DNA-based and RNA-based assays of HPV. The cellular material can also be used in proteomic studies of biomarkers that investigate overexpression of cell-cycle regulating proteins, such as cyclin-dependent kinases and other proteins involved in cervical neoplasia pathogenesis with viral oncogenes.

Examples of population-based studies are those investigating long-term and short-term HPV genotype changes seen in the years following the introduction of HPV vaccination. Other areas of interest include changes in patterns of screening effectiveness, and general questions on the natural history of HPV infection and HPV-related dysplasias and cancers.[27]

FUTURE OF THE CYTOLOGY LABORATORY

In these challenging times for medicine, the cytology laboratory will not be immune to significant changes. The new recommendations for screening intervals across different age groups is leading to a diminished role for the cytology laboratory and an increased role for the HPV testing laboratory. One recent projection is an expectation of approximately 20 to 30 million fewer Pap tests annually if there is adherence to the current recommendations.[28] Alternatively, as the US Affordable Care Act is implemented, an increase in cervical screening cytology may be seen with the anticipated expansion of health care coverage.

Cytology laboratories will adapt to this changing environment as they will to the different demands emerging in other current trends in medicine. The inclusion of cytology in electronic medical records (EMR) is ongoing in many laboratories, producing a demand for electronic interfaces between laboratory information systems and the EMRs. One may expect to see a movement away from paper requisitions for Pap and hrHPV tests toward computerized order entry.

In addition, patient access and connectivity to their medical records is increasing, including access to their laboratory results. Many health care systems already offer patient portals to access their own laboratory information. With such access, it is critical for laboratories to provide patients with accurate and understandable information to facilitate understanding of their laboratory results. The laboratory also has an important role in protecting patient confidentiality issues that can be problematic with this increased access.

REFERENCES

1. Castle PE, Cremer M. HPV testing in cervical cancer screening. In: Waxman A, editor. Obstetrics and gynecology clinics of North America. New York: Elsevier; 2013.
2. Zhao C, Huaitao Y. Approved assays for detecting HPV DNA-design, indications, and validation. CAP Today January 2012. Available at: http://captoday.epubxp.com/i/52881/39.
3. Darragh TM, Colgan TJ, Cox JT, et al. LAST project work groups. The lower anogenital squamous terminology standardization project for HPV-associated lesions: background and consensus recommendations from the College of American Pathologists and the American Society for Colposcopy and Cervical Pathology. J Low Genit Tract Dis 2012;16:205–42.
4. Roelens J, Reuschenbach M, von Knebel Doeberitz M, et al. p16INK4a Immunocytochemistry versus human papillomavirus testing for triage of women with minor cytologic abnormalities. Cancer Cytopathol 2012;120:294–307.
5. Edgerton N, Cohen C, Siddiqui MT. Evaluation of CINtec PLUS testing as an adjunctive test in ASC-US diagnosed SurePath preparations. Diagn Cytopathol 2011. http://dx.doi.org/10.1002/dc 21757.
6. Schmidt D, Bergeron C, Denton KJ, et al. p16/Ki-67 dual-stain cytology in the triage of ASCUS and LSIL Papanicolaou cytology. Cancer Cytopathol 2011; 119:158–66.
7. Petry KU, Schmidt D, Scherbring S, et al. Triaging pap cytology negative, HPV positive cervical cancer screening results with p16/Ki-67 dual-stained cytology. Gynecol Oncol 2011;121:505–9.

8. Ravarino A, Nemolato S, Macciocu E, et al. CINtec PLUS immunocytochemistry as a tool for the cytologic diagnosis of glandular lesions of the cervix uteri. Am J Clin Pathol 2012;138:652–6.
9. Singh M, Mockler D, Akalin A, et al. Immunocytochemical colocalization of p16^{INK4a} and Ki-67 predicts CIN2/3 and AIS/Adenocarcinoma. Cancer Cytopathol 2012;120:26–34.
10. Badr RE, Walts AE, Chung F, et al. BD ProEx C: a sensitive and specific marker of HPV-associated squamous lesions of the cervix. Am J Surg Pathol 2008;32: 899–906.
11. Siddiqui MT, Hornaman K, Cohen C, et al. ProEx C Immunocytochemistry and high-risk human papillomavirus DNA testing in Papanicolaou tests with atypical squamous cell (ASC-US) cytology: correlation study with histologic biopsy. Arch Pathol Lab Med 2008;132:1648–52.
12. Siddiqui MT, Cohen C, Nassar A. Detecting high-grade cervical disease on ASC-H cytology, Role of BD ProEx C and Digene hybrid capture II HPV DNA testing. Am J Clin Pathol 2008;130:765–70.
13. Oberg TN, Kipp BR, Vrana JA, et al. Comparison of p16^{INK4a} and ProEx C immunostaining on cervical ThinPrep cytology and biopsy specimens. Diagn Cytopathol 2010;38:564–72.
14. Mayrand MH, Duarte-Franco E, Rodrigues I, et al. Human papillomavirus DNA versus Papanicolaou screening tests for cervical cancer. N Engl J Med 2007; 357:1579–88.
15. Naucler P, Ryd W, Törnberg S, et al. Efficacy of HPV DNA testing with cytology triage and/or repeat HPV DNA testing in primary cervical cancer screening. J Natl Cancer Inst 2009;101:88–99.
16. Goldie SJ, Kim JJ, Wright TC. Cost-effectiveness of human papillomavirus DNA testing for cervical cancer screening in women aged 30 years or more. Obstet Gynecol 2004;103:619–31.
17. Saslow D, Solomon D, Lawson HW, et al. Screening guidelines for the prevention and early detection of cervical cancer. CA Cancer J Clin 2012;62(3):147–72.
18. Check W. HPV testing—proceed with cautions. CAP Today October 2010. Available at: http://tinyurl.com/caphpvtesting.
19. Katki HA, Kinney WK, Fetterman B, et al. Cervical cancer risk for women undergoing concurrent testing for human papillomavirus and cervical cytology: a population-based study in routine clinical practice. Lancet Oncol 2011;12:663–72.
20. Zaibo L, Austin RM, Guo M, et al. Screening test results associated with cancer diagnoses in 287 women with cervical squamous cell carcinoma. Arch Pathol Lab Med 2012;136:1533–40.
21. Parkin DM, Bray F. Chapter 2: the burden of HPV-related cancers. Vaccine 2006; 24(Suppl 3):S3/11-25.
22. Sankaranarayanan R, Nene BM, Shastri SS, et al. HPV screening for cervical cancer in rural India. N Engl J Med 2009;360:1385–94.
23. Zhao FH, Lewkowitz AK, Chen F, et al. Pooled analysis of a self-sampling HPV DNA test as a cervical cancer primary screening method. J Natl Cancer Inst 2012;104:178–88.
24. Qiao YL, Sellors JW, Eder PS, et al. A new HPV-DNA test for cervical-cancer screening in developing regions: a cross-sectional study of clinical accuracy in rural China. Lancet Oncol 2008;9:929–36.
25. ASCUS-LSIL Triage Study (ALTS) Group. Results of a randomized trial on the management of cytology interpretations of atypical squamous cells of undetermined significance. Am J Obstet Gynecol 2003;188:1383–92.

26. Cuzick J, Thomas Cox J, Zhang G, et al. Human papillomavirus testing for triage of women with low-grade squamous intraepithelial lesions. Int J Cancer 2012. http://dx.doi.org/10.1002/ijc.27723.
27. Arbyn M, Andersson K, Bergeron C, et al. Cervical cytology biobanks as a resource for molecular epidemiology. Methods Mol Biol 2011;675:279–98.
28. Check W. New guidelines could jump-start hrHPV testing. CAP Today July 2012. Available at: http://tinyurl.com/guideline-jumpstarthrHPV.

New Cervical Cancer Screening Guidelines, Again

Nicole Karjane, MD, David Chelmow, MD*

KEYWORDS

- Pap smear • HPV • Cervical cancer screening • Cervical cytology • Guidelines

KEY POINTS

- Several major organizations, including the American Cancer Society, the US Preventative Services Task Force, and the American College of Obstetricians and Gynecologists, have recently revised their guidelines for cervical cancer screening and prevention.
- Cervical cancer screening should begin at 21 years of age, regardless of risk factors.
- Women aged 21 to 29 years should be screened with cytology alone at 3-year intervals.
- Women aged 30 to 65 years should be screening with cytology and high-risk human papilloma virus cotesting at 5-year intervals or cytology alone every 3 years, with cotesting specifically preferred by all but the US Preventative Services Task Force.
- Women older than 65 years with adequate negative prior screening should not undergo further screening for cervical cancer.

INTRODUCTION

Over the past year, cervical cancer screening guidelines have undergone a series of important revisions by major organizations. In March, the American Cancer Society (ACS), the American Society for Colposcopy and Cervical Pathology (ASCCP), and the American Society for Clinical Pathology revised their recommendations (referred to as *ACS guidelines* in this article).[1] At the same time, the US Preventive Service Task Force (USPSTF)[2] (referred to here as *USPSTF guidelines*) revised their guidelines. In addition, the American College of Obstetricians and Gynecologists (ACOG) released a revised practice bulletin in November 2012 (ACOG practice bulletin). Each of these major organizations used slightly different methodologies to arrive at their recommendations. This article discusses and summarizes these recommendations and the rationale for them.

Disclosures: D. Chelmow and N. Karjane have no relationship with any commercial companies with direct financial interest in the article.

Department of Obstetrics and Gynecology, Virginia Commonwealth University School of Medicine, 1250 East Marshall Street, PO Box 980034, Richmond, VA 23298, USA

* Corresponding author.

E-mail address: dchelmow@mcvh-vcu.edu

RATIONALE FOR REVISIONS

Each of the organizations listed earlier recognized the need to revise existing re-commendations. Cervical cancer screening has been a true preventative medicine success. The introduction of cervical cancer screening programs has resulted in marked reductions in cervical cancer incidences whenever and wherever they have been implemented.[3,4] Cervical cytology was initially recommended arbitrarily on an annual basis as early as the 1940s. This recommendation was done without support-ive data and without understanding the pathophysiology of cervical carcinogenesis. By the 1960s, annual Papanicolaou screening became the basis for the annual well-woman visit. Given the extraordinary success in cancer reduction and tradition of annual visits, annual screening became deeply entrenched in medical practice and patient expectations.

Guideline revisions are not new and, in fact, have occurred regularly over the last 25 years. Given the importance of cervical cancer screening and prevention, major societies have developed screening recommendations and guided their evolution as new data has become available. The frequency of screening has been a major focus. As early as 1976, the Walton report from Canada suggested that every 3-year screening was as effective as annual screening. The ACS included every 3-year testing in their guidelines in 1987. The ACOG first suggested an increased interval in their practice bulletin revision in 2003.

The need to yet again revise the guidelines came from new data in several areas. First, when cytology was initially implemented, it was without the knowledge of the role of the human papilloma virus (HPV). It has become clear that HPV is necessary for the development of squamous cell carcinoma of the uterine cervix. HPV infection, however, is incredibly common; most people who are infected are unaware of their infection and do not suffer any consequences, let alone develop cancer. The current model[5,6] assumes that HPV infection of the cervix behaves in 2 different ways. Most infections are transient. In women with transient infections, the immune system clears the virus; these women are not at an increased risk for cervical cancer. These infec-tions may be manifested by low-grade squamous intraepithelial lesion (LSIL) cytology and cervical intraepithelial neoplasia (CIN) 1 histology. In a second, much smaller group of women, the virus persists. These persistent infections are manifested by high-grade squamous intraepithelial lesion (HSIL) cytology and CIN 2 and 3 histology. These patients do have appreciable risk of developing cervical cancer if the precur-sors are not detected and treated. In a tragically misguided observational study of women with high-grade cervical dysplasia who were observed without treatment, 31.3% went on to develop cervical cancer over 30 years of follow-up.[7] Second, it has been recognized that there are harms related to screening. These harms include discomfort from examinations, anxiety, and potential morbidity. There is emotional impact from labeling patients with sexually transmitted infections. In addition, there is evidence[8] that women treated with excisional procedures for neoplasia may have an increased risk for premature birth. Although some recent evidence has begun to question this risk,[9,10] treatment that does not lead to a reduction in cancer risk should still clearly be avoided. Although all of the major organizations explicitly did not consider costs in their recommendations, costs would inevitably be reduced if the same cancer reduction could be reached with less intensive testing and treatment. Given the current health care environment, it is extremely important that we avoid unnecessary screening. Third, the understanding of the role of HPV in cervical carci-nogenesis has led to the Food and Drug Administration (FDA) approval of tests for high-risk HPV types. Prior screening recommendations did not effectively integrate

HPV testing. Guideline revision was necessary, therefore, to integrate the understanding of HPV in carcinogenesis and the ability to test for HPV, while minimizing harms of testing too frequently.

Since the last set of revisions, vaccines for the prevention of infection with high-risk HPV subtypes have been approved and recommended by the Advisory Committee on Immunization Practices.[11–13] However, given the pathogenesis of HPV infection and cervical cancer, it is expected that a significant impact on cervical cancer incidence will not occur until approximately 20 or more years after widespread vaccination begins. Both the ACS and the ACOG explicitly state that HPV vaccination should not alter cervical cancer screening at this time.

DIFFERENCES BETWEEN GUIDELINES

In the past, the guideline updates occurred at different times unrelated to one another. This year, the USPSTF and the ACS released guidelines almost simultaneously; the ACOG released their guidelines immediately after reviewing both.

It is important to realize that there are some noteworthy differences between each organization's guidelines. These differences stem from the differing goals and methodologies of the organizations developing them. In the past, guidelines from the USPSTF, ACS, and ACOG have differed significantly in several important areas. The USPSTF makes recommendations about the effectiveness of specific clinical preventative services. These recommendations are extremely important because under the Affordable Care Act, new private insurance plans and Medicare are required to cover USPSTF-recommended preventative services without patient cost sharing. The USPSTF's guidelines focus on effectiveness, however, and are not intended to contain adequate detail for implementation in clinical settings. The ACS provides a much greater level of detail, with the intent to provide guidance for the implementation of cervical screening for typical patients. Although they provide evidence-based guidelines for the populations and situations within the scope of the guidelines, they make no comment about the areas outside the guidelines. The ACOG, which adopted the ACS guidelines, provides additional guidance to providers based on expert opinion for some areas outside the scope of the ACS's guidelines. All of the guidelines are evidence based, but the ACOG provides a larger amount of expert opinion to fill the gaps between evidence to allow for more complete implementation. Despite the differences in methodologies and aims, all 3 guidelines ended up with very similar recommendations.

INITIATION OF SCREENING

The USPSTF explicitly recommends against screening for cervical cancer in women younger than 21 years. They base this recommendation on a decision analysis that they commissioned.[14] The ACS and ACOG make the same recommendation, stipulating that women younger than 21 years should not be screened regardless of the age of sexual initiation or other behavior-related risk factors. Of note, this differs from the Centers for Disease Control and Prevention's (CDC) recommendations for women who are human immunodeficiency virus (HIV) positive,[15] which states that women who are HIV positive should be screened starting at the time of diagnosis, with no exception for adolescents. The ACS's recommendations were carried forward from the Practice Improvement in Cervical Screening and Management Symposium[16] and were not actually new recommendations.

The recommendations for age at initiation of cervical cancer screening make sense in light of the extreme rarity of cervical cancer before 21 years of age, which is estimated at 1 to 2 cases per million girls aged 15 to 19 years.[5] In addition, studies examining the initiation of screening in younger populations have not shown a decrease in cervical cancer rates.[17,18] In light of the lack of evidence for the prevention of cancer and that abnormal screening tests are incredibly common in this age group, screening leads to harm without benefit. Cervical cancer prevention efforts in this age group should be directed at compliance with the ACIP's recommendations for HPV vaccination, not screening.

APPROPRIATE TESTS FOR SCREENING

The FDA has approved several tests for high-risk HPV types over the past several years. The use of these tests in addition to cervical cytology (cotesting) was not included in the USPSTF's prior guidelines. The ACS's earlier guidelines recommended screening with either cytology alone every 2 to 3 years or cotesting every 3 years in women older than 30 years. The addition of HPV testing in women aged 30 years or older makes sense in light of HPV's role in cervical carcinogenesis. Previous recommendations were arbitrary, however, and incompletely guided by evidence. It is known that HPV testing increases the sensitivity for high-grade lesions while decreasing specificity.[19,20] Given this trade-off, the rationale for the ACS's prior guidelines recommending either testing with cytology or cotesting at similar intervals was not optimal.

The ACS, USPSTF, and ACOG are all in agreement regarding using cytology alone in women aged 20 to 29 years. Each of the guidelines specifically states that cytology and HPV cotesting should not be performed in women younger than 30 years for screening purposes. The rationale for avoiding the use of cotesting in women younger than 30 years is that the prevalence of high-risk HPV infection is high, and the incidence of cervical cancer is extremely low in sexually active women in this age group. Because HPV testing is so much more sensitive and less specific than cervical cytology,[19] cotesting women younger than 30 years would largely detect transient HPV infections that have little to no clinical significance. Detecting infections that do not have carcinogenic potential would lead to large amounts of additional testing and potential treatment with minimal to no impact on cervical cancer prevention.[21]

The selection of appropriate tests for women aged 30 to 65 years is the area in which the major society guidelines have the most significant difference. The ACS's guidelines specifically state that HPV and cytology cotesting is preferred in women aged 30 years and older. They state that cytology alone every 3 years is acceptable.[1] The ACS argues that HPV testing is more sensitive but less specific than cytology for identifying women with CIN 3 or greater.[19] In addition, women with negative HPV tests have a lower subsequent risk of CIN 3 or greater[22,23] as well as a lower subsequent risk of cervical cancer.[24]

Since the previous guideline update, no less than 4 randomized trials have compared cytology with cotesting. Three of them focused on women aged 30 to 65.[25–27] Each of the studies used slightly different protocols and evaluation schemes for abnormal cotests, but all had similar results. In all 3 trials, cotesting detected a greater proportion of high-grade dysplasia in the first round of screening, and lower rates in subsequent testing compared with cytology alone. Rijkaart[26] demonstrated a statistically significant reduction in cancer in the second round of screening (4 of 19 579 in the cotesting group vs 14 of 19 731 cytology alone; RR 0.29, 95% confidence interval [CI] 0.10–0.87), and Ronco[21] showed a statistically significant reduction from .03% to 0%. Naucler[25] did not report the difference in cancer detection.

The ACS states that "While co-testing is preferred to cytology alone based on risks and harms assessment, such a strategy might not be feasible in all clinical settings in the United States due to a lack of payment for co-testing or due to local policies."[1] Cytology alone is acceptable in circumstances when it is the only option; but when available, cotesting is clearly preferred.

The initial draft of the USPSTF's guidelines posted on the Internet for public comment gave cotesting a grade I statement, meaning, "Current evidence is insufficient to assess the balance of benefits and harms of the service. Evidence is lacking, poor quality, or conflicting and the benefits of benefits and harms cannot be determined."[28] Their rationale was that current evidence was insufficient to assess the relevant benefits and harms for cotesting with HPV. This decision would have had profound implications because without a grade A or B rating of effectiveness by the USPSTF, cotesting would not have been on the list of approved preventative services covered without cost sharing by the Affordable Care Act. Fortunately, additional data became available, and cotesting was given a grade A recommendation in the final document.

Even in their final document, however, the USPSTF does not distinguish between the two alternatives. They recommend cytology every 3 years or cotesting every 5 years equally. They specify cotesting as an option for women aged 30 to 65 years "who want to lengthen the screening interval."[2] They state that both strategies administered with the appropriate intervals provide a reasonable balance between benefits and harms. They caution that women who choose cotesting should be counseled that "positive screening results are more likely with co-testing than with cytology alone, and that some women may require prolonged surveillance with additional frequent testing if they have persistently positive HPV results."

The formal incorporation of cotesting into both the USPSTF's and the ACS's guidelines was likely the most profound change in this set of revisions. The ACS's guidelines, which are more likely to be widely followed, specifically prefer cotesting, unlike their prior recommendations, which offered cytology or cotesting equally. In light of the randomized evidence suggesting decreased cancer in subsequent screening rounds, the availability of cotesting and its routine use should be a significant step forward in cervical cancer prevention. Even with the USPSTF's change in their final guidelines, this remains the area of most significant difference between the USPSTF and the ACS. In its latest practice bulletin on cervical cancer screening, the ACOG adopted the ACS's recommendation that cotesting be used whenever available and agreed that cotesting should be the preferred screening method for women aged 30 to 65 years.

AT WHAT INTERVAL SHOULD PATIENTS BE TESTED?

The USPSTF, ACS, and ACOG all agree on the interval at which patients should be screened. Women without special risk factors should be tested with cytology alone every 3 years from 21 years of age until they reach 30 years of age. Women aged from 30 to 65 years should be tested with cotesting every 5 years, assuming negative results for both tests. If cotesting is not available, cytology alone should be performed every 3 years. This guideline represents a significant change from the ACS's and ACOG's prior guidelines, which specified either cotesting or cytology alone every 3 years after 30 years of age. Between 21 and 30 years of age, prior guidelines recommended screening every 2 years.

The choice of a screening interval is a balance between benefits and harms. Testing needs to be sufficiently frequent to detect high-grade lesions before the development of cervical cancer. Conversely, it should be infrequent enough that transient infections of no risk to patients can be allowed to resolve, avoiding unnecessary diagnostic tests and treatments that will not decrease patients' cancer risk. Both the USPSTF and the ACS acknowledged the need to balance screening risks and benefits and to decrease the harms from overtesting compared with previously recommended screening intervals and, most importantly, to stop annual screening.

The interval is particularly important with cotesting. The initiation of HPV testing significantly increases the sensitivity of HPV detection while decreasing specificity.[19] Repeating cotesting too frequently will result in the detection of large numbers of transient infections and result in much additional testing. There are a few studies specifically addressing intervals at any age. Both organizations relied heavily on a modeling study by Kulasingam and colleagues[14] in making their recommendations. Stout[29] modeled outcomes for women 20 years of age screened over 10 years and predicted that screening every 3 years compared with 1 year would reduce colposcopy by half (187 vs 403 per 1000) while only slightly changing lifetime cancer risks (0.69% vs 0.33%). Kulasingam and colleagues[14] compared outcomes for screening every 1, 2, or 3 years. Compared with intervals of every 2 years, screening every 3 years negligibly changed cancer risks (37 vs 39 cancer cases per 100,000 women) and led to significantly more colposcopies (176 vs 134 per 100 000). Sasieni[30] studied women in the United Kingdom who had been screened every 2 or 3 years after negative test results and noted no difference in risk. Given the compelling evidence that screening annually in this age group leads to significantly greater colposcopies with only a slight advantage for cancer risk and that every-2-year and every-3-year intervals seem to behave similarly and were both a better balance than annual screens, all organizations recommended every-3-year testing with cytology alone in this age group.

In women aged 30 to 65 years, all 3 organizations again recommended every 3 years as the appropriate interval for screening with cytology alone. Previously, the ACS recommended screening every 2 to 3 years without specifying a preference for one interval versus the other. At least 4 studies[30–33] compared annual to every-2-year or every-3-year interval screening in organized programs and noted no advantage to annual screening. Both the Stout[29] and Kulasingam[14] modeling studies again noted very low cervical cancer rates with either 1- or 2-year screening and significantly more testing with more frequent screening. Screening with cytology every 3 years yielded a slightly higher cancer rate but required much less diagnostic testing.

In developing their guidelines, the ACS used a principle that women at similar cancer risk should be managed similarly. Further, they acknowledged that the cancer risk achieved with every-3-year screening was the accepted standard and should be the benchmark. They chose every-5-year cotesting as optimal because it has the same or lower cancer risk as compared with testing with cytology alone every 3 years. Cotesting achieved slightly lower cancer rates with less screening and fewer follow-up colposcopies than cytology alone in both a pooled analysis of small studies and a single large population study. Dillner and colleagues[22] pooled 7 studies conducted in Europe and reported a 0.28% risk of CIN 3 + 5 years after negative cotesting compared with 0.51% 3 years after negative cytology alone. In an analysis of the Kaiser Permanente of Northern California database, Katki[23] noted a 0.016% risk of cervical cancer in women 5 years after a negative cotest compared with 0.037% after negative cytology alone. Using modeling, Kulasingam[14] noted cotesting every 5 years had similar or fewer cancer cases, cancer deaths, and colposcopy than cytology performed every 3 years.

There is abundant evidence that despite recommendations to stop annual testing made by the ACS years ago and by the ACOG in 2003, many providers are still performing annual cytology testing or cotesting more frequently than every 3 years.[34] This practice has the potential to cause significant harm, particularly by detecting low-grade lesions of no appreciable risk of becoming cancer. Detecting these low-grade lesions generates further unnecessary testing and treatment of lesions that will likely spontaneously resolve. Although all 3 organizations explicitly did not consider cost in their recommendations, extra testing clearly leads to extra cost, which is of significant concern in today's health care economic environment. The ACOG and the ACS explicitly state that annual testing should not be performed.

CESSATION OF SCREENING

All 3 major society guidelines are in agreement that under usual circumstances, screening should stop at 65 years of age. The USPSTF recommends against screening for cervical cancer in women older than 65 years who have had adequate prior screening and are not otherwise at a high risk for cervical cancer. In a separate clinical consideration section, they state that the clinician should base the decision to end screening on whether patients meet criteria defined by established guidelines and specifically cite the ACS's guidelines, reiterating their criteria.

The ACS's guidelines state women older than 65 years with evidence of adequate prior screening and no history of CIN 2 or greater within the last 20 years should not be screened for cervical cancer with any modality. Once screening is discontinued, it should not resume for any reason, even if a woman reports having a new sexual partner. In addition, the ACS's guidelines state that adequate negative prior screening is defined as 3 consecutive negative cytology results or 2 consecutive negative cotests within the 10 years before ceasing screening, with the most recent test performed within the past 5 years. Women older than 65 years with a history of CIN 2, CIN 3, or adenocarcinoma in situ (AIS) should continue routine screening for at least 20 years, even if this extends screening past 65 years of age. These guidelines state that the 20 years should start after spontaneous regression or completion of appropriate management for the abnormality. The ACOG adopted this component of the ACS's guidelines without change.

The rationale for ceasing screening is twofold. First, there is little benefit of screening older women. Given the natural history of cervical cancer, which requires a median of 15 to 25 years after acquisition of HPV to develop, it is tremendously unlikely that someone who has not developed cytologic abnormalities by 65 years of age will live long enough to develop cervical cancer.[14] The study included 3 separate models. These models suggest that in women who were well screened, defined as cytology every 3 years until 65 years of age, only approximately 1.6 cancers per 1000 women and 0.5 cancer deaths per 1000 women would be prevented by continuing screening to 90 years of age. Over the course of this continued testing, many colposcopies and additional testing would be required without evidence of benefit. The rationale for not restarting screening, even when new risk factors are identified, is again motivated by the natural history of cervical cancer. Even if patients were infected with carcinogenic HPV strains at 65 years of age, they would be unlikely to live long enough to develop cervical cancer.

In addition to scant benefit of continued screening beyond 65 years of age, there is risk and inconvenience. Epithelial atrophy makes interpreting cervical cytology much more difficult after menopause; and there are many false-positive lesions, particularly low-grade lesions. Sawaya and colleagues[33] studied women from the Heart and Estrogen/Progestin Replacement Study and noted a rate of 23 new cytologic abnormalities per 1000 person years of women studied. Of the 130 women in the study with known histologic diagnoses, only one had confirmed mild to moderate dysplasia for a positive predictive value of 0.9% over 2 years. Thus, although a significant amount of abnormal cytology was diagnosed, only a tiny fraction had true histologic abnormalities. The combination of low yield and high false positives makes screening in older women ineffective; therefore, it is not recommended.

SPECIAL CIRCUMSTANCES

All of the major society guidelines are intended for typical women without special risk factors. Certain groups have been excluded from each of the major society guidelines. The USPSTF specifically states that their recommendations do not apply to "women who have received a diagnosis of high-grade precancerous cervical lesion or cervical cancer, women with in utero exposure to Diethylstilbestrol (DES), or women who are immunocompromised (such as those who are HIV positive)."[2] The ACS's guidelines do address women with a prior diagnosis of high-grade lesions but do not address women with a history of cervical cancer, exposed to in utero DES, or who are immunocompromised. The ACS recommends that women with a history of prior CIN 2, CIN 3, or AIS should first have completion of surveillance after treatment or documentation of spontaneous lesion regression according to the 2006 consensus guidelines for the management of women with CIN or AIS.[35] For women with a history of CIN 2, CIN 3, or AIS, they recommend that routine age-based screening continue for at least 20 years after spontaneous regression or completion of appropriate management, even if this extends the screening until after 65 years of age. The reason for continued screening in this population is that these women have a residual risk of significant recurrent disease that extends for this time period. Soutter[36] performed a meta-analysis and showed that women who had prior treatment of CIN 2 or CIN 3 had a 2.8-fold increased risk of invasive disease that persisted for up to 20 years after treatment. Although these patients do need continued screening, once they are out of the immediate surveillance period, they do not need increased frequency of testing; the recommendation is to follow the general age-based screening recommendations.

The CDC makes recommendations for women infected with HIV.[15] They recommend that women infected with HIV be screened every 6 months for the first year after HIV diagnosis, then annually thereafter. Screening should be with cytology alone. They recommend performing colposcopy for any abnormal cytology. They do not state an age at which screening should be stopped. They also do not stipulate a minimum age at which to start. If read literally, these recommendations are impractical. For instance, according to the recommendations, a female child who had vertical transmission of HIV would be screened at 6 and 12 months of life and then annually thereafter. If following the CDC's guidelines, clinical judgment should be used regarding when to start screening adolescents with HIV. The ACS's guidelines do make a specific statement that may apply to other populations, including those with HIV. They specifically recommend against screening anyone before 21 years of age, regardless of risk factors; therefore, the ACS's recommendations would suggest 21 years as a reasonable age to begin testing women infected with HIV.

The ACOG does provide some guidance for women with DES exposure and for those who are immunocompromised, such as solid organ transplant recipients. They comment that characteristics of HPV testing have not been determined for these populations and recommend against cotesting. They recommend screening with cytology alone annually starting at 21 years of age and do not specify an age at which to cease.

SCREENING AFTER HYSTERECTOMY

The USPSTF specifically states that their recommendations apply only to women who have a cervix. ACS states that women who have undergone hysterectomy and have had no history of CIN 2 or greater should not be screened for vaginal cancer using any modality. They specify that evidence of adequate negative prior screening is not required and that once screening is discontinued, it should not resume for any reason, including a woman's report of having a new sexual partner. They do not make recommendations for women who had a history of CIN 2 or greater before their hysterectomy. The ACOG adopted the ACS's recommendations but provide additional guidance for patients with a prior history of CIN 2 or greater.

The rationale for discontinuing screening in women without a cervix and with no history of CIN 2 or greater is that vaginal cancer is exceedingly rare. As with extremely rare diseases, screening is ineffective. A systematic review of 19 studies including 6543 women with prior hysterectomy and with no history of CIN[37] noted that 1.8% had abnormal vaginal cytology screening after hysterectomy and only 0.12% had vaginal intraepithelial neoplasia (VAIN) on biopsy. In 5822 women with CIN 3 before their hysterectomy, 14.1% had abnormal cytology, but VAIN was confirmed by biopsy only in 1.7%, and there was only one case of cancer. Screening after hysterectomy generates significant additional testing with negligible impact on the detection of an extremely rare disease. The few lesions that are detected seem confined to women with a history of prior high-grade disease. The ACOG's guidance reflects these observations. They recommend routine screening with cytology alone for up to 20 years after spontaneous regression of the lesion or completion of the ASCCP's recommended posttreatment surveillance period.[35] Because there is no data for cotesting in this setting, they recommend testing with cytology alone. The choice of a 20-year time period is a generalization of the data from which the recommendation was made for patients who still have their cervix and have a history of prior high-grade lesion.[36]

MANAGING COTESTING RESULTS

The use of cotesting will yield several combinations of results. The USPSTF does not include management of test results at all within their recommendations. The ACS does provide some guidance. Cytologic abnormalities with a significant risk of CIN 3 are managed as per the ASCCP's 2006[38] recommendations. These recommendations include results such as atypical squamous cells–cannot exclude high grade squamous intraepithelial lesion, LSIL, HSIL, and AIS, which all merit colposcopy regardless of the HPV test result. The ASCCP's 2006 recommendations are currently being revised. The consensus meeting took place in September 2012, and the publication of the recommendations is anticipated in March 2013. The ACS does make recommendations for common screening test results with low risk for CIN 3, particularly atypical squamous cells of uncertain significance (ASC-US) with negative HPV test results and cytology that showed no intraepithelial lesion or malignancy (NILM) with a positive HPV test. Although management of these test results was included in the screening guidelines, they could also be considered elements of management. Draft revisions of the ASCCP's 2006 guidelines for the management of abnormal screening tests posted for comment on the Internet included revised management recommendations for HPV-negative ASC-US cytology, which may supersede the ACS's recommendations.

The ACS recommended that women with ASC-US cytology with negative HPV test results should be managed the same as women with negative cotesting, with continued follow-up as per age-appropriate recommended screening. This recommendation was based on the risk of CIN 3 at the time of colposcopy and over 5 years of follow-up, both of which are extremely low. In the Addressing THE Need for Advanced HPV Diagnostics trial, the risk of CIN 3 at colposcopy was 0.28%.[39] In the Kaiser Permanente of Northern California Database, the incidence of CIN 3 was

0.54% over 5 years of follow-up. For comparison, women with NILM cytology alone had a risk of 0.36%, which is only slightly smaller. Thus, ASC-US with a negative HPV cotest has similar risk to normal cytology; if it has higher risk, the increment is small, leading to recommendations to manage both the same way. The draft revisions to the ASCCP's 2006 guidelines posted for public comment on the Internet included a recommendation to repeat age-appropriate screening 3 years after this finding. Although the final revised guidelines are not available at the time of this writing, if the draft recommendation is adopted, the recommendations discussed here will change.

The larger challenge with cotesting is the management of NILM cytology with a positive HPV cotest. The ACS recommends that these women should be followed as per the ASCCP's recommendations,[38,40] which offer 2 options. One option is to repeat cotesting in 1 year, with colposcopy if either repeat test is abnormal. Alternatively, HPV-16 or HPV-16/18 genotyping can be performed with immediate colposcopy if either HPV-16 or -18 is present. They also clearly state that colposcopy should not be performed at the initial cotest. The ACOG adopted this recommendation.

This recommendation is particularly important because these results will be common when cotesting is performed. In the Kaiser Permanente Northern California Database,[23] NILM cytology with positive HPV testing occurred in 4.7% of screenings. In their guideline document (2011), the ACS summarized the results of 11 prospective studies that followed patients up to 16 years and noted that the risk of developing CIN 3 in the year after this finding ranged from 0.8% to 4.1%. These risks are much lower than typical thresholds for recommending colposcopy. Data for the recommendation are based on expert opinion and extrapolation from other data. In particular, data suggest that most HPV will clear, and the risk of having a significant pathologic condition occurs in the small fraction where the HPV persists. Two studies[24,41] noted approximately two-thirds of patients with NILM cytology and positive HPV cotest were HPV negative by 6 to 12 months. In the study by Rodriguez and colleagues,[24] 21% of women who had persistent HPV at 12 months developed CIN 2 or CIN 3 by 30 months. The selection of 1 year as the interval to wait before repeating the cotest was based on expert opinion and was the balance of allowing time for low-risk lesions to resolve while testing soon enough that high-risk lesions did not progress. The rationale for HPV-16 or HPV-16/18 genotype testing is that the risk of CIN 3 is significantly higher with these types than other HPV types. Several studies[42–45] noted an approximately 10% risk of CIN 3 over several years after the detection of HPV-16 or -18. Because a 10% risk of having a high-grade lesion is the threshold typically chosen for colposcopy, proceeding to immediate colposcopy in the presence of HPV-16 or -18 was thought to be reasonable. Logistic difficulties and limited availability of genotyping, however, have limited the use of this triage option.

IMPLICATIONS OF LESS FREQUENT TESTING

In the decades since its introduction, the annual Papanicolaou test became a ritual to which patients and providers have become deeply attached. This tradition has allowed the development of the annual well-woman visit, which is routinely covered by insurance and allows women better access to preventative care. With the recommendations by all major societies that annual cervical cytology is no longer required, concerns have been expressed that the annual visit is threatened. Increasing the interval of cervical cancer screenings is clearly the right thing to do because it decreases the harms of testing without negatively impacting cancer rates. Rather than posing a threat to women or the annual well-woman visit, the decrease in cervical cancer screening requirements presents an opportunity to further enhance the annual visit.[46] There are many other preventative screening and counseling requirements recommended by other guidelines from the ACS, ACOG, and USPSTF. It is difficult to cover them effectively in the limited time available. The time previously devoted to cervical cancer screening can instead be devoted to these other important issues. The ACOG[12] has clearly stated that the well-woman visit remains important despite the diminished need for cervical cancer screening.

REFERENCES

1. Saslow D, Solomon D, Lawson HW, et al. American Cancer Society, American Society for Colposcopy and Cervical Pathology, and American Society for Clinical Pathology Screening Guidelines for the Prevention and Early Detection of Cervical Cancer. J Low Genit Tract Dis 2012;16(3):175–204.
2. Moyer VA, for the U.S. Preventive Services Task Force. Screening for cervical cancer: U.S. preventive services task force recommendation statement. Ann Intern Med 2012;156(12):880–91.
3. Gustafsson L, Pontén J, Bergström R, et al. International incidence rates of invasive cervical cancer before cytological screening. Int J Cancer 1997;71(2): 159–65.
4. Gustafsson L, Pontén J, Zack M, et al. International incidence rates of invasive cervical cancer after introduction of cytological screening. Cancer Causes Control 1997;8(5):755–63.
5. Schiffman M, Kjaer SK. Chapter 2: natural history of anogenital human papillomavirus infection and neoplasia. J Natl Cancer Inst Monographs 2003;31:14–9 SEER 2012 Section 5, Table 7. Available at: http://seer.cancer.gov/csr/1975_2008/browse_csr.php?section=5&page=sect_05_table.07.html. Accessed September 23, 2012.
6. Wright TC, Schiffman M. Adding a test for human papillomavirus DNA to cervical-cancer screening. N Engl J Med 2003;6:489–90.
7. McCredie MR, Sharples KJ, Pual C, et al. Natural history of cervical neoplasia and risk of invasive cancer in women with cervical intraepithelial neoplasia 3: a retrospective cohort study. Lancet Oncol 2008;9:425–34.
8. Kyrgiou M, Koliopoulos G, Martin-Hirsch P, et al. Obstetric outcomes after conservative treatment for intraepithelial or early invasive cervical lesions: systematic review and meta-analysis. Lancet 2006;367:489–98.
9. Bruinsma FJ, Quinn MA. The risk of preterm birth following treatment for precancerous changes in the cervix: a systematic review and meta-analysis. BJOG 2011;118:1031–41.
10. Macones GA, Cahill A, Stamilio D, et al. Pregnancy after LEEP: results of a multicenter study. Am J Obstet Gynecol 2012;206(Suppl):S3–4.
11. Centers for Disease Control and Prevention (CDC). ACIP. FDA licensure of bivalent human papillomavirus vaccine (HPV2, Cervarix) for use in females and updated HPV vaccination recommendations from the Advisory Committee on Immunization Practices (ACIP). MMWR Morb Mortal Wkly Rep 2010;59(20):626–9.
12. American College of Obstetrics and Gynecology. Well-woman visit. ACOG Committee Opinion No. 534. Obstet Gynecol 2012;120(2 Pt 1):421–4.
13. Anttila A, Kotaniemi TL, Leinonen M, et al. Rate of cervical cancer, severe intraepithelial neoplasia, and adenocarcinoma in situ in primary HPV DNA screening with cytology triage: randomised study within organised screening programme. BMJ 2010;340:c1804.

14. Kulasingam SL, Havrilesky L, Ghebre R, et al. Screening for cervical cancer: a decision analysis for the U.S. Preventive Services Task Force. Rockville (MD): Agency for Healthcare Research and Quality; 2011. AHRQ Publication No. 11-05157-EF-1.

15. Kaplan JE, Benson C, Holmes KH, et al. Guidelines for prevention and treatment of opportunistic infections in HIV-infected adults and adolescents: recommendations from CDC, the National Institutes of Health, and the HIV Medicine Association of the Infectious Diseases Society of America. Centers for Disease Control and Prevention (CDC); National Institutes of Health; HIV Medicine Association of the Infectious Diseases Society of America. MMWR Recomm Rep 2009; 58(RR-4):1–207.

16. Moscicki AB, Cox JT. Practice improvement in cervical screening and management (PICSM): symposium on management of cervical abnormalities in adolescents and young women. J Low Genit Tract Dis 2010;14:73–80.

17. Barnholtz-Sloan J, Patel N, Rollison D, et al. Incidence trends of invasive cervical cancer in the United States by combined race and ethnicity. Cancer Causes Control 2009;20:1129–38.

18. Sasieni P, Castanon A, Cuzick J. Effectiveness of cervical screening with age: population based case-control study of prospectively recorded data. BMJ 2009;339:2968.

19. Arbyn M, Sasieni P, Meijer CJ, et al. Chapter 9: clinical applications of HPV testing: a summary of meta-analyses. Vaccine 2006;24(Suppl 3):S3/78–89.

20. Arbyn M, Bergeron C, Klinkhamer P, et al. Liquid compared with conventional cervical cytology. Obstet Gynecol 2008;111:167–77.

21. Ronco G, Segnan N, Giorgi-Rossi P, et al. Human papillomavirus testing and liquid-based cytology: results at recruitment from the New Technologies for Cervical Cancer randomized controlled trial. J Natl Cancer Inst 2006;98:765–74.

22. Dillner J, Rebolj M, Birembaut P, et al. Long term predictive values of cytology and human papillomavirus testing in cervical cancer screening: joint European cohort study. BMJ 2008;337:a1754.

23. Katki HA, Kinney WK, Fetterman B, et al. Cervical cancer risk for women undergoing concurrent testing for human papillomavirus and cervical cytology: a population-based study in routine clinical practice. Lancet Oncol 2011;12:663.

24. Rodriguez AC, Schiffman M, Herrero R, et al. Rapid clearance of human papillomavirus and implications for clinical focus on persistent infections. J Natl Cancer Inst 2008;100:513–7.

25. Naucler P, Ryd W, Tornberg S, et al. Human papillomavirus and Papanicolaou tests to screen for cervical cancer. N Engl J Med 2007;357:1589–97.

26. Rijkaart DC, Berkhof J, Rozendaal L, et al. Human papillomavirus testing for the detection of high-grade cervical intraepithelial neoplasia and cancer: final results of the POBASCAM randomised controlled trial. Lancet Oncol 2012;13:78–88.

27. Ronco G, Giorgi-Rossi P, Carozzi F, et al. Efficacy of human papillomavirus testing for the detection of invasive cervical cancers and cervical intraepithelial neoplasia: a randomised controlled trial. Lancet Oncol 2010;11:249–57.

28. US Preventive services. Available at: http://www.uspreventiveservicestaskforce.org/uspstf/grades.htm.

29. Stout NK, Goldhaber-Fiebert JD, Ortendahl JD, et al. Trade-offs in cervical cancer prevention: balancing benefits and risks. Arch Intern Med 2008 Sept 22;168(17): 1881–9.

30. Sasieni P, Adams J, Cuzick J. Benefit of cervical screening at different ages: evidence from the UK audit of screening histories. Br J Cancer 2003;89:88–93.

31. Eddy DM. The frequency of cervical cancer screening. Comparison of a mathematical model with empirical data. Cancer 1987;60:1117–22 (Level III).
32. IARC Working Group on evaluation of cervical cancer screening programmes. Screening for squamous cervical cancer: duration of low risk after negative results of cervical cytology and its implication for screening policies. Br Med J (Clin Res Ed) 1986;293:659–64.
33. Sawaya GF, Kerlikowske K, Lee NC, et al. Frequency of cervical smear abnormalities within 3 years of normal cytology. Obstet Gynecol 2000;96:219–23.
34. Saraiya M, Berkowitz Z, Yabroff KR, et al. Cervical cancer screening with both human papillomavirus and Papanicolaou testing vs Papanicolaou testing alone: what screening intervals are physicians recommending? Arch Intern Med 2010; 170:977–85.
35. Wright TC Jr, Massad LS, Dunton CJ, et al. 2006 consensus guidelines for the management of women with cervical intraepithelial neoplasia or adenocarcinoma in situ. Am J Obstet Gynecol 2007;197:340–5.
36. Soutter WP, Sasieni P, Panoskaltsis T. Long-term risks of invasive cervical cancer after treatment of squamous cervical intraepithelial neoplasia. Int J Cancer 2006 April 15;118(8):2048–55.
37. Stokes-Lampard H, Wilson S, Waddell C, et al. Vaginal vault smears after hysterectomy for reasons other than malignancy: a systematic review of the literature. BJOG 2006;113:1354–65.
38. Wright TC Jr, Massad LS, Dunton CJ, et al. 2006 consensus guidelines for the management of women with abnormal cervical cancer screening tests. Am J Obstet Gynecol 2007;197:346–55 B.
39. Stoler MH, Wright TC Jr, Sharma A, et al. High-risk human papillomavirus testing in women with ASC-US cytology: results from the ATHENA HPV study. Am J Clin Pathol 2011;135(3):468–75.
40. ASCCP, HPV genotyping clinical update. Available at: http://www.asccp.org/Portals/9/docs/pdfs/Consensus%20Guidelines/clinical_update_20090408.pdf. Accessed September 24, 2012.
41. Clavel C, Masure M, Bory JP, et al. Human papillomavirus testing in primary screening for the detection of high-grade cervical lesions: a stud of 7932 women. Br J Cancer 2001;89:1616–23.
42. Khan MJ, Castle PE, Lorincz AT, et al. The elevated 10-year risk of cervical precancer and cancer in women with human papillomavirus (HPV) type 16 or 18 and the possible utility of type-specific HPV testing in clinical practice. J Natl Cancer Inst 2005;97(14):1072–9.
43. Kjaer SK, Frederiksen K, Munk C, et al. Long-term absolute risk of cervical intraepithelial neoplasia grade 3 or worse following human papillomavirus infection: role of persistence. J Natl Cancer Inst 2010;102:1478–88.
44. Wright TC, Stoler MH, Sharma A, et al. Evaluation of HPV-16 and HPV-18 genotyping for the triage women with high-risk HPV+ cytology-negative results. Am J Clin Pathol 2011;136:578–86.
45. Kjaer SK, Frederiksen K, Iftner T. Long-term absolute risk of cervical intraepithelial neoplasia grade 3 or worse following human papillomavirus infection: role of persistence. J Natl Cancer Inst 2010 Oct 6;102(19):1478–88.
46. Chelmow D, Waxman A, Cain JM, et al. The evolution of cervical screening and the specialty of obstetrics and gynecology. Obstet Gynecol 2012;119:695–9.

The Lower Anogenital Squamous Terminology Project and Its Implications for Clinical Care

Tomas Nuño, PhD[a], Francisco García, MD, MPH[b],*

KEYWORDS

- Squamous intraepithelial lesion • Human papillomavirus • Lower anogenital tract
- Terminology

KEY POINTS

- Terminology for lower anogenital tract-associated premalignant disease historically developed along 2 separate paths depending on whether the epithelial lesion was mucosal or cutaneous.
- The LAST (Lower Anogenital Squamous Terminology) Project was designed to reassess and harmonize the terminology used to describe human papillomavirus-associated squamous lesions of the lower anogenital tract.
- The clarification of this terminology is relevant to clinicians and patients.

INTRODUCTION

Terminology for lower anogenital tract (LAT)-associated premalignant disease historically developed along 2 separate paths depending on whether the epithelial lesion was mucosal or cutaneous.[1] The terminology of mucosal cervical, vaginal, and anal lesions was developed by general pathologists, gynecologic pathologists, and gynecologists. By contrast, terminology for cutaneous vulvar, penile, and perianal lesions was mostly developed by dermatologists and dermatopathologists. These conventions evolved over more than a century and certainly antedate our improved

This article was written using funding provided by the Racial and Ethnic Approaches to Community Health (REACH) program, the Arizona Area Health Education Center (AzAHEC) Clinical Outcomes and Comparative Effectiveness Research (COCER) Fellowship program, and the National Cancer Institute of the National Institutes of Health under Award Number R25CA078447. The content is solely the responsibility of the authors and does not necessarily represent the official views of the National Institutes of Health.

[a] The Clinical Outcomes and Comparative Effectiveness Research Fellowship Program, The Arizona Cancer Center, Center of Excellence in Women's Health, University of Arizona, 1515 North Campbell Avenue, PO Box 245024, Tucson, AZ 85724-5024, USA; [b] Center of Excellence in Women's Health, University of Arizona, 1295 North Martin Avenue, PO Box 245209, Tucson, AZ 85724-5209, USA
* Corresponding author.
E-mail address: fcisco@email.arizona.edu

Obstet Gynecol Clin N Am 40 (2013) 225–233
http://dx.doi.org/10.1016/J.ogc.2013.02.008
0889-8545/13/$ – see front matter © 2013 Elsevier Inc. All rights reserved.

understanding of the etiologic role of human papillomavirus (HPV), related disease processes, and a broader range of treatment options. These differing terminologies, for lesions now recognized to be biologically similar, create the potential for miscommunication between and among pathologists seeking to reconcile the various terminologies with clinically identified lesions; clinicians must make patient management decisions based on pathologic assessments.

Since Zur Hausen first proposed the etiologic link between HPV and cervical cancer, there has been a growing recognition of the role of this viral infection in other epithelial neoplasias, including those of the vagina, vulva perineum, and anus, as well as the penis and scrotum. It is now generally accepted that HPV infection in most end organs may follow 2 possible pathways. One supports virion production but may or may not lead to the development of transient lesions not destined for invasion. These processes may be known by a variety of terms, including cervical intraepithelial neoplasia 1 (CIN1), mild dysplasia, low-grade squamous lesions, or in specific cases condyloma. In the alternative preneoplastic pathway, there is a loss of control between viral oncogene expression and epithelial differentiation. The products of this viral oncogene overexpression lead to cell proliferation and clonal expansion of relatively undifferentiated cells by viral replication and the development of the truly premalignant lesion. These processes are similar across tissue types and regardless of sex of the individual and support a unified cause for HPV-related squamous neoplasia.

Despite the histologically identical nature of these lesions, multiple complex terminologies and historically meaningful eponyms have been developed to describe this pathologic and clinical spectrum of disease for the purpose of patient management.

Historical Context

Intraepithelial precancer was first described in 1888 by Sir John Thomas.[2] With subsequent descriptions as surface carcinoma or intraepithelial carcinoma and later carcinoma in situ (CIS), treatment became increasingly dependent of histopathologic assessment.[3–5] The term CIS led to a clinical management approach of hysterectomy for women with CIS, reserving more conservative approaches for those without CIS. By the 1950s, other terms came into use for surface lesions that had less risk of progressing to cancer than CIS. Initially termed anaplasia and atypical hyperplasia, these terms were subsequently replaced by the more widely accepted dysplasia.

The largest change in cervical histologic terminology came in 1969, when cervical carcinogenesis was proposed as a continuum of disease ranging from mild dysplasia to invasive cervical cancer.[6] CIN was coined to emphasize its status as a precursor to invasive cervical cancer. Under this nomenclature, dysplasias were termed: mild dysplasia–CINI; moderate dysplasia–CINII; and severe dysplasia–CINIII.

As the biology of HPV infection and its relationship to cervical oncogenesis became increasingly understood by the 1980s, the subjectivity of the differentiation between CIN2 and CIN3 became more apparent. This situation led to numerous proposals to replace the 3-tiered CIN system with a 2-tiered system of low-grade intraepithelial lesions (LSIL) and high-grade intraepithelial lesions (HSIL), similar to cytology terminology of the 1988 Bethesda System.[7,8] However, such a 2-tiered nomenclature for histopathology was not widely adopted in the 1990s and lacked the support of most professional organizations.[1]

The 2001 and 2006 American Society for Colposcopy and Cervical Pathology (ASCCP) Consensus Guidelines for the clinical management of cervical histologic abnormalities began to move toward a 2-tiered nomenclature for cervix using the terms CIN1 and CIN2, 3. The exception was for disease in adolescent and young women, for whom where the differentiation between CIN2 and CIN3 was preserved.[9,10]

In the 1990s, 2 important changes occurred in the management of CIN. Expectant management became the primary follow-up for CIN1. This situation was based largely on increasing appreciation for the transient nature of most of these lesions. By contrast, in-office excision of the transformation zone using the loop electrosurgical excision procedure became the principal management for precancer lesions (CIN2, 3) across the United States and much of the developed world.[11] During the last decade, there has again been a renewed interest in 2-tiered low-grade and high-grade nomenclature that better reflects the natural history of LAT HPV-associated intraepithelial lesions. The Lower Anogenital Squamous Terminology (LAST) Conference was an attempt to systematically reassess the latest data in an effort to develop a consensus across specialty groups and stakeholders for this change in nomenclature.

THE LAST PROCESS

Based on a growing recognition of a need for unified terminology the ASCCP and the College of American Pathologists (CAP) Pathology and Laboratory Quality Center jointly convened a process to tackle this challenge (the details of which can be found at http://links.lww.com). This 14-month process brought together a broad array of 53 experts and opinion leaders from a variety of clinical and scientific disciplines. Five Working Groups (WGs) (**Box 1**) were assembled to conduct systematic reviews of the relevant literature and discussions of the relevant issues, and the process culminated in a consensus conference in March, 2012.

The LAST Project, conceived and sponsored by the CAP and the ASCCP, was designed to reassess and harmonize the terminology used to describe HPV-associated squamous lesions of the LAT as manifested in a variety of end organs, including the cervix, the vagina, the vulva, the perianus, the anus, the penis, and the scrotum.[1]

The primary goals of the last process were following: (1) to standardize the terminology used for reporting histopathology diagnoses of HPV-related mucocutaneous squamous lesions of the lower genital tract, including intraepithelial lesions and minimally invasive cancers (but excluding non-HPV-related dermatologic and vulvar lesions); (2) to harmonize terminology across the various LAT sites using current evidence-based knowledge regarding the biology of HPV-related squamous lesions and their clinical management; (3) to harmonize the terminology for histopathology with the Bethesda System for reporting gynecologic and anal cytology (if applicable); (4) to assess the use of new technologies to validate proposed terminology standards

---

Box 1
LAST WGs

WG1: historical review of lower anogenital track HPV-associated squamous lesion terminology

WG2: squamous intraepithelial lesions; subgrouped as:

   a. Cervix and vagina

   b. Vulva, penis, and scrotum

   c. Anal canal and perianus

WG3: SISCCA (SCC)

WG4: biomarkers in HPV-associated lower anogenital squamous lesions

WG5: implications and implementation of standardized terminology

and provide guidelines for appropriate use. This work was conducted primarily by 5 WGs comprising content experts and representatives from a range of professional societies and stakeholder groups (see **Box 1**).

The recommendations of the LAST Conference and the background documentation are detailed in a pair of simultaneously published papers in the October, 2012 issues of *Lower Genital Tract Disease*[1] and *Archives of Pathology*.[12] Supporting documentation and related material are included in electronic appendices that can be accessed from the journal Web sites.

FINDINGS AND RECOMMENDATIONS OF THE LAST CONFERENCE

The LAST Conference findings support a single unified histopathologic 2-tiered nomenclature with a single set of diagnostic terms, specifically LSIL and HSIL. This nomenclature can be further qualified using the -IN terminology to facilitate clinical management. Immunohistochemistry p16 testing is recommended when there is a diagnosis of -IN2 under the old terminology or to help adjudicate cases of disagreement between pathologists. A strong diffuse positive staining pattern is consistent with the HSIL diagnosis, whereas negative staining supports the LSIL diagnosis or a non-HPV cause. Another clinically important innovation is the development of the term superficially invasive squamous cell carcinoma (SISCCA) for minimally invasive squamous cancers of the lower anogenital track that are completely excised and potentially amenable to conservative therapy. In the cervix, this terminology describes a lesion that is not grossly visible, has invaded 3 mm or less from the basement membrane, has a horizontal spread of 7 mm or less, and has been completely excised. Relevant variations of this terminology are described for the anal canal, vulva, and perianus (**Box 2**).

Box 2 lists the recommendations of WGs2, 3, and 4. WG2 issued 3 recommendations. Their first recommendation supports a unified histopathologic nomenclature with a single set of diagnostic terms recommended for all HPV-associated preinvasive squamous lesions of the LAT. Their comprehensive literature review and expert opinion support the biological and morphologic equivalence of HPV-associated squamous proliferations across the LAT. Given this equivalence, a unified histopathologic nomenclature is recommended for all HPV-associated preinvasive intraepithelial squamous lesions in the LAT. Biomarker characteristics, as noted by WG4, are also consistent across LAT sites, lending further support to this recommendation.

WG2's second recommendation was for a 2-tiered nomenclature for noninvasive HPV-associated squamous proliferations of the LAT, which may be further qualified with the appropriate -IN terminology (-IN refers to the generic intraepithelial neoplasia terminology, without specifying the location. For a specific location, the appropriate complete term should be used. Thus, for an -IN 3 lesion: cervix = CIN3, vagina = VaIN3, vulva = VIN3, anus = AIN3, perianus = PAIN3, and penis = PeIN3). The rationale for this recommendation is that current understanding of HPV biology does not support a progressive 3-tiered system of mild, moderate, severe dysplasia/CIS or -IN1, 2, 3. Rather, there is support for a dichotomous separation of morphologic designations that reflect transient active HPV replication and persistent HPV-associated precancer. From the comprehensive literature review by WG4, no biomarker data supported a 3-tiered system (see later discussion). Instead, data are consistent with a 2-tiered system with low-grade lesions that are generally self-limited HPV infection and high-grade lesions that have the potential to progress to invasive carcinoma. The equivocal nature of the diagnosis of -IN2, an intermediate category that has no biological correlate, is believed to represent a mixture of low-grade and precancerous disease that cannot

---

Box 2
Summary of recommendations

Squamous Intraepithelial Lesions (WG2)

1. A unified histopathologic nomenclature with a single set of diagnostic terms is recommended for all HPV-associated preinvasive squamous lesions of the LAT.

2. A 2-tiered nomenclature is recommended for noninvasive HPV-associated squamous proliferations of the LAT, which may be further qualified with the appropriate -IN terminology.

3. The recommended terminology for HPV-associated squamous lesions of the LAT is LSIL and HSIL, which may be further classified by the applicable -IN subcategorization.

SISCCA (WG3)

1. The term SISCCA is recommended for minimally invasive SCC of the LAT that has been completely excised and is potentially amenable to conservative surgical therapy.

2. For cases of invasive squamous carcinoma with positive biopsy/resection margins, the pathology report should state whether:

   The examined invasive tumor exceeds the dimensions for a SISCCA (defined later)

   or

   The examined invasive tumor component is less than or equal to the dimensions for a SISCCA and conclude that the tumor is "at least a superficially invasive squamous carcinoma."

3. In cases of SISCCA, the following parameters should be included in the pathology report:

   The presence or absence of lymph-vascular invasion (LVI).

   The presence, number, and size of independent multifocal carcinomas (after excluding the possibility of a single carcinoma).

4. Cervix: SISCCA of the cervix is defined as an Invasive squamous carcinoma that:

   Is not a grossly visible lesion, and

   Has an invasive depth of 3 mm or less from the basement membrane of the point of origin, and

   Has a horizontal spread of 7 mm or less in maximal extent, and

   Has been completely excised.

5. Vagina: no recommendation is offered for early invasive squamous carcinoma of the vagina. Because of the rarity of primary SCC of the vagina, there are insufficient data to define early invasive squamous carcinoma in the vagina.

6. Anal canal: the suggested definition of SISCCA of the anal canal is an invasive squamous carcinoma that:

   Has an invasive depth of 3 mm or less from the basement membrane of the point of origin, and

   Has a horizontal spread of 7 mm or less in maximal extent, and

   Has been completely excised.

7. Vulva: vulvar SISCCA is defined as an American Joint Committee on Cancer (AJCC) T1a (International Federation of Gynecology and Obstetrics [FIGO] IA) vulvar cancer. No change in the current definition of T1a vulvar cancer is recommended.

8. Penis: penile SISCCA is defined as an AJCC T1a. No change in the current definition of T1a penile cancer is recommended.

9. Scrotum: no recommendation is offered for early invasive squamous carcinoma of the scrotum.

10. Perianus: the suggested definition for SISCCA of the perianus is an invasive squamous carcinoma that:

   Has an invasive depth of 3 mm or less from the basement membrane of the point of origin, and

   Has a horizontal spread of 7 mm or less in maximal extent, and

   Has been completely excised.

Biomarkers in HPV-Associated Lower Anogenital Squamous Lesions (WG4)

1. p16 immunochemistry (IHC) is recommended when the hematoxylin-eosin morphologic differential diagnosis is between precancer (-IN2 or -IN3) and a mimic of precancer (eg, processes known to be not related to neoplastic risk, such as immature squamous metaplasia, atrophy, reparative epithelial changes, tangential cutting).

2. If the pathologist is entertaining a hematoxylin-eosin morphologic interpretation of -IN2 (under the old terminology, which is a biologically equivocal lesion falling between the morphologic changes of HPV infection [low-grade lesion] and precancer), p16 IHC is recommended to help clarify the situation. Strong and diffuse block-positive p16 results support a categorization of precancer. Negative or non–block-positive staining strongly favors an interpretation of low-grade disease or a non-HPV-associated disease.

3. p16 is recommended for use as an adjudication tool for cases in which there is a professional disagreement in interpretation of histologic specimen, with the caveat that the differential diagnosis includes a precancerous lesion (-IN2 or -IN3).

4. WG4 recommends against the use of p16 IHC as a routine adjunct to histologic assessment of biopsy specimens with morphologic interpretations of negative, -IN1, and -IN3.

Special circumstance: p16 IHC is recommended as an adjunct to morphologic assessment for biopsy specimens interpreted as -IN1 that are at high risk for missed high-grade disease, which is defined as a previous cytologic interpretation of HSIL, ASC-H (atypical squamous cells of high grade), ASC-US (atypical squamous cells of undetermined significance)/HPV-16+, or Atypical Glandular Cells (Not Otherwise Specified).

be reliably distinguished based on hematoxylin-eosin morphology.[13,14] The -IN2 category is not a reproducible histologic category among pathologists. Studies of diagnostic concordance show considerable interobserver variability reflected in very low [κ] statistics.[13] As might be expected from this mixture of high-grade and low-grade lesions, the risk of progression for lesions classified as -IN2 is intermediate between -IN1 and -IN3. In addition, a substantial proportion of CIN2 is found to represent CIN3 on follow-up.[15] The recommendation for a 2-tiered system also harmonizes LAT terminology with other published systems, including those of recent textbooks and professional societies.[16–20]

WG2's third recommendation was that the terminology for HPV-associated squamous lesions of the LAT as LSIL and HSIL, may be further classified by the applicable -IN subcategorization. This recommendation harmonizes the descriptive terminology for cytology and histopathology for biologically similar HPV-associated squamous lesions of the LAT. This terminology is also the one used for 2-tiered histologic systems in recent textbooks published in the field.[18–20] In addition, this terminology was the most widely supported by responses during the open comment period and at least a 67% supermajority of the participants at the consensus conference.

WG3 reviewed data across LAT sites to recommend specific terminology for minimally invasive SCC. They delineated 10 recommendations. As described earlier, a key recommendation was the term SISCCA for minimally invasive SCC of the LAT that has been completely excised and is potentially amenable to conservative surgical therapy.

Recommendations 2 and 3 deal with specific parameters of defining a case of SISCCA. Recommendation 2 is for cases of invasive squamous carcinoma with positive biopsy/resection margins. It is recommended that the pathology report state whether the examined invasive tumor exceeds the dimensions for SISCCA or the tumor component is less than or equal to the dimensions of SISCCA and conclude that the tumor is at least a superficially invasive carcinoma. Recommendation 3 is for cases of SISCCA; parameters should be included in the pathology that report the presences or absence of LVI and the presence, number, and size of independent multifocal carcinoma.

Recommendations 4, 5, 6, 7, 8, 9, and 10 provide site-specific recommendations. Specifically, SISCCA of the cervix, vagina, anal canal, vulva, penis, scrotum, and perianus. It is generally believed that all SCCs of the cervix are attributable to HPV.[21] SISCCA of the cervix is defined as an invasive SCC that is not a grossly visible lesion and has an invasive depth of 3 mm or less from the basement membrane of the point of origin and has a horizontal spread of 7 mm or less in maximal extent and has been completely excised. Recommendations 5 and 9 are that there is no recommendation for early invasive squamous carcinoma of the vagina and scrotum, respectively. This Situation is because of the rarity of primary SCC of the vagina and scrotum, and insufficient data to define early invasive squamous carcinoma in this site. Recommendation 6, 7, 8, and 10 provide parameters for site-specific definitions of SISCCA for anal canal, vulva, penis, and perianus, respectively.

WG4 described 4 recommendations dealing with the use of molecular biomarkers in HPV-associated lower anogenital squamous lesions. Recommendation 1 stated that p16 IHC is recommended when the hematoxylin-eosin morphologic differential diagnosis is between precancer and a mimic of precancer. Strong and diffuse block-positive p16 results provide support in a categorization of precancerous disease. Recommendation 2 was that if the pathologist is entertaining a hematoxylin-eosin morphologic interpretation of -IN2 under the old terminology, p16 IHC is recommended to help clarify the diagnosis. Recommendation 3 states that p16 is recommended for use as an adjudication tool for cases in which there is a professional disagreement in interpretation of a histologic specimen, with the caveat that the differential diagnosis includes a precancerous lesion. Recommendation 4 is a recommendation against the use of p16 IHC as a routine adjunct to histologic assessment of biopsy specimens with interpretations of negative, -IN1, and -IN3.

WG5 was tasked with communication strategies to disseminate the work of the LAST terminology and promote the uptake of its recommendations. Communities of interest were identified for the LAST Project. These communities included patients and patient advocacy groups, pathologists, gynecologists, primary care providers, dermatologists, infectious disease specialists, colorectal surgeons, urologists, nurse practitioners, and other allied health professionals and government, regulatory, and nomenclature agencies. Specific actions recommended by WG5 include support for guideline publications, promotion of editorial commentaries for journals in related fields, presentation of summary recommendations at scientific meetings, educational materials, and development of a Web site that would include reference images, sample reports, and a self-test.

SUMMARY

The clarification of this terminology is not simply an esoteric exercise but instead it is critical to clinicians and patients alike. The historical heterogeneity of clinical and histopathologic terminology has led to inevitable diagnostic variation and miscommunication between those taking the biopsies and those interpreting the findings; this in turn has important implications for the treatment, follow-up, and prognosis of these lesions. The clear unambiguous distinction between cancer precursors and those without malignant potential inevitably leads to greater consistency in the interpretation of management guidelines and the therapeutic options offered to patients. However, the new terminology formally acknowledges a common cause of this disease grouping and opens up the possibility of novel preventive and therapeutic approaches across tissue types.

REFERENCES

1. Darragh TM, Colgan TJ, Cox JT, et al. The lower anogenital squamous terminology standardization project for HPV-associated lesions: background and consensus recommendations from the College of American Pathologists and the American Society for Colposcopy and Cervical Pathology. J Low Genit Tract Dis 2012;16(3):205–42.
2. Williams J. On cancer of the uterus: being the Harveian lectures for 1886. London: H.K. Lewis; 1888.
3. Cullen T. Cancer of the uterus: its pathology, symptomatology, diagnosis, and treatment. New York: Appleton; 1900.
4. Rubin I. The pathological diagnosis of incipient carcinoma of the cervix. Obstet Gynecol 1910;62:668–76.
5. Broders A. Carcinoma in situ contrasted with benign penetrating epithelium. JAMA 1932;99:1670–4.
6. Richart R, Barron B. A follow-up study of patients with cervical dysplasia. Am J Obstet Gynecol 1969;105:386–93.
7. Richart R. A modified terminology for cervical intraepithelial neoplasia. Obstet Gynecol 1990;75:131–3.
8. The 1988 Bethesda System for reporting cervical/vaginal cytological diagnoses. JAMA 1989;262:931–4.
9. Wright TC Jr, Cox JT, Massad L, et al. 2001 consensus guidelines for the management of women with cervical intraepithelial neoplasia. Am J Obstet Gynecol 2003; 189:295–304.
10. Wright TC Jr, Massad L, Dunton C, et al. 2006 consensus guidelines for the management of women with cervical intraepithelial neoplasia. Am J Obstet Gynecol 2007;197:340–5.
11. Cox JT. Management of cervical intraepithelial neoplasia. Lancet 1999; 353(9156):857–9.
12. Darragh TM, Colgan TJ, Cox JT, et al. The lower anogenital squamous terminology standardization project for HPV-associated lesions: background and consensus recommendations from the College of American Pathologists and the American Society for Colposcopy and Cervical Pathology. Arch Pathol Lab Med 2012;136(10):1266–97.
13. Stoler M, Schiffman M. Interobserver reproducibility of cervical cytologic and histologic interpretations: realistic estimates from the ASCUS-LSIL triage study. JAMA 2001;285:1500–5.
14. Castle P, Stoler M, Solomon D, et al. The relationship of community biopsy-diagnosed cervical intraepithelial neoplasia grade 2 to the quality control pathology-reviewed diagnoses: an ALTS report. Am J Clin Pathol 2007;127: 805–15.

15. Stoler MH, Vichnin MD, Ferenczy A, et al. The accuracy of colposcopic biopsy: analyses from the placebo arm of the Gardasil clinical trials. Int J Cancer 2011; 128(6):1354–62.
16. Heller DS. Report of a new ISSVD classification of VIN. J Low Genit Tract Dis 2007;11(1):46–7.
17. Scurry J, Wilkinson EJ. Review of terminology of precursors of vulvar squamous cell carcinoma. J Low Genit Tract Dis 2006;10(3):161–9.
18. Witkiewicz A, Wright T, Ferenczy A, et al. Carcinoma and other tumors of the cervix. In: Kurman R, Ellenson L, Ronnett B, editors. Blaustein's pathology of the female genital tract. New York: Springer; 2011. p. 253–303.
19. Crum C, Lee K. Diagnostic gynecologic and obstetric pathology. Philadelphia: Saunders; 2005.
20. Kurman R, Ronnett J, Sherman M, et al. Atlas of tumor pathology: tumors of the cervix, vagina, and vulva. Washington, DC: Armed Forces Institute of Pathology, American Registry of Pathology; 2010.
21. Parkin D, Bray F. The burden of HPV-related cancer. Vaccine 2006;24:S11–25.

Colposcopy: A Global Perspective

Introduction of the New IFCPC Colposcopy Terminology

Silvio Tatti, MD, MSc, PhD[a], Jacob Bornstein, MD, MPA[b],
Walter Prendiville, FRCOG[c],*

KEYWORDS

- Nomenclature • Colposcopy • Preinvasive cervical intraepithelial neoplasia
- Vulvovaginal

KEY POINTS

- It is incumbent on colposcopists to become as objective and clear as possible in publications and practice.
- It is hoped the current classification improves clarity in colposcopic practice and research and helps make progress toward better patient care in the future.
- The latest IFCPC nomenclature attempts to bring greater clarity to terminology in diagnostic and therapeutic colposcopy practice.

INTRODUCTION

In any branch of scientific endeavor, progress evolves from a clear understanding of previous research and experience. Clarity of terminology and practice is fundamental to understanding published research and reports of experience in similar and in different clinical circumstances. When no agreed nomenclature exists it is difficult to accurately compare existing practice or to evaluate new evidence. The latest International Federation for Cervical Pathology and Colposcopy (IFCPC) nomenclature attempts to bring greater clarity to terminology in diagnostic and therapeutic colposcopy practice.

Screening programs for cervical precancer have reduced the incidence of cervical cancer especially in those countries with properly organized and quality assured call and recall systems.[1] It is not the screening itself that reduces the risk of cancer, but rather it is the treatment of screen-positive women who are found to be at significant risk of developing cancer. Most screen-positive women are, however, at very low risk

[a] Buenos Aires University Hospital de Clinicas, Austria 2640, Caba 1425, Argentina;
[b] Department of Obstetrics and Gynecology, Western Galilee Hospital, PO Box 21, Nahariya 22100, Israel; [c] The Gynae Clinic, Mount Carmel Hospital, Braemor Park, Braemor Road, Churchtown, Dublin 14, Ireland
* Corresponding author.
E-mail address: prendiville.walter@gmail.com

Obstet Gynecol Clin N Am 40 (2013) 235–250
http://dx.doi.org/10.1016/j.ogc.2013.02.002
0889-8545/13/$ – see front matter © 2013 Elsevier Inc. All rights reserved.

obgyn.theclinics.com

of progression to cancer. These women may be reassured and followed-up appropriately. Colposcopic assessment of the grade of abnormality and therefore the risk of progression is key to the process of managing screen-positive women. This is also true of colposcopic assessment of other transformation zone (TZ) characteristics, such as the size, site, and visibility of the entire TZ. Most importantly, when properly undertaken, colposcopy reduces the risk of overtreatment and undertreatment. For those women with a relatively high risk of progression to cancer and who do need to be treated, precise excision of the TZ zone is associated with the lowest risk of pregnancy-related morbidity[2] and the highest chance of achieving successful eradication of all precancer epithelium[3,4] Although colposcopic image recognition of high-grade disease is not of a consistently high quality[5] and it has not performed uniformly well across the globe,[6,7] there is very good evidence that routine colposcopy performed by properly trained colposcopists in a quality assured clinical environment performs effectively in terms of disease recognition and negative predictive value, even in the context of women who have low-grade cytologic abnormality (ie, suspected LSIL [low grade squamus intraepithelial neoplasia] or ASCUS [atypical squamus cells of uncertain significance] smears).[8,9]

EVOLUTION OF COLPOSCOPY AND TERMINOLOGY

The first reported use of a colposcope came from Hamburg as a result of collaboration between the University of Hamburg and the German microscope manufacturer Leitz, whose technicians built the first colposcope in the very early 1920s. The early work published in the 1930s from Hamburg described the origins of cervical cancer being in a sheet of epithelium (ie, intraepithelial) as opposed to arising from a single focal lesion. During the 1930s and 1940s colposcopy practice spread and evolved throughout Europe (Mestwert, Limburg, Wespi, Navratil, Ganze, Antoine, Coupez, and Kolstad) and South America (Jakob and Reipert). It was not until the 1960s and 1970s that colposcopy became established in the English-speaking world, again through individual experts. These included Jordan in the United Kingdom, Coppelson and Pixley in Australia, and Stafl in the United States. The IFCPC was founded in Mar del Plata in 1972. There have been four nomenclature committees since that time.[10–13] The most recent built on the work of the three previous publications and introduced a classification of excision types in the treatment of cervical intraepithelial neoplasia (CIN) (**Figs. 1–3**). For the first time, this nomenclature includes vulval and vaginal terminology. The Nomenclature Committee of the IFCPC met over the triennium 2008 to 2011 and reported its' findings to the Board of the IFCPC. The Nomenclature Committee and the Board of the IFCPC unanimously endorsed the new nomenclature, which was again unanimously endorsed at the Annual General Meeting of the IFCPC at its' World Congress in Rio de Janeiro in 2011.

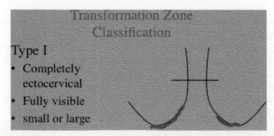

Fig. 1. Classification of excision types in the treatment of CIN. The type 1 TZ.

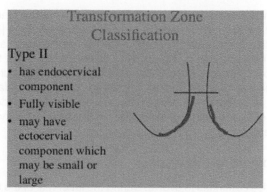

Fig. 2. Classification of excision types in the treatment of CIN. The type 2 TZ.

PRACTICE VARIATION

Clinical practice across the spectrum of medicine varies enormously around the world. Stark examples in obstetrics include the threshold for performing caesarean section and management of the third stage of labor. Another example is vaginal examination at antenatal visits, which is routine in many parts of France and yet rarely performed in any part of the United Kingdom. Gynecologic practice is similarly dissimilar. Dilatation and curettage under general anesthesia is still the standard investigation for abnormal uterine bleeding in some centers, whereas office hysteroscopy with or without directed sampling is the norm in others. In many European hospitals endometrial cancer is treated by way of a simple total hysterectomy and bilateral salpingo-oophorectomy either at laparotomy or laparoscopy, whereas an extended hysterectomy and lymphadenectomy is also commonly offered to women with the same disease in much of the United States and also in many European centers. Another example is the management of ectopic pregnancy, which may be and is managed by laparoscopy or laparotomy depending on where a patient presents.

Colposcopic practice varies dramatically across the globe. A colposcopic examination is considered necessary for every woman attending a gynecologist in some European countries, quite independent of the clinical presentation. In the United Kingdom, Australia, and much of North and South America colposcopic examination is performed only for women with an abnormal screening test or because of symptoms or signs that suggest cervical disease. So-called cone biopsy, using a cold knife, is the most common treatment of women with an abnormal smear in much of France and Germany and is often performed without any preliminary colposcopic examination and may be undertaken by a general surgeon rather than a gynecologist or

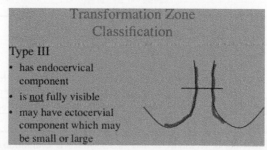

Fig. 3. Classification of excision types in the treatment of CIN. The type 3 TZ.

colposcopist. In the United Kingdom, Australian, and Canadian practices large loop excision of the TZ (large loop excision of the transformation zone [LLETZ]),[14] which became loop electrosurgical excision procedure (loop electrosurgical excision procedure [LEEP])[15] on its introduction to the United States, is the usual treatment choice for women for whom treatment is indicated, and the procedure would usually be performed in the outpatient clinic as part of a thorough colposcopic examination, sometimes at the first or assessment visit. Hysterectomy is also widely used as the primary treatment of CIN despite the associated increased morbidity and without any benefit to the patient.

EVOLUTION OF COLPOSCOPIC PRACTICE

Colposcopic practice continues to evolve. During the latter half of the twentieth century colposcopic expertise focused on very precise image recognition skills and the ability to discriminate between the grades of abnormality within a particular lesion. The threshold for treatment was placed at the higher end of the spectrum of precancer disease and the ability to recognize microinvasive disease was highly respected. Today diagnostic acumen is largely focused at the lower end of the spectrum of intraepithelial abnormality. Indeed, the decision to excise the TZ in the presence of cytologic and colposcopic evidence of high-grade disease is no longer always dependent on biopsy. In selected cases the TZ may reasonably be excised at the initial assessment.

The decision to treat or monitor women with the cytologic suspicion of low-grade or borderline smear reports is much more difficult and is the more common dilemma for colposcopists today. In this circumstance, especially in young women, the ability to discriminate between low-grade dysplasia and normal epithelium from high-grade disease is paramount. Furthermore, once the decision to treat has been made it is important to remove the entire TZ and only the TZ to adequately treat and to reduce the risk of unnecessary longer-term pregnancy-related morbidity. To this end several attempts to make colposcopic examination more reliable and more objective have been implemented over the last decade.[16–20] Perhaps the best of these is the Swede score, detailed in **Table 1**. The Swede score differs from previous scores in that it includes

Table 1 The Swede score			
Swede Score	**0**	**1**	**2**
Aceto uptake	Zero or transparent	Shady, milky Neither transparent nor opaque	Distinct Opaque White
Margins/surface	Diffuse	Sharp but irregular, jagged, geographic satellites	Sharp, even difference in surface level, includes cuffing
Vessels	Fine, regular	absent	Coarse or Atypical
Lesion size	<5 cm	5–15 cm or Two quadrants	>15 cm or Three to four quadrants or undefined endocervically
Iodine staining	Brown	Faintly or patchy yellow	Distinct yellow
Total score			

Data from Bowring J, Strander B, Young M, et al. The Swede score: evaluation of a scoring system designed to improve the predictive value of colposcopy. J Low Genit Tract Dis 2010;14:301–5.

lesion size, which is now known to be an important predictor of high-grade dis-ease.[21–23] The Swede score is also very simple to understand and easy to use.

Recently Tidy and colleagues[24] produced evidence that biophysical devices are able to discriminate between high- and low-grade intraepithelial lesions or normal tis-sue. This technique, which uses electrical impedance spectroscopy, may aid the col-poscopist and the patient in two ways. First, it is an objective technique and, in association with colposcopic assessment, seems to improve predictive recognition of high-grade lesions. Second, it may allow the colposcopist to avoid biopsy. If verified by further clinical research these findings should reduce rates of undertreatment and overtreatment and unnecessary biopsies.

RATIONALE

One might reasonably ask why there is a need to modify existing and accepted nomen-clature classifications. Variation in practice is inevitable given the diversity of clinical and socioeconomic conditions across the globe. So, why bother to try to standardize terminology? The most cogent arguments for trying to achieve global consensus in col-poscopy terminology is that without agreed terminology it is impossible to truly compare practice, whether it be diagnostic or therapeutic. Currently, the same term may mean different things to different clinicians. The classic example of this is the term "cone biopsy" or "conization." To most colposcopists in the United Kingdom a cone biopsy means excision of a significant portion of the endocervical canal and the term is reserved for those cervices where the lesion is thought to be out of colposcopic view in the endocervical canal, either wholly or in part. However, to many colposcopists in the United States and Europe conization means excision of any type of TZ no matter how much of the endocervical canal has been excised. Again, confused understanding of terminology of the excised specimen can get in the way of valid comparison of exci-sion techniques. The terms height and depth are used almost interchangeably in different publications and this leads to invalid comparison in the published literature.

In producing this nomenclature the IFCPC Nomenclature Committee reviewed those publications that had examined the value of colposcopic signs such that an evidential terminology might evolve. **Table 2** presents a summary of the 2012 Nomen-clature. It is divided into the following sections:

General assessment including the TZ types
Normal colposcopic findings
Abnormal colposcopic findings
Suspicious for invasion
Miscellaneous findings
Addendum: excision treatment types and excision specimen dimensions

GENERAL ASSESSMENT

A general and initial assessment of the cervix allows the colposcopist to determine whether or not examination of the cervical epithelium is adequate, whether it is compromised by inflammation, bleeding, atrophy, scar tissue, or subepithelial fibrotic change. Assessing whether or not the TZ is fully visible and where it is situated allows determination of the TZ type.

TZ AND TZ EXCISION TYPES

The classification of TZ type has not changed since that described by Walker's Nomen-clature Committee in 2003. The old term of unsatisfactory colposcopy has been

Table 2
Summary of the new Nomenclature. 2011 IFCPC Colposcopic Terminology of the Cervix

Basic definitions		SCJ visualization: complete/partial/none Adequate/inadequate for the reason... (ie, cervix obscured by inflammation, bleeding, scar)	
Normal colposcopic findings		Original squamous epithelium Columnar epithelium Including ectopy Transformation zones types 1, 2, 3	Deciduosis in pregnancy Atrophic epithelium Nabothian cyst Gland (crypt) openings
Abnormal colposcopic findings	General principles	Inside or outside the TZ Number of cervical quadrants the lesion covers Size of the lesion in percentage of cervix Lugol staining (Schiller test): stained/nonstained	
	Grade 1 (minor)	Fine acetowhite epithelium	Fine mosaic Fine punctation
	Grade 2 (major)	Dense acetowhite epithelium Sharp border Exophytic lesion Coarse mosaic Inner border sign Coarse Ridge sign punctuation Leukoplakia	Rapid appearance of acetowhitening Cuffed gland (crypt) openings
Suspicious for invasion		Atypical vessels, fragile vessels, irregular surface Necrosis, ulceration (necrotic) tumor/gross neoplasm	

Miscellaneous finding		Erosion
		(traumatic)
		Inflammation Endometriosis
		                Condyloma
		                Polyp (ectocervical/
		                endocervical)
			Stenosis
			Congenital anomaly
			Posttreatment
			consequence

Abbreviation: SCJ, squamo columnar junction.

Data from Bornstein J, Bentley J, Bösze P, et al. The 2011 Colposcopic Terminology of the International Federation for Cervical Pathology and Colposcopy. Obstet Gynecol 2012;120(1):166.

abandoned because of its relative ambiguity. The TZ type is usually the first examination finding that is documented at a competent colposcopic examination. A fully visible ectocervical TZ is a type 1 TZ, a TZ that is partially or totally endocervical but yet fully visible is a type 2 TZ, and one that is partially or completely endocervical but is not fully visible is a type 3 TZ. Whether the TZ is fully visible or not and where it is situated influences the diagnostic completion of the examination and the method of treatment. In this nomenclature excision types have been introduced. A fully visible ectocervical and small TZ is easy to assess and simple to treat either by destruction or simple excision. A large type 3 TZ, however, is not possible to completely assess colposcopically because all or part of it is situated out of colposcopic view. Treatment is associated with greater difficulty and the likelihood of long-term morbidity[2] and an increased risk of failure to eradicate the disease.[3,4] The TZ excision types are illustrated in **Figs. 4–6** and detailed in **Table 3**.

THE EXCISED SPECIMEN

Several studies have shown that the size of the excised specimen of the cervix has implications for future pregnancy outcome. Therefore, there is a need to standardize the description of the excised specimen dimensions. The committee recognized that there is a lack of consensus in the published literature concerning the terms "length,"

Type 1 Excision

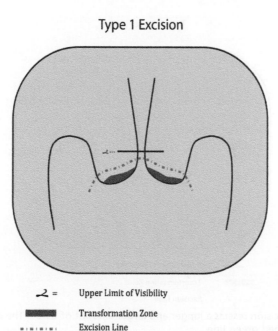

⊿ = Upper Limit of Visibility

■■■ Transformation Zone

■⋅■⋅■⋅■ Excision Line

Fig. 4. The type 1 TZ resects a completely ectocervical or type 1 TZ. The large loop excision of the TZ (LLETZ) procedure need not encroach the endocervical canal nor be greater than 8 mm thick throughout the resection. The excision margin is depicted by a dashed green line.

Type 2 Excision

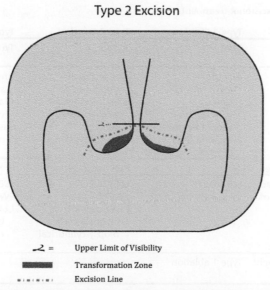

⊿ = Upper Limit of Visibility

■■■ Transformation Zone

■⋅■⋅■⋅■ Excision Line

Fig. 5. A type 2 excision resects a type 2 TZ (has an endocervical component but is fully visible). The excision margin is depicted by a dashed green line.

Type 3 Excision

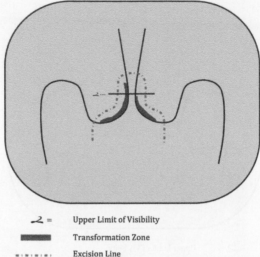

◿ =	Upper Limit of Visibility
▬	Transformation Zone
▪ ▪ ▪	Excision Line

Fig. 6. A type 3 excision resects a longer and larger amount of tissue. The excision margin is depicted by a dashed green line.

"depth," and "height" of the specimen. To clarify this, the proposed terminology advises abandoning the terms "depth" and "height" and instead proposes the terms "length" and "thickness," which are clear and more universally understood. When multiple excision specimens are obtained, as is the case with the so-called "top-hat"

Table 3
Classification of excisional treatment

Excision Type	Type 1 Excision	Type 2 Excision	Type 3 Excision
Transformation Zone type	Type 1	Type 2	Type 3
Condition	Any grade of squamous CIN, serious consideration should be given to excising CIN3 disease	Any grade of squamous CIN Glandular disease in women <36 y Suspected microinvasion	Any grade of squamous CIN Glandular disease in women >36 y Suspected microinvasion
Other circumstances		Previous treatment	Previous treatment
Techniques included in this category of excision	LLETZ/LEEP Laser excision	LLETZ/LEEP SWETZ Laser excision Cold knife cone biopsy/cylindrical excision	LLETZ/LEEP SWETZ Cold knife cone biopsy/cylindrical excision
Alternative treatment choices	Type 1 ablation		

Abbreviations: LEEP, loop electrosurgical excision procedure; LLETZ, large loop excision of the transformation zone; SWETZ, straight wire excision of the transformation zone.

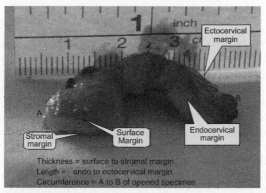

Fig. 7. Opened LLETZ specimen after removal with dimensions used to determine thickness, length, and circumference in this study.

specimen, each specimen should be measured separately. **Figs. 7** and **8** illustrate TZ excision types and the dimensions length and thickness.

The first two excision types relate exactly to the TZ types 1 and 2. A type 3 excision, however, may be used in several circumstances not dictated purely by TZ type. For example, excision of a glandular lesion usually warrants a type 3 excision. Some clinicians may wish to perform a type 3 excision in the presence of severe dysplasia or microinvasive disease where a woman has completed her family. Because of the difficulty of comprehensively assessing the TZ in a patient who has previously been treated a type 3 excision may again be considered appropriate.

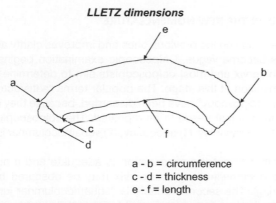

Fig. 8. Line drawing of opened LLETZ specimen after removal with dimensions used to determine thickness, length, and circumference used in this study

COLPOSCOPIC FINDINGS
Normal Colposcopic Findings

Normal epithelial variations that may be recognized at colposcopic examination of the cervix include original squamous epithelium; nabothian follicles, also known as nabothian cysts; metaplastic squamous epithelium; crypt or gland openings; and decidual changes associated with pregnancy.

Abnormal Colposcopic Findings

Where a lesion is present it may be found either proximal or distal to the original squamocolumnar junction (ie, it may be inside or outside the TZ). The lesion may be small or large and occupy from one to four quadrants of the TZ. The size of the lesion and the proportion of the TZ that it covers seem to be important predictors of lesion grade and is included as one of the indices of severity in Strander's scoring system (see **Table 1**).

Minor-grade changes include fine vascular patterns (mosaic or punctate); thin white epithelial uptake after the application of 3% or 5% acetic acid; irregular or geographic borders; and satellite lesions. Major-grade changes include sharp lesion borders; inner borders (within the TZ); the ridge sign; dense or rapid uptake of acetic acid; coarse vascular patterns (mosaic or punctate); and cuffed crypt or gland openings.

Nonspecific findings include leukoplakia (keratosis or hyperkeratosis) and erosion. Features that might raise the suspicion of invasive disease include atypical vessels, fragile vessels, an irregular epithelial surface, exophytic lesions, necrosis, ulceration, tumor formation, or gross neoplasm. Miscellaneous findings included in this classification are the congenital or original TZ, condyloma, polyps, inflammation, stenosis, congenital anomaly, posttreatment epithelial changes, and endometriosis.

Some of these terms are open to subjective interpretation. For example, it is difficult to define in words the difference between irregular or geographic margins and straight ones. However, margin status has been found to be important in predicting high-grade abnormality. Furthermore, rolled or peeling edges have also been found to be associated with high-grade lesions.[16,25] The inner border sign is a sharp demarcation between two areas of different acetowhite uptake within the same lesion.[26] The ridge sign is a relatively new sign described by Scheungraber and coworkers[27] and is a protuberance of acetowhite epithelium within the TZ. The IFCPC is currently creating an atlas of images to correlate with this terminology of colposcopic findings, which may allow easy reference and will be available on its' Web site (www.ifcpc.org) later in 2013.

INDIVIDUAL TERMS IN THE NEW NOMENCLATURE

This nomenclature builds on the previous ones and improves clarity around some terminology that has become vague. Colposcopic examination begins with a general assessment of the cervix and most colposcopists aim to determine the level of reliability of the examination at this stage. The popular terms "satisfactory colposcopy" and "unsatisfactory colposcopy" have been discarded, because they have the connotation of an examination that needs to be repeated. The colposcopic examination is now assessed by three variables: (1) adequacy, (2) squamocolumnar junction visibility, and (3) TZ type.

The first is whether or not the examination is adequate and if not why not. The reason should be documented (eg, the cervix may be obscured by inflammation, bleeding, or scarring). The second variable is "squamocolumnar junction visibility," which can be described as "completely visible," "partially visible," or "not visible." The reason that the visibility and site of the squamocolumnar junction are so important is that it influences the ability to do a satisfactory examination and, when treatment is indicated, the extent and type of excision. The terms "adequacy" and "squamocolumnar junction visibility" are not mutually exclusive; the squamocolumnar junction may be "partially visible" because a portion of its inner margin is located high in the endocervical canal, whereas the test is still "adequate" because the cervix is not obscured by blood or inflammation. The third parameter is the TZ type. It overlaps to some degree, but not completely, with the visibility of the squamocolumnar junction. The TZ and the squamocolumnar junction are not the same thing: the squamocolumnar junction is the "inner" margin of the TZ. Both types 1 and 2 TZ are "completely visible," and the difference between the two is important, mainly for planning treatment. The TZ type defines the site and visibility of the squamocolumbar junction. The localization of the lesion within or without the TZ has been reintroduced, having been omitted from the 2003 publication. This is because a lesion within the TZ zone, as opposed to one outside, has been shown to be an independent predictor of a high-grade lesion or carcinoma (odds ratio, 8.60; 95% confidence interval, 1.2–63.4).[25] Lesion size has also been shown to be an independent predictor of high-grade disease (odds ratio, 3.6; 95% confidence interval, 2.1–6.3).[21,22] The size may be quantified as (1) the number of cervical quadrants the lesion covers, (2) the size of the lesion as a percentage of the cervix, or (3) the size of the lesion as depicted by its' clock position.

This nomenclature sees the introduction of two new colposcopic image signs, the "inner border sign" and the "ridge sign," to the grade 2 (major lesions) section. Published work validated their worth as markers of high-grade CIN.[26,27] A sharp border around a lesion has also been reported as being associated with a more severe lesion. The term leukoplakia has previously been classified as a major grade finding and a miscellaneous one. In this nomenclature it is included in the nonspecific abnormal finding category. This is because it has been reported to have a 25% independent predictive value of containing high-grade or invasive neoplasia.[25] In truth leukoplakia may cover innocent or pathologic epithelium and colposcopic examination cannot determine which. Uptake of Lugol iodine has moved from the minor category of previous nomenclature to the nonspecific one because several publications have suggested relatively poor reliability of the test.[28–30] Cervical polyps have remained in the miscellaneous finding category. They may be ectocervical or endocervical in origin.

VULVOVAGINAL NOMENCLATURE

Women affected by diseases of the vulva are frequently referred for care to colposcopy clinics, especially in areas where vulvar experts are unavailable. However, for many colposcopists, examination of vulvar lesions presents an enigma. Furthermore, the terminology for vulvar disease of the International Society for the Study of Vulval Diseases (ISSVD), the guardian organization of vulvar diseases, has not, until lately, included pattern recognition terminology but was rather a classification according to disease pathophysiology.[31,32] Indeed, recently the ISSVD has prepared new ISSVD terminology[33]; however, this ISSVD terminology requires some in-depth knowledge of vulvar disease. For this reason, it does not contain a section on "basic definitions" and "normal findings." These may be redundant for expert vulvologists but essential for the novice clinician inexperienced in dealing with vulvar lesions.

In addition, the ISSVD terminology does not include a colposcopic terminology. However, many members of the IFCPC believe that although the finding of acetowhitening alone is not specific on the vulva, there is still a use for the colposcope in vulvar examination. Colposcopic examination after the application of acetic acid (vulvoscopy, anoscopy) helps to delineate the lesion and choose the biopsy site. For example, it can be used to clearly delineate cases suspected of vulvar intraepithelial neoplasia (VIN) or early stromal invasion. Also, the ISSVD terminology does not have specific terminology for anal lesions, but covers only vulvar lesions. Recently, there has been an increase in the incidence of the diagnosis of anal intraepithelial neoplasia, a precursor of anal carcinoma.[34] The high-resolution anoscopy examination, used to detect intraepithelial and invasive anal neoplasia, is basically colposcopy of the anus. For these reasons, it became apparent that vulvar terminology should be introduced into the IFCPC nomenclature. Colposcopists need a terminology of vulvar colposcopic findings.

To reach a consensus with the ISSVD, we introduced to the vulvar terminology[35] the terms of vulvar pattern recognition from the new ISSVD terminology into the "abnormal findings" section of the IFCPC nomenclature. In addition, only the last section of the IFCPC terminology describes colposcopy of the vulva and anus. The first part of the vulvar nomenclature (**Table 4**) deals with basic definitions. It describes the various structures of the vulva and anus and their composition. Although some conditions affect both skin and mucosa, many diseases are unique to the skin alone or to the mucosa alone. We further divided the skin into hairy (eg, labia majora) and nonhairy (eg, clitoris), because hairy skin harbors skin appendages, which may be involved in a variety of diseases, affecting their treatment, such as VIN. This may affect the question of excisional treatment of VIN in hair-bearing areas in contrast to CO_2 laser vaporization in non–hair-bearing areas.

The normal findings section includes micropapillomatosis; sebaceous glands (Fordyce spots); and vestibular redness. These may have been mistakenly diagnosed as genital condylomata acuminata and treated by CO_2 laser vaporization. Therefore, the IFCPC nomenclature committee considered that micropapillomatosis and Fordyce

Table 4
The 2011 IFCPC Clinical/Coloscopic Terminology of the Vulva (including the Anus)

Section	Pattern		
Basic definitions	*Various structures* Urethra, Skene duct openings, clitoris, prepuce, frenulum, pubis, labia majora, labia minora, interlabial sulki, vestibule, vestibular duct openings, Bartholin duct openings, hymen, fourchette, perineum, anus, anal squamocolumnar junction (dentate line) *Composition* Squamous epithelium, hairy/nonhairy, mucosa		
Normal findings	Micropapillomatosis, sebaceous glands (Fordyce spots), vestibular redness		
Abnormal findings	General principles: size in centimeters, location		
	Lesion type:	Lesion color:	Secondary morphology
	Macule	Skin-colored	Eczema
	Patch	Red	Lichenification
	Papule	White	Excoriation
	Plaque	Dark	Purpura
	Nodule		Scarring
	Cyst		Ulcer
	Vesicle		Erosion
	Bulla		Fissure
	Pustule		Wart
	Trauma		
	Malformation		
	Gross neoplasm, ulceration, necrosis, bleeding, exophytic lesion, hyperkeratosis With or without white, gray, red, or brown discoloration Acetowhite epithelium, punctuation, atypical vessels, surface irregularities Abnormal and squamocolumnar junction (note location about the dentate line)		

Data from Bornstein J, Sideri M, Tatti S, et al. 2011 Terminology of the Vulva of the International Federation for Cervical Pathology and Colposcopy. J Lower Genital Tract Dis 2012;16(3):292.

Table 5 Definitions of primary lesion types	
Term	**Definition**
Macule	Small (<1.5 cm) area of color change; no elevation and no substance on palpation
Patch	Large (>1.5 cm) area of color change; no elevation and no substance on palpation
Papule	Small (<1.5 cm) elevated and palpable lesion
Plaque	Large (>1.5 cm) elevated, palpable, and flat-topped lesion
Nodule	A large papule (>1.5 cm); often hemispherical or poorly marginated; may be located on the surface, within, or below the skin; nodules may be cystic or solid
Vesicle	Small (<0.5 cm) fluid-filled blister; the fluid is clear (blister: a compartmentalized, fluid-filled elevation of the skin or mucosa)
Bulla	A large (>0.5 cm) fluid-filled blister; the fluid is clear
Pustule	Pus-filled blister, the fluid is white or yellow

Data from Bornstein J, Sideri M, Tatti S, et al. 2011 Terminology of the Vulva of the International Federation for Cervical Pathology and Colposcopy. J Lower Genital Tract Dis 2012;16(3):292.

spots are normal findings. Similarly, vestibular redness alone is not a sign of dermatitis or inflammation. The remainder of the terminology table (see **Table 4**) is composed of pattern recognition nomenclature that can be made with a colposcope or a magnifying lens. After the pattern has been recognized, further evaluation and differential diagnosis may be performed.

The abnormal findings of the vulvar terminology include variables that characterize each lesion by its size, location, type, color, and secondary morphology, if present. These definitions are detailed in **Tables 5** and **6**. The miscellaneous findings may describe various traumatic insults to the vulva, such as hematoma. A biopsy should be performed whenever there is a suspicion of malignancy.

The last section of the terminology describes the abnormal colposcopic findings and contains the terms for colposcopic recognition of intraepithelial neoplasia of the vulva, perineum, perianal, and anal areas.

Table 6 2011 Terminology of the vulva of the International Federation for Cervical Pathology and Colposcopy. Definitions of secondary morphology presentation	
Term	**Definition**
Eczema	A group of inflammatory diseases that are characterized by the presence of itchy, poorly marginated red plaques with minor evidence of microvesiculation or subsequent surface disruption
Lichenification	Thickening of the tissue and increased prominence of skin markings. Scale may or may not be detectable in vulvar lichenification. Lichenification may be bright-red, dusky-red, white, or skin colored in appearance
Excoriation	Surface disruption (notably excoriations) occurring as a result of the "itch-scratch cycle"
Erosion	A shallow defect in the skin surface; absence of some, or all, of the epidermis down to the basement membrane; the dermis is intact
Fissure	A thin, linear erosion of the skin surface
Ulcer	Deeper defect; absence of the epidermis and some, or all, of the dermis

Data from Bornstein J, Sideri M, Tatti S, et al. 2011 Terminology of the Vulva of the International Federation for Cervical Pathology and Colposcopy. J Lower Genital Tract Dis 2012;16(3):292.

SUMMARY

This nomenclature builds on previous IFCPC classifications. However it introduces some new concepts: the discontinuation of the use of the term "unsatisfactory" colposcopy, bringing back the size and location of the lesion, and for the first time includes a classification of excisional treatment types. They complement the previous TZ type classification introduced in 2003. This nomenclature introduces new terms: the "inner border" and "ridge sign." It changes the weight given to patterns, such as "leukoplakia" and iodine staining. It is hoped that the current classification improves clarity in colposcopic practice and research and helps make progress toward better patient care in the future. It should at least allow more valid comparison of published clinical research data. As the microscope of critical review turns to colposcopic performance so should clinicians try to improve and objectify colposcopic image recognition and therapeutic intervention. Objective immunochemical and immunocytochemical tests may replace more subjective morphologic assessments used in the laboratory. It is incumbent on colposcopists to become as objective and clear as possible in publications and practice. The current IFCPC nomenclature may help in this ambition.

REFERENCES

1. National Health Service, Cervical Cancer Screening Programme. October 2012. Profile of cervical cancer in England: incidence, mortality and survival. Available at: www.cancerscreening.nhs.uk/cervical/. Accessed October 1, 2012.
2. Khalid S, Dimitriou E, Conroy R, et al. The thickness and volume of LLETZ specimens can predict the relative risk of pregnancy-related morbidity. BJOG 2012 May;119(6):685–91.
3. Manchanda R, Baldwin P, Crawford R, et al. Effect of margin status on cervical intraepithelial neoplasia recurrence following LLETZ in women over 50 years. BJOG 2008;115:1238–42.
4. Ghaem-Maghami S, Sagi S, Majeed G, et al. Incomplete excision of cervical intraepithelial neoplasia and risk of treatment failure: a meta-analysis. Lancet Oncol 2007;8:985–93.
5. Jeronimo J, Schiffman M. Colposcopy at crossroads. Am J Obstet Gynecol 2006; 195:349–53.
6. Pretorius RG, Peterson P, Azizi F, et al. Subsequent risk and presentation of cervical intraepithelial neoplsia (CIN) 3 or cancer after a colposcopic diagnosis of CIN 1 or less. Am J Obstet Gynecol 2006;195:1260–5.
7. Ferris DG, Litaker MS. Cervical biopsy sampling variability in ALTS. J Low Genit Tract Dis 2011;15(2):163–8.
8. Kelly RS, Walker P, Kitchener H, et al. Incidence of CIN grade 2 or worse in colposcopy-negative women with low grade cytological abnormalities. BJOG 2011;1471:20–4.
9. Cruickshank M, on behalf of the TOMBOLA study. Poster presentation, British Society for Colposcopy and Cervical Pathology. Liverpool, UK. April, 2013.
10. Stafl A. New nomenclature for colposcopy. Report of the Committee on Terminology. Obstet Gynecol 1976;48:123–4.
11. Stafl A, Wilbanks GD. An international terminology of colposcopy: report of the Nomenclature Committee of the International Federation of Cervical Pathology and Colposcopy. Obstet Gynecol 1991;77:313–4.
12. Walker PG, Dexeus S, De Palo G, et al. International terminology of colposcopy: an updated report from the International Federation for Cervical Pathology and Colposcopy. Obstet Gynecol 2003;101:175–7.

13. Bornstein J, Bentley J, Bösze P, et al. The 2011 Colposcopic Terminology of the International Federation for Cervical Pathology and Colposcopy. Obstet Gynecol 2012 Jul;120(1):166–72.
14. Prendiville W, Cullimore J, Norman S. Large loop excision of the transformation zone (LLETZ). A new method of management for women with cervical intraepithelial neoplasia. Br J Obstet Gynaecol 1989;96(9):1054–60.
15. Ferenczy A, Choukroun D, Arseneau J. Loop electrosurgical excision procedure for squamous intraepithelial lesions of the cervix: advantages and potential pitfalls. Obstet Gynecol 1996;87(3):332–7.
16. Reid R, Scalzi P. Genital warts and cervical cancer. VII. An improved colposcopic index for differentiating benign papillomaviral infections from high-grade cervical intraepithelial neoplasia. Am J Obstet Gynecol 1985;153:611–8.
17. Mousavi AS, Fakour F, Gilani MM, et al. A prospective study to evaluate the correlation between Reid colposcopic index impression and biopsy histology. J Low Genit Tract Dis 2007;11:147–50.
18. Seidl S. Reflections on the international colposcopic nomenclature. Geburtshilfe Frauenheilkd 2005;65:1028–30.
19. Bowring J, Strander B, Young M, et al. The Swede score: evaluation of a scoring system designed to improve the predictive value of colposcopy. J Low Genit Tract Dis 2010;14:301–5.
20. Strander B, Ellstrom-Andersson A, Franzen S, et al. The performance of a new scoring system for colposcopy in detecting high-grade dysplasia in the uterine cervix. Acta Obstet Gynecol Scand 2005;84:1013–7.
21. Shaw E, Sellors J, Kaczorowski J. Prospective evaluation of colposcopic features in predicting CIN: degree of acetowhite change most important. J Low Genit Tract Dis 2003;7:6–10.
22. Sideri M, Spolti N, Spinaci L, et al. Inter-observer variability of colposcopic interpretations and consistency with final histologic results. J Low Genit Tract Dis 2004;8:212–6.
23. Kierkegaard O, Byrjalsen C, Hansen KC, et al. Association between colposcopic findings and histology in cervical lesions: the significance of the size of the lesion. Gynecol Oncol 1995;57:66–71.
24. Tidy JA, Brown BH, Healey TJ, et al. Accuracy of detection of high-grade cervical intraepithelial neoplasia using electrical impedance spectroscopy with colposcopy. BJOG 2013;120(4):400–11.
25. Hammes LS, Naud P, Passos EP, et al. Value of the International Federation for Cervical Pathology and Colposcopy (IFCPC) Terminology in predicting cervical disease. J Low Genit Tract Dis 2007;11:158–65.
26. Scheungraber C, Glutig K, Fechtel B, et al. Inner border: a specific and significant colposcopic sign for moderate or severe dysplasia (cervical intra- epithelial neoplasia 2 or 3). J Low Genit Tract Dis 2009;13:1–4.
27. Scheungraber C, Koenig U, Fechtel B, et al. The colposcopic feature ridge sign is associated with the presence of cervical intraepithelial neoplasia 2/3 and human papillomavirus 16 in young women. J Low Genit Tract Dis 2009; 13:13–6.
28. Ferris DG, Litaker MS, ALTS Group. Prediction of cervical histologic results using an abbreviated Reid Colposcopic Index during ALTS. Am J Obstet Gynecol 2006;194:704–10.
29. El-Shalakany AH, Saeed MM, Abdel-Aal MR, et al. Direct visual inspection of the cervix with Lugol iodine for the detection of premalignant lesions. J Low Genit Tract Dis 2008;12:193–8.

30. Rubio CA, Thomassen P. A critical evaluation of the Schiller test in patients before conization. Am J Obstet Gynecol 1976;125:96–9.
31. Lynch PJ, Moyal-Barracco M, Bogliatto F, et al. 2006 ISSVD classification of vulvar dermatoses: pathologic subsets and their clinical correlates. J Reprod Med 2007; 52:3–9.
32. Moyal-Barracco M, Lynch PJ. 2003 ISSVD terminology and classification of vulvo-dynia: a historical perspective. J Reprod Med 2004;49:772–7.
33. Lynch PJ, Moyal-Barracco M, Scurry J, et al. 2011 ISSVD Terminology and Clas-sification of Vulvar Dermatological Disorders: an approach to clinical diagnosis. J Low Genit Tract Dis 2012;16:339–44.
34. Swedish KA, Lee EQ, Goldstone SE. The changing picture of high-grade anal in-traepithelial neoplasia in men who have sex with men: the effects of 10 years of experience performing high-resolution anoscopy. Dis Colon Rectum 2011;54: 1003–7.
35. Bornstein J, Sideri M, Tatti S, et al. Nomenclature Committee of International Federation for Cervical Pathology and Colposcopy. J Low Genit Tract Dis 2012; 16:290–5.

Cervical Cancer Prevention
New Guidelines in the United States and New Opportunities for Low- and Middle-Income Countries

Alan G. Waxman, MD, MPH

KEYWORDS

- Cervical cancer prevention • Consensus conference • Cancer prevention
- Low- and middle-income countries

KEY POINTS

- New cervical guidelines in the United States focus on reducing unnecessary testing and bringing diagnostic terminology into line with current understanding of the natural history of human papillomavirus (HPV) disease.
- Implementation of new cervical screening and management guidelines will likely decrease the number of young women requiring colposcopy.
- As colposcopists see fewer cases, and as increasing immunization decreases the impact of HPV-16, the diagnostic skills of colposcopists will be challenged.
- In resource-poor countries, newer non–cytology-based tests offer the possibility of significantly reducing the burden of cervical cancer.

The events of the past 18 months may well signal a watershed for cervical cancer screening in the United States and also in low-resource countries. The changes wrought perhaps do not compare with 2006, when the first human papillomavirus (HPV) DNA vaccine was approved, but all of us will be practicing differently as a result of recent events.

March 2012 saw the publication of the recommendations of the November 2011 Consensus Conference sponsored jointly by American Cancer Society (ACS), the American Society for Colposcopy and Cervical Pathology (ASCCP), and the American Society for Clinical Pathology (ASCP).[1] These professional organizations for the first time recommended the use of cotesting, that is, screening with cytology and HPV testing, as preferable to screening with cytology alone in women aged 30 to 65 years. The US Preventive Services Task Force, in a coordinated release of publications, also

Department of Obstetrics and Gynecology, University of New Mexico School of Medicine, MSC 10 5580, 1 University of New Mexico, Albuquerque, NM 87131-0001, USA
E-mail address: awaxman@salud.unm.edu

Obstet Gynecol Clin N Am 40 (2013) 251–255
http://dx.doi.org/10.1016/j.ogc.2013.03.006
0889-8545/13/$ – see front matter © 2013 Elsevier Inc. All rights reserved.

recommended cotesting, but gave it equal weight to cytology.[2] Several months later the American College of Obstetricians and Gynecologists (ACOG), in its updated Practice Bulletin on cervical cancer screening, endorsed the ACS/ASCCP/ASCP recommendations.[3] Based on European and American studies, these professional organizations recommended screening intervals of 3 years for those women screened with cytology alone and 5 years when cotesting is used. Metaphorically speaking, this is the last nail in the coffin of the annual Papanicolaou (Pap) test. ACOG, while recognizing that annual cervical cytology screening in the United States population has the potential to lead to more harms than benefits, has reminded its members of the potential benefits of routine gynecologic visits independent of the Pap test.[4]

Also in March the ASCCP, in collaboration with the College of American Pathologists (CAP), convened the Lower Anogenital Squamous Terminology (LAST) Standardization Project consensus conference. Its purpose was to harmonize the nomenclature of HPV-associated squamous intraepithelial lesions across multiple tissues of the lower anogenital tract. Their recommendations were published in July 2012.[5] These recommendations will not have as much direct impact on clinicians as the new screening guidelines, but they will change the way biopsies of squamous tissues of the cervix, vulva, vagina, perianus, penis, and anus are interpreted and reported. These guidelines move from the accustomed 3-tiered nomenclature, intraepithelial neoplasia (-IN) grades 1, 2, and 3, to a 2-tiered terminology of low-grade or high-grade squamous intraepithelial lesion (LSIL, HSIL), similar to cytology. It has long been recognized that CIN 2 is a poorly reproducible diagnosis. The LAST guidelines recommend the use of the immunostain p16 to increase the reliability of determining which should be called LSIL and which HSIL. This recommendation has been controversial, especially as it relates to the potential for overuse of p16 and its impact on the management of young women with HSIL on biopsy.[6] Although there are no long-term studies evaluating the natural history of lesions that are morphologically called CIN 2, but are p16 negative, classification of equivocal high-grade lesions based on p16 staining has been shown to correlate well with interpretation on adjudicated histology review.[7] The LAST nomenclature will necessitate greater clinical skill in managing young women with HSIL on biopsy. The ASCCP Consensus Guidelines since 2006 have allowed for conservative management of CIN 2 and CIN 3, but have recommended treatment at a diagnostic threshold of CIN 3.[8] In the case of a diagnosis of HSIL not otherwise specified, young women can still be managed conservatively with semi-annual cytology and colposcopy, so long as the transformation zone remains fully visualized, and the lesion is not large with widespread HSIL or becomes clinically more severe in appearance during the observation period.[6]

The first ASCCP Consensus Conference on the management of women with abnormal cytology and histology took place in 2001. Its recommendations[9] were updated in 2006 based on studies published in the intervening years.[8,10] In September 2012, relying largely on data from the extensive Kaiser Permanente of Northern California (KPNC) database, the management guidelines were again updated.[11] These new recommendations built on the previous ASCCP guidelines, but recognized that cervical cancer screening results will now include the outcomes of HPV tests for most women aged 30 years and older. The KPNC group has used cotesting and has maintained its database of outcomes since 2003.[11]

Primary prevention of HPV-related cancers is being adopted in many countries around the world. Australia and Great Britain, for example, have incorporated HPV vaccines in national immunization programs, and report that greater than 72% and 84% of 12- to 13-year-old girls, respectively, have received all 3 doses of vaccine. Mexico and Rwanda have also recently started a national HPV immunization program.

By contrast, in the United States only 32% of 13- to 17-year-olds had been adequately immunized as of 2010.[12]

More widespread immunization against HPV and the new screening and management guidelines will have a profound impact on the practice of colposcopy. With the recommendations to no longer screen women younger than 21 years and to only selectively use colposcopy to examine those younger than 25 with atypical squamous cells of undetermined significance or LSIL on cytology, the number of colposcopies performed in America will decline. With a decline in disease associated with HPV types 16 and 18, the high-risk types covered by the vaccines, the pool of women needing colposcopy will shrink further. One result of immunization is that colposcopists will see fewer high-grade lesions. Clinical trials of the bivalent vaccine showed a 59% reduction in HSIL cytology in those young women, aged 15 to 25 years, who had been vaccinated before exposure to HPV-16 or HPV-18, and a 30% reduction in the total vaccine cohort of the same ages.[13] Furthermore, HPV-16 appears to present the colposcopist with more easily recognized lesions and is diagnosed earlier than lesions caused by other HPV types.[14,15] These factors will lead to fewer colposcopies being indicated, fewer high-grade lesions, and greater difficulty recognizing those high-grade lesions that present. As the number of true high-grade lesions decreases, we can expect to see an increase in false-positive colposcopy examinations with negative or LSIL biopsies. This change will pose the great challenge to colposcopists to hone their skills and also to be more liberal in taking biopsies of suspicious areas.

In the industrialized world, the age-old threat of cervical cancer is being reduced through immunization and new efficient regimens of screening. In low- and middle-resource countries it is still a challenge to provide any form of prevention of cervical cancer. Whereas cervical cancer has been reduced to a rarity in much of Europe and North America, it remains a common cancer and one of the greatest causes of death by cancer in women in much of the developing world,[16] largely due to the lack of prevention programs. In many of these countries, recent screening projects have emerged that do not rely on the inefficient 3-visit model of cytology, colposcopy, and treatment. A single-visit "see-and-treat" model using visual inspection with dilute acetic acid (VIA) has been in use in parts of Asia, Latin America, and Sub-Saharan Africa for much of the past decade. The cervix is washed with 5% acetic acid (table vinegar) and inspected, generally without magnification, often by a nurse or trained community health worker. Treatment with cryotherapy is often used at the same visit if a distinct acetowhite lesion is seen. This low-tech methodology has sensitivity comparable with or better than that of the Pap test, although its specificity is lower[17,18]; this results in the inherent overtreatment of many women and undertreatment of a few.

An increasing body of literature has shown the high sensitivity and negative predictive values of screening with HPV testing alone in comparison with cytology and VIA.[19,20] A large Indian study[21] showed that a population of women screened just once with an HPV test had a lower cervical cancer mortality and a lower incidence of advanced-stage invasive disease compared with women undergoing a single cytology or VIA. In the past year a low-cost, rapid-result (2 hours) HPV test has become available in some low-resource countries. As described in article elsewhere in this issue by Castle and Cremer, HPV testing has the potential to reduce the incidence and mortality from cervical cancer if a cytology-based program is not feasible. As in so many other areas of public health, the difference in focus between rich and resource-poor countries is stark.

There have indeed been significant developments in the prevention of cervical cancer over recent months. In low- and middle-income countries, there is now increased potential for primary prevention with immunization, and relatively sensitive and specific secondary prevention with HPV testing. In the United States and much of Europe, the recommendation for increased use of HPV testing in the screening, post-colposcopy, and postmanagement process will help increase the early diagnosis of cervical precancer and adenocarcinoma in situ in comparison with cytology alone. On the other hand, the decline in the number of young women needing colposcopy and the ultimate elimination of 3-tiered CIN nomenclature will challenge us to be better colposcopists.

REFERENCES

1. Saslow D, Solomon D, Lawson HW, et al. American Cancer Society, American Society for Colposcopy and Cervical Pathology, and American Society for Clinical Pathology screening guidelines for the prevention and early detection of cervical cancer. J Low Genit Tract Dis 2012;16(3):175–204.
2. Moyer VA, U.S. Preventive Services Task Force. Screening for cervical cancer: U.S. Preventive Services Task Force recommendation statement. Ann Intern Med 2012;156:880–91.
3. Committee on Practice Bulletins–Gynecology. ACOG practice bulletin 131: screening for cervical cancer. Obstet Gynecol 2012;120(5):1222–38.
4. Chelmow D, Waxman A, Cain JM, et al. The evolution of cervical screening and the specialty of obstetrics and gynecology. Obstet Gynecol 2012;119:695–9.
5. Darragh TM, Colgan T, Cox JT, et al. The Lower Anogenital Squamous Terminology Standardization Project for HPV-Associated Lesions: background and consensus recommendations from the College of American Pathologists and the American Society for Colposcopy and Cervical Pathology. J Low Genit Tract Dis 2012;16: 205–42.
6. Waxman AG, Chelmow D, Darragh TM, et al. Revised terminology for cervical his-topathology and its implications for management of high-grade squamous intra-epithelial lesions of the cervix. Obstet Gynecol 2012;120:1465–71.
7. Bergeron C, Ordi J, Schmidt D, et al, European CINtec Histology Study Group. Conjunctive p16INK4a testing significantly increases accuracy in diagnosing high-grade cervical intraepithelial neoplasia. Am J Clin Pathol 2010;133:395–406.
8. Wright TC Jr, Massad LS, Dunton CJ, et al. 2006 consensus guidelines for the management of women with cervical intraepithelial neoplasia or adenocarcinoma in situ. J Low Genit Tract Dis 2007;11:223–39.
9. Wright TC Jr, Cox JT, Massad LS, et al. 2001 Consensus Guidelines for the management of women with cervical cytological abnormalities. JAMA 2002; 287(16):2120–9.
10. Wright TC Jr, Massad L, Dunton CJ, et al. 2006 consensus guidelines for the management of women with abnormal cervical screening tests. J Low Genit Tract Dis 2007;11(4):201–22.
11. Massad LS, Einstein MH, Huh WK, et al. 2012 Updated consensus guidelines for the management of abnormal cervical cancer screening tests and cancer precur-sors. J Low Genit Tract Dis 2013;17(5):S1–27.
12. Wheeler CM. Less is More: a step in the right direction for human papillomavirus (HPV) vaccine implementation. J Natl Cancer Inst 2011;103(19):1424–5.
13. Lehtinen M, Paavonen J, Wheeler CM, et al. Overall efficacy of HPV-16/18 AS04-adjuvanted vaccine against grade 3 or greater cervical intraepithelial neoplasia: 4-year end-of-study analysis of the randomised, double-blind PATRICIA trial. Lan-cet Oncol 2012;13(1):89–99.

14. Jeronimo J, Massad S, Castle P, et al, National Institutes of Health (NIH)–American Society for Colposcopy and Cervical Pathology (ASCCP) Research Group. Inter-observer agreement in the evaluation of digitized cervical images. Obstet Gynecol 2007;110:833–40.
15. Safaeian M, Schiffman M, Gage J, et al. Detection of precancerous cervical lesions is differential by human papillomavirus type. Cancer Res 2009;69(8): 3262–6.
16. Ferlay J, Shin HR, Bray F, et al. GLOBOCAN 2008 v2.0, cancer incidence and mortality worldwide: IARC CancerBase No. 10 [Internet]. Lyon (France): International Agency for Research on Cancer; 2010. Available at: http://globocan.iarc.fr. Accessed January 25, 2013.
17. Sritipsukho P, Thaweekul Y. Accuracy of visual inspection with acetic acid (VIA) for cervical cancer screening: a systematic review. J Med Assoc Thai 2010; 93(Suppl 7):S254–61.
18. Sauvaget C, Fayette JM, Muwonge R, et al. Accuracy of visual inspection with acetic acid for cervical cancer screening. Int J Gynaecol Obstet 2011;113(1): 14–24.
19. Denny L, Kuhn L, Hu CC, et al. Human papillomavirus-based cervical cancer prevention: long-term results of a randomized screening trial. J Natl Cancer Inst 2010;102:1557–67.
20. Mayrand MH, Duarte-Franco E, Rodrigues I, et al. Human papillomavirus DNA versus Papanicolaou screening tests for cervical cancer. N Engl J Med 2007; 357(16):1579–88.
21. Sankaranarayanan R, Nene BM, Shastri SS, et al. HPV screening for cervical cancer in rural India. N Engl J Med 2009;360(14):1385–94.

Screening Adolescents and Young Women

Lori A. Boardman, MD, ScM[a],*, Katina Robison, MD[b]

KEYWORDS

- Cervical cancer screening • Adolescents • Young women • Abnormal cytology
- HPV testing • HPV vaccination

KEY POINTS

- Cervical cancer screening should begin at age 21 years regardless of a young woman's risk factors for human papillomavirus (HPV) acquisition.
- For young women between the ages of 21 and 29 years with normal cytology, screening should be repeated after no sooner than 3 years. Cervical cytology alone should be used for screening in this population.
- The addition of HPV testing to routine cervical cancer screening is not indicated in women aged 21 to 29 years because of the high prevalence of high-risk HPV infection in this population.
- The impact of HPV vaccination in real-world settings is under way in the United States, vaccination status does not change screening guidelines.

INTRODUCTION

In 2009 and again in 2012, recommendations changed for both the age at which to begin cervical cancer screening and the optimal screening intervals for young women.[1–5] In late 2012, the 2006 American Society for Colposcopy and Cervical Pathology (ASCCP) Consensus Guidelines were also revised and recommendations regarding the management of abnormal cervical cytology and histology in young women, and particularly for those in their early 20s, have been recently published.[6] The impetus for these changes included data showing an exceedingly low risk of

Funding Sources: None (L.A. Boardman); Brown/Women and Infants' Women's Reproductive Health Research Career Development Program (K. Robison).
Conflict of Interest: None.
[a] Departments of Clinical Sciences and Medical Education, Health Sciences Campus at Lake Nona, University of Central Florida College of Medicine, 6850 Lake Nona Boulevard, Orlando, FL 32827, USA; [b] The Program in Women's Oncology, Women and Infants' Hospital of Rhode Island, The Warren Alpert Medical School of Brown University, 101 Dudley Street, Providence, RI 02905, USA
* Corresponding author.
E-mail address: Lori.Boardman@ucf.edu

Obstet Gynecol Clin N Am 40 (2013) 257–268
http://dx.doi.org/10.1016/j.ogc.2013.02.007
0889-8545/13/$ – see front matter © 2013 Elsevier Inc. All rights reserved.

cervical cancer in these populations,[7] evidence that screening is less effective in women younger than 25 years, as well as the potential for increased risk of harm, including not only anxiety but adverse pregnancy outcomes for those young women undergoing excisional procedures.[8,9]

Adolescents, defined as women aged 20 years and younger, represent a unique population of patients. Incident oncogenic human papillomavirus (HPV) infection and mild cytologic abnormalities are commonly seen in this age group. Rates of sexually transmitted infections (STIs), including HPV, are highest in younger women. In a recent meta-analysis of women with normal cytology, 23% of those younger than 25 years compared with 9% of those aged 25 to 34 years and less than 5% of those aged 35 years and older were found to be HPV positive.[10] Although acquisition of HPV is often associated with risk factors such as a higher number of new sexual partners and younger age at first intercourse, young age remains a significant risk even after adjustment for other known behavioral factors. The biological vulnerability of young women to HPV and other STIs has often been attributed to the extent of cervical ectopy in younger women. However, recent prospective data showed that the key factor involved in HPV 16 acquisition and the development of a clinical cervical lesion was not amount of ectopy, but rather the rate of observed metaplastic change.[11]

Although at risk to develop high-grade disease, many adolescents experience regression of both cytologic and histologic disease. Despite the high incidence of HPV infection among newly sexually active women, such infections in adolescents and young women are often transient. In numerous studies, approximately 50% of HPV infections in young women persist in the short-term, but fewer than 10% remain at 24 months.[12–15]

HPV-related low-grade cytologic abnormalities, in particular, are frequently detected in sexually active adolescents.[16] For example, in a cohort of 1075 sexually active teens between 15 and 19 years of age with normal cytology and negative HPV tests at recruitment, 407 (38%) became HPV positive over the 3-year study period, and 246 (23%) developed abnormal cervical cytology.[17] Similar rates of incident HPV infection were documented in a longitudinal cohort study of more than 500 college-aged women in Washington State.[18] The 36-month cumulative incidence of squamous intraepithelial lesions in this population was 47%. Of the 112 women who developed incident low-grade squamous intraepithelial lesions (LSIL), 96 (87%) became cytologically normal while enrolled in the study.[19] Moscicki and colleagues[20] similarly reported high rates of resolution of LSIL among teens and young women, with regression rates more than 60% at 12 months of follow-up and 91% at 36 months.

Regression has also been noted in young women with high-grade squamous intraepithelial lesions (HSIL), as well as biopsy-proven cervical intraepithelial neoplasia 2 (CIN2). Over a median follow-up period of 18 months, Moore and colleagues[21] found regression in 65% of a cohort of young women aged 20 years and younger with CIN2. In another retrospective study of expectantly managed adolescents and young women (aged 21 years and younger) with CIN2, Fuchs and colleagues[22] reported that 50% of CIN2 lesions regressed within 2 years and 75% regressed within 3 years. Progression to CIN3 occurred in 8% of this cohort. Moscicki and colleagues[23] documented similar rates of regression of CIN2 (68% by 3 years) among a cohort of 95 adolescents and women aged 13 to 24 years. In none of the above studies was invasive cancer detected.

Similar to adolescents, women in their early 20s commonly present with mild cytologic abnormalities, the optimal management of which has remained unclear. Data in adolescent populations have clearly shown that cervical cancer is rare, and rates of high-grade neoplasia in teens and in young women younger than 25 years with atypical squamous cells of undetermined significance (ASC-US) and LSIL seem to be lower than rates found in adult populations.[24,25] Women in their late 20s, on the other hand, have been found to have significantly higher rates of CIN2+ compared with their younger counterparts, and thus immediate colposcopy remains the standard of care for this population. For these reasons, recommendations for conservative management of mildly abnormal cervical cytology and histology (including CIN2) in women in their early 20s have recently been made.[6]

SCREENING OF WOMEN AGED 20 YEARS AND YOUNGER
Recommendation

Cervical cancer screening should begin at age 21 years. Factors such as age of sexual initiation or number of sexual partners should not be used to initiate screening before age 21 years.[3–5] This recommendation does not apply to HIV-seropositive young women, women with known immunocompromise, or young women previously treated for CIN2, CIN3, or cancer.

In the Past

Over the past 2 decades, guidelines have steadily moved away from screening young women younger than 21 years. In 2002, the American Cancer Society (ACS) recommended initiating cervical cancer screening at age 21 years or at 3 years after sexual debut (whichever came first).[26] However, this recommendation was difficult to follow and raised concern about doing harm with little evidence of benefit. Beginning in the late 2000s, multiple organizations, including the American College of Obstetricians and Gynecologists (ACOG)[1] and ASCCP,[2] moved to the recommendation to begin screening at age 21 years regardless of a patient's past sexual or behavioral history. This recommendation was recently reaffirmed in guidelines published by the United States Preventive Services Task Force (USPSTF), the ACS/ASCCP/American Society for Clinical Pathology (ASCP) and ACOG.[3–5]

Rationale and Evidence

A low incidence of cervical cancer and a lack of data showing the effectiveness of screening in young women support the most recent recommendations to initiate screening at age 21 years. In the developed world, cervical cancer is not common, and it is even rarer in younger women. Based on combined data from the National Program of Cancer Registries and the SEER (Surveillance Epidemiology and End Results) program, Benard and colleagues[7] documented an average of 3063 cases of invasive cervical carcinomas annually from 1999 to 2008, with an average of 14 carcinomas per year among those aged 15 to 19 years and 125 cases among those aged 20 to 24 years. The rate of cervical cancer in 15-year-olds to 19-year-olds (approximately 0.1 per 100,000) has remained unchanged from that reported nearly 40 years ago (1973–1977).[7,27]

As with teens, screening in younger women has not been shown to reduce the rate of cervical cancer. For example, in a population-based case-control study in the United Kingdom, investigators found that cervical screening in women aged 20 to 24 years had no detectable impact on rates of cervical cancer at ages 25 to 29 years.[28] Reasons for why screening seems to be ineffective in young women include the presence of cancers in this age group that are less detectable by current screening methods or are more aggressive and therefore more likely to arise during screening intervals.[29] In the analysis by Benard and colleagues[7] discussed earlier, more noncarcinomas were detected among the youngest age groups. These noncarcinomas were often childhood cancers (eg, embryonal rhabdomyosarcoma), which would not have been detected through cervical cancer screening.

Recommendation

Because some younger women will continue to be screened, it is reasonable to follow the 2006 Consensus Guidelines for the management of adolescents with abnormal cervical screening tests.

Rationale and Evidence

Although providers often continue to screen and treat younger women,[30,31] recent evidence from the Behavioral Risk Factor Surveillance System (BRFSS) does point to both less frequent screening initiation and screening frequency in women younger than 21 years. In 2010, 52.5% of young women aged 18 to 21 years reported having been screened (compared with 73.7% in 2000), and 41.5% reported having had a Papanicolaou (Pap) test in the past 12 months (compared with 65% in 2000). Early adoption of the 2009 cervical cancer screening guidelines or increased awareness of the potential harms of screening were likely associated with these observed changes in screening behaviors.[32]

Although this evidence is reassuring, more than 25% of women younger than 21 years in the BRFSS were still screened in 2010. The consequences of both screening and treating adolescents include not only the emotional effect of telling a teen that she has both an STI and a potential precancer and the anxiety associated with colposcopy but also the potential risk of preterm delivery should she be overtreated.[5] Evidence that excisional therapy poses long-term obstetric risks is particularly salient in adolescents, many of whom have not yet begun or completed childbearing. Cervical conization, including loop electrosurgical excision procedures (LEEP), has been shown to increase the risk of pregnancy complications such as preterm premature rupture of the membranes[33] and preterm delivery.[34] Treatment with LEEP has been estimated to result in an approximately 2-fold to 3-fold increased risk of preterm birth.[34,35] Increasing cone depth as well as multiple procedures have both been shown in several studies to be associated with a further increase in the risk of preterm delivery.[8,36]

On the other hand, in a recent population-based record linkage study of nearly 175,000 Welsh women, Reilly and colleagues[37] found that women referred for colposcopy had an increased and similar risk of preterm delivery whether or not they received excisional therapy compared with women with negative cytology. Ablative therapy, often suggested as an alternative to excisional procedures in young or nulliparous women, has also recently been found to be associated with an increase in preterm delivery rates, although the magnitude of this effect was less pronounced.[9] Although avoiding unnecessary excision or ablation is advisable in young women, the long-accepted association between LEEP and adverse pregnancy outcomes continues to be challenged.

To reduce the risk of such complications, several special populations were identified, including adolescent women (defined as those aged 20 years and younger) in the 2006 Consensus Guidelines. Given the high rates of HPV infection and concomitant mild cytologic abnormalities in young women that are highly likely to regress, immediate colposcopy was discouraged. For young women with ASC-US or LSIL, repeat cytology in 12 months is recommended. If repeat cytology test at that time reveals HSIL or greater, colposcopy is indicated. If repeat cytology is ASC-US or LSIL, cytology should be repeated again in 12 months, and any cytologic abnormality at the second visit should prompt colposcopic evaluation.[38]

In 2006, HPV DNA testing was found to be unacceptable for adolescents with ASC-US (again based on reports of a high prevalence of HPV among adolescents with this cytologic diagnosis[39]) and if inadvertently performed was not to be used in management decisions. Immediate colposcopic examination continues to be advised for all women, including adolescents, with atypical squamous cells, cannot exclude HSIL (ASC-H), HSIL, and atypical glandular cells on cervical cytologic testing.[38]

SCREENING OF 21-YEAR-OLD TO 29-YEAR-OLD WOMEN
Recommendation

Screening with cytology (either conventional or liquid based) alone should be performed every 3 years. This recommendation does not apply to human immunodeficiency virus–seropositive young women, immunocompromised women, or women previously treated for CIN2, CIN3, or cancer.[3–5]

In the Past

Screening was previously recommended annually for women in this age group.[1]

Rationale and Evidence

Few studies specifically address the optimal screening interval for women aged 21 to 29 years. Data from several modeling studies have assessed the impact of different screening regimens and intervals in this age group. Although the likelihood of high-grade cervical neoplasia increases with age, most women have neither CIN2 nor CIN3 at the time of screening. More than 95% of referrals to colposcopy are either false positive (no lesion detected) or potentially excessive (CIN1 only). For example, among a cohort of 1000 20-year-old women screened for a 10-year period with cytology and triage HPV testing for ASC-US, screening every 5 years, compared with annually or every 3 years, resulted in the fewest number of excessive colposcopies (defined as CIN1 or less) but at the cost of missing 2 of 7 expected cases of high-grade neoplasia. Screening annually compared with every 3 years confers no additional benefit (both result in detection of 7 cases of CIN2 or CIN3), but results in 396 compared with 180 excessive referrals to colposcopy, respectively.[40]

Kulasingam and colleagues[41] looked specifically at cervical cancer screening performed annually, every 2 years, and every 3 years and found little additional benefit between the 2-year and 3-year screening regimens. The trade-off between a negligibly increased risk of cancer (37 cases per 100,000 screened vs 39 cases per 100,000) and unnecessary colposcopies (176 vs 134 procedures per 100,000 women) favored the 3-year screening recommendation. Based on such results, screening women aged 21 to 29 years with cervical cytology every 3 years provided the best balance between the benefits and harms of screening.

Recommendation

HPV testing, either in the setting of cotesting or as a stand-alone test, should not be performed in women younger than 30 years.[3–5]

Rationale and Evidence

As with younger women, the high prevalence of HPV in women aged 21 to 29 years precludes the addition of HPV testing to primary screening with cervical cytology or the use of HPV testing as a primary screening test alone. For example, analysis of the 2003 to 2006 National Health and Nutrition Examination Surveys indicated that HPV infection, both overall and with types 6, 11, 16, and 18, is highest among young women aged 20 to 24 years.[42,43] Detecting largely transient HPV infection in this population would result in marked increases in referral to colposcopy with no benefit in the detection of high-grade cervical disease. For instance, Stout and colleagues[40] assessed the impact of screening 20-year-old women over the course of 10 years. Comparing screening with cytology and HPV triage testing for ASC-US to cotesting with cytology and HPV testing would result in a 5-fold increase in the number of excessive referrals to colposcopy, with no change in the detection of CIN2 or CIN3.

Recommendation

For women with unsatisfactory Pap tests, early repeat cytology at 2 to 4 months is recommended. If repeat cytology is again unsatisfactory, colposcopy is indicated.[6]

Rationale and Evidence

Because most women are now screened with liquid-based cytology, unsatisfactory tests are largely a result of obscuring factors, scant cellularity, and technical problems. In a recent study of 226 unsatisfactory tests, the presence of lubricant (96 cases) and blood (64 cases) was most commonly encountered. Cases affected by blood or technical problems showed significant improvement after reprocessing (56% and 91%, respectively), whereas only 17% of those affected by lubricant improved after reprocessing.[44]

However, studies performed in clinical practice have not consistently confirmed an increased rate of unsatisfactory tests among conventional cytologic samples when water-soluble lubricants have been used.[45] In a randomized trial of a small amount (3 mL) of lubricating gel compared with water used to cover both speculum blades, use of the gel resulted in significantly lower pain scores with speculum insertion and digital examination and did not affect the interpretability of liquid-based cytologic specimens.[46]

Among adolescents and young women, barriers to cervical screening include most commonly pain or discomfort with speculum insertion, along with embarrassment, fear, poor rapport with the provider, and the advice of their peers.[47] For those adolescents inadvertently screened and who now require a speculum examination, application of a small amount of water-soluble lubricating gel to the exterior bills of the speculum should have little to no impact on the interpretability of cervical cytology. Although water is often used to make speculum insertion more comfortable, evidence shows that gel is superior in this regard.

To ensure adequate collection of cells, all women should be cautioned to avoid intercourse, tampons, intravaginal medication, and douching for at minimum 48 hours before screening. If using the combination of spatula and brush, use of the spatula first minimizes bleeding. In general, avoidance of specimen collection during menses is advised, although women with irregular bleeding should be sampled, because these symptoms could indicate a more concerning lesion.[6]

Recommendation

For women aged 21 to 29 years with cytology reported as negative for intraepithelial lesion or malignancy (NILM) but with absent or insufficient endocervical cells or transformation zone (EC/TZ) component, routine screening with repeat cytology in 3 years is indicated. HPV testing in this age group is unacceptable.[6]

Rationale and Evidence

Although interpretable, these cytologic samples lacking in metaplastic cells indicate inadequate sampling of the squamocolumnar junction (SCJ). This situation in turn increases concern for missed cancers that often arise at or above the SCJ and may have led to previous recommendations for early repeat cytology.[48] However, More recent data demonstrate that women missing these components are not at higher risk for CIN3+.[49]

HPV VACCINATION
Recommendation

Recommended screening practices should not change based on HPV vaccination status.[3–5]

Rationale and Evidence

Despite recommendations in 2006 to vaccinate girls aged 11 to 12 years (as young as 9 years, with catch-up vaccination of those aged 13–26 years), and in 2011 to vaccinate young boys and men aged 11 to 12 years (with catch-up for those aged 13–21 years), vaccination rates remain low in the United. States compared with other developed nations.[50] Many factors play a role in ensuring high participation in vaccination, cost and acceptability being primary. In the United States, the Vaccines for Children Program supplies private and public health care providers with federally purchased vaccines for use among children aged 18 years and younger. Despite availability, coverage with at least 1 dose of HPV vaccine among 13-year-old to 17-year-old girls has increased slowly, from 25% in 2007 to only 53% in 2011. Vaccination with all 3 doses increased to 35% from 32% in 2010. Geographic disparities in HPV vaccine rates, with the lowest rates seen in the southeastern United States, where cancer rates are higher, continue to exist, as do even lower vaccination rates among the target population of 11-year-olds to 12-year-olds. Vaccination with all 3 doses of vaccine occurred in 16% of eligible adolescents in Arkansas and was highest in Rhode Island, where 57% of eligible girls were fully vaccinated.[50] Acceptability of the vaccines remains problematic as well. Data from the 2008 and 2009 National Immunization Survey-Teen, for example, revealed that one-third of parents of unvaccinated girls did not intend to have their daughters vaccinated, a decision driven by lack of knowledge about the disease risks and benefits of the HPV vaccine as well as failure of providers to recommend vaccination.[51]

HPV vaccine trial data (both with the quadrivalent vaccine approved by the US Food and Drug Administration in 2006 and the bivalent vaccine approved in 2009) have consistently shown that rates of subsequent vaccine-type HPV infection, as well as related CIN2+, are markedly reduced in per-protocol populations as well as intention-to-treat populations.[52,53] Both vaccines target oncogenic HPV 16 and 18, and the quadrivalent is also directed against 2 nononcogenic types, HPV 6 and 11. Data continue to emerge showing the long-term impact of vaccination on CIN3 and cervical cancer as well as genital warts (quadrivalent vaccine only). In a linkage study of 18-year-old to 19-year-old Finns vaccinated in a multinational phase 3 HPV 6/11/16/18 vaccine (Females United to Unilaterally Reduce Endo/Ectocervical Disease II) trial and the Finnish Cancer Registry, Rana and colleagues[54] reported a CIN3 incidence rate of 0/100,000 among vaccinated women after 4 years of passive follow-up. In both the placebo and unvaccinated groups, the corresponding rates were 87.1/100,000 and 93.8/100,000, respectively. In Australia, where vaccination rates exceed 80%, dramatic declines in the number of young women and men presenting with genital warts occurred within 4 years of beginning a program of free quadrivalent vaccines to adolescent girls.[55]

Recent modeling data have shown that vaccinating 12-year-old girls with the bivalent or quadrivalent vaccine is predicted to reduce the cumulative incidence of CIN2 and CIN3 by 51% for the bivalent vaccine and 46% for the quadrivalent.[56] However, to achieve significant reductions, at least 80% of sexually naive females need to be vaccinated,[57] and it will likely take decades to recognize the effect of vaccination.[58] Continuation of cervical cancer screening remains critical. However, understanding the impact of vaccination on cervical cytology is equally important in determining future guidelines for screening.[59]

Current recommendations for screening young women include almost exclusively cervical cytology, with little role played by HPV testing except in the triage of ASC-US. However, cytology has several limitations, including a low sensitivity (51% in a systematic review by Nanda and colleagues[60]) as well as a lower specificity for high-grade disease than low-grade, leading potentially to overtreatment.[60,61] Such limitations are predicted to increase with the implementation of HPV vaccination. As vaccination rates increase, the prevalence of cytologic abnormalities will decrease, thus limiting the effectiveness of cytology as a screening tool. For example, estimates indicate that widespread vaccination would result in a reduction from the current 50% to 70% positive predictive value to approximately 10% to 20%. Interobserver variability in cytologic interpretation will also increase, leading to more false-negative diagnoses and further reductions in the sensitivity of cytology.[62]

As regards the impact of HPV vaccination on screening algorithms in younger women (including potentially increasing the age at which to initiate screening), considerable uncertainty remains as to changing current recommendations. More data are needed regarding the effect of vaccination on the development of non-HPV 16/18 lesions (ie, type replacement), the timing and impact of vaccination relative to sexual initiation, and adherence to screening guidelines after vaccination, as well as duration of immunity. It has been difficult in the United States to evaluate the impact of vaccination because of the lack of a national HPV vaccine registry. Linkage of a vaccination registry with screening and HPV testing databases would allow for comparison of HPV types, screening behaviors, and histologic outcomes between vaccinated and unvaccinated populations.[63] Surveillance mechanisms have been established by both the US Centers for Disease Control and Prevention in sentinel sites (HPV-IMPACT including sites in California, Connecticut, New York, Oregon, and Tennessee)[64] and in New Mexico[65] and will allow for linkage of vaccination histories to screening practices and clinical outcomes. Clinical trials of a nonavalent vaccine (addition of HPV 31/33/45/52/58) as well as immunogenic studies of L2-based vaccines (which would confer broader protection) are under way, and, if successful, may further decrease the risk for CIN2/3 lesions and affect screening decisions.[66,67]

SUMMARY

Recent guidelines from multiple organizations, including the USPSTF, ACS/ASCCP/ASCP, ACOG, and most recently the 2013 Update to the 2006 ASCCP Consensus Guidelines, all stress screening initiation no sooner than the age of 21 years and conservative management of both cytologic and histologic abnormalities in young women. Adherence to these guidelines should help to not only decrease the number of unnecessary diagnostic procedures in this specific population of women but also to reduce the anxiety associated with repeat screening and colposcopy and the long-term obstetric risks of excisional or ablative therapy and help prevent the potential negative impact on future screening behaviors.

Primary prevention with HPV vaccination has the potential to significantly affect the development of high-grade cervical lesions, including cancer. In the United States, linkage studies are under way to assess the impact and timing of vaccination with clinical outcomes in young women, findings that will help tailor future changes to current guidelines for screening and management of abnormal cervical testing in women. Expanded coverage with a nonavalent vaccine is likely, and will result in the need for continued evaluation before consideration of its impact on screening strategies. The use of cervical cytology as a primary screening tool in younger women remains unchanged, and it is important for providers to convey adherence to this recommendation to their patients. With screening starting at the age of 21 years, it remains equally important that adolescents continue to have access to family planning services as well as prevention and treatment services for STIs, including HPV vaccination. Maximizing vaccination uptake and assessing clinical outcomes among vaccinated and unvaccinated women will allow for development of screening strategies that lead to significant reductions in cancer risk, health care costs, and patient harm.

REFERENCES

1. Committee on Adolescent Health Care. ACOG Committee Opinion No. 436: evaluation and management of abnormal cervical cytology and histology in adolescents. Obstet Gynecol 2009;113:1422–5.
2. Moscicki AB, Cox JT. Practice improvement in cervical screening and management (PICSM): symposium on management of cervical abnormalities in adolescents and young women. J Low Genit Tract Dis 2010;14:73–80.
3. Moyer VA, US Preventive Services Task Force. Screening for cervical cancer: U.S. Preventive Services Task Force recommendations statement. Ann Intern Med 2012;156:880–91, W312.
4. Saslow D, Solomon D, Lawson HW, et al. American Cancer Society, American Society for Colposcopy and Cervical Pathology, and American Society for Clinical Pathology screening guidelines for the prevention and early detection of cervical cancer. CA Cancer J Clin 2012;62:147–72.
5. Committee on Practice Bulletins-Gynecology. ACOG Practice Bulletin Number 131: screening for cervical cancer. Obstet Gynecol 2012;120:1222–38.
6. Massad LS, Einstein MH, Huh WK, et al. Updated guidelines for the management of abnormal cervical cancer screening tests and cancer precursors. J Low Genit Tract Dis 2013;17:S1–S27. http://dx.doi.org/10.1097/LGT.0b013c318287d329.
7. Benard VB, Watson M, Castle PE, et al. Cervical carcinoma rates among young females in the United States. Obstet Gynecol 2012;120:1117–23.
8. Kyrgiou M, Koliopoulos G, Martin-Hirsch P, et al. Obstetric outcomes after conservative treatment for intraepithelial or early invasive cervical lesions: systematic review and meta-analysis. Lancet 2006;367:489–98.
9. Bruinsma FJ, Quinn MA. The risk of preterm birth following treatment for precancerous changes in the cervix: a systematic review and meta-analysis. BJOG 2011;118:1031–41.
10. Bruni I, Diaz M, Castellsague X, et al. Cervical human papillomavirus prevalence in 5 continents: meta-analysis of 1 million women with normal cytological findings. J Infect Dis 2010;202:1789–90.
11. Hwang LY, Ma Y, Shiboski SC, et al. Active squamous metaplasia of the cervical epithelium is associated with subsequent acquisition of human papillomavirus 16 infection among healthy young women. J Infect Dis 2012;206:504–11. http://dx.doi.org/10.1093/infdis/jis398.
12. Evander M, Edlund K, Gustaffson A, et al. Human papillomavirus infection is transient in young women: a population based cohort study. J Infect Dis 1995;171:1026–30.

13. Moscicki AB, Shiboski S, Broering J, et al. The natural history of human papillomavirus infection as measured by repeated DNA testing in adolescent and young women. J Pediatr 1998;132:277–84.
14. Ho GY, Bierman R, Beardsley L, et al. Natural history of cervicovaginal papillomavirus infection in young women. N Engl J Med 1998;338:423–8.
15. Winer RL, Hughes JP, Feng Q, et al. Early natural history of incident, type-specific human papillomavirus infections in newly sexually active young women. Cancer Epidemiol Biomarkers Prev 2011;20:699–707.
16. Moscicki AB, Hills N, Shiboski S, et al. Risks for incident human papillomavirus infection and low-grade squamous intraepithelial lesion development in young females. JAMA 2001;285:2995–3002.
17. Woodman CB, Collins S, Winter H, et al. Natural history of cervical human papillomavirus infection in young women: a longitudinal cohort study. Lancet 2001; 357:1831–6.
18. Winer RL, Lee SK, Hughes JP, et al. Genital human papillomavirus infection: incidence and risk factors in a cohort of female university students. Am J Epidemiol 2003;157:218–26.
19. Winer RL, Kiviat NB, Hughes JP, et al. Development and duration of human papillomavirus lesions, after initial infection. J Infect Dis 2005;191:731–8.
20. Moscicki AB, Shiboski S, Hills NK, et al. Regression of low-grade squamous intra-epithelial lesions in young women. Lancet 2004;364:1678–83.
21. Moore K, Cofer A, Elliot L, et al. Adolescent cervical dysplasia: histologic evaluation, treatment, and outcomes. Am J Obstet Gynecol 2007;197:141.e1–6.
22. Fuchs K, Weitzen S, Wu L, et al. Management of cervical intraepithelial neoplasia 2 in adolescents. J Pediatr Adolesc Gynecol 2007;20:269–74.
23. Moscicki AB, Ma Y, Wibbelsman C, et al. Rate of and risks for regression of cervical intraepithelial neoplasia 2 in adolescents and young women. Obstet Gynecol 2010;116:1373–80.
24. Clements AB, Raker CA, Cooper AS, et al. Prevalence and patient characteristics associated with CIN 3 in adolescents. Am J Obstet Gynecol 2011;204: 128.e1–7.
25. Moore G, Fetterman B, Cox JT, et al. Lessons from practice: risk of CIN 3 or cancer associated with an LSIL or HPV-positive ASC-US screening result in women aged 21 to 24. J Low Genit Tract Dis 2010;14:97–102.
26. Saslow D, Runowicz CD, Solomon D, et al. American Cancer Society guidelines for the early detection of cervical cancer. CA Cancer J Clin 2002;52:342–62.
27. Castle PE, Fetterman B, Cox JT, et al. The age-specific relationships of abnormal cytology and human papillomavirus DNA results to the risk of cervical precancer and cancer. Obstet Gynecol 2010;116:76–84.
28. Sasieni P, Castanon A, Cuzick J. Effectiveness of cervical screening with age: population based case-control study of prospectively recorded data. BMJ 2009;339:b2968. http://dx.doi.org/10:1131/bmj.b2968.
29. Hildesheim A, Hadjimichael O, Schwartz PE, et al. Risk factors for rapid-onset cervical cancer. Am J Obstet Gynecol 1999;180:571–7.
30. Yabroff KR, Saraiya M, Meissner HI, et al. Specialty differences in primary care physician reports of Papanicolaou test screening practices: a national survey, 2006-2007. Ann Intern Med 2009;151:602–11.
31. Saraiya M, Berkowitz Z, Yabroff KR, et al. Cervical cancer screening with both human papillomavirus and Papanicolaou testing vs Papanicolaou testing alone: what screening intervals are physicians recommending? Arch Intern Med 2010; 170:977–85.

32. Centers for Disease Control and Prevention (CDC). Cervical cancer screening among women aged 18-30 years–United States, 2000-2010. MMWR Morb Mortal Wkly Rep 2013;61:1038–42.

33. Sadler L, Saftlas A, Wang W, et al. Treatment for cervical intraepithelial neoplasia and risk of preterm delivery. JAMA 2004;291:2100–6.

34. Samson SL, Bentley JR, Fahey TJ, et al. The effect of loop electrosurgical excision procedure on future pregnancy outcome. Obstet Gynecol 2005;105: 325–32.

35. Jakobsson M, Gissler M, Paavonen J, et al. Loop electrosurgical excision procedure and the risk of preterm birth. Obstet Gynecol 2009;114:504–10.

36. Noehr B, Jensen A, Frederiksen K, et al. Depth of cervical cone removed by loop electrosurgical excision procedure and subsequent risk of spontaneous preterm delivery. Obstet Gynecol 2009;114:1232–8.

37. Reilly R, Paranjothy S, Beer H, et al. Birth outcomes following treatment for precancerous changes to the cervix: a population-based record linkage study. BJOG 2012;119:236–44.

38. Wright TC Jr, Massad LS, Dunton CJ, et al. 2006 consensus guidelines for the management of women with abnormal cervical cancer screening tests. Am J Obstet Gynecol 2007;197:346–55.

39. Boardman LA, Stanko C, Weitzen S, et al. Atypical squamous cells of undetermined significance: human papillomavirus testing in adolescents. Obstet Gynecol 2005;105:741–6.

40. Stout NK, Goldhaber-Fiebert JD, Ortendahl JD, et al. Trade-offs in cervical cancer prevention: balancing benefits and risks. Arch Intern Med 2008;168: 1881–9.

41. Kulasingam SL, Havrilesky L, Ghebre R, et al. Screening for cervical cancer: a decision analysis for the U.S. Preventive Services Task Force. Rockville (MD): Agency for Healthcare Research and Quality; 2011. AHRQ Publication No. 11-05157-EF-1. Available at: http://www.uspreventiveservicestaskforce.org/uspstf11/cervcancer/cervcancerdecan.pdf. Accessed January 2, 2013.

42. Dunne EF, Unger ER, Sternberg M, et al. Prevalence of HPV infection among females in the United States. JAMA 2007;297:813–9.

43. Dunne EF, Sternberg M, Markowitz LE, et al. Human papillomavirus (HPV) 6, 11, 16 and 18 prevalence among females in the United States–National Health and Nutrition Examination Survey, 2003-2006: opportunity to measure HPV vaccine impact? J Infect Dis 2011;204:562–5.

44. Rosa M, Pragasam P, Saremian J, et al. The unsatisfactory ThinPrep Pap Test™: analysis of technical aspects, most common causes, and recommendations for improvement. Diagn Cytopathol 2012. http://dx.doi.org/10.1002/dc.22904.

45. Pawlik M, Martin FJ. Does a water-based lubricant affect Pap smear and cervical microbiology results? Can Fam Physician 2009;55:376–7.

46. Hill DA, Lamvu G. Effect of lubricating gel on patient comfort during vaginal speculum examination: a randomized controlled trial. Obstet Gynecol 2012; 119:227–31.

47. Kahn JA, Chiou V, Allen JD, et al. Beliefs about Papanicolaou smears and compliance with Papanicolaou smear follow-up in adolescents. Arch Pediatr Adolesc Med 1999;153:1046–54.

48. Davey DD, Cox JT, Austin M, et al. Cervical cytology specimen adequacy: updated patient management guidelines. J Low Genit Tract Dis 2008;12:71–81.

49. Elumir-Tanner L, Doraty M. Management of Papanicolaou test results that lack endocervical cells. CMAJ 2011;183:563 8.

50. Centers for Disease Control and Prevention (CDC). National and state vaccination coverage among adolescents aged 13-17 years–United States, 2011. MMWR Morb Mortal Wkly Rep 2012;61:671–7.
51. Dorrell CG, Yankey D, Santibanez TA, et al. Human papillomavirus vaccination series intitiation and completion, National Immunization Survey-Teen, 2008-2009. Pediatrics 2011;128:830–9.
52. Munoz N, Kraer SK, Sigurdsson K, et al. Impact of human papillomavirus (HPV)-6/11/16/18 vaccine on all HPV-associated genital diseases in young women. J Natl Cancer Inst 2010;102:325–39.
53. Lu B, Kumar A, Castellsague X, et al. Efficacy and safety of prophylactic vaccines against cervical HPV infection and diseases among women: a systematic review and meta-analysis. BMC Infect Dis 2011;11:13.
54. Rana MM, Huhtala H, Apter D, et al. Understanding long-term protection of human papillomavirus vaccination against cervical carcinoma: cancer registry-based follow-up. Int J Cancer 2012. http://dx.doi.org/10.1002/ijc.27971.
55. Read TR, Koching JS, Chen MY, et al. The near disappearance of genital warts in young women 4 years after commencing a national human papillomavirus (HPV) vaccination programme. Sex Transm Infect 2011;87:544–7.
56. Van de Velde N, Boily MC, Drolet M, et al. Population-level impact of the bivalent, quadrivalent and nonavalent human papillomavirus vaccines: a model-based analysis. J Natl Cancer Inst 2012;104:1712–23.
57. Poljak M. Prophylactic human papillomavirus vaccination and primary prevention of cervical cancer: issues and challenges. Clin Microbiol Infect 2012;18:64–9.
58. de Blasio BF, Neilson AR, Klemp M, et al. Modeling the impact of screening policy and screening compliance on incidence and mortality of cervical cancer in the post-HPV vaccination era. J Public Health (Oxf) 2012;34:539–47.
59. Boone JD, Erickson BK, Huh WK. New insights into cervical cancer screening. J Gynecol Oncol 2012;23:282–7.
60. Nanda K, McCrory DC, Myers ER, et al. Accuracy of the Papanicolaou test in screening for and follow-up of cervical cytologic abnormalities: a systematic review. Ann Intern Med 2000;132:810–9.
61. Elfgren K, Rylander E, Radberg T, et al. Colposcopic and histopathologic evaluation of women participating in population-based screening for human papillomavirus deoxyribonucleic acid persistence. Am J Obstet Gynecol 2005;193:650–7.
62. Franco EL, Cuzick J, Hildesheim A, et al. Issues in planning cervical cancer screening in the era of HPV vaccination. Vaccine 2006;24(Suppl 3):S3/171-7.
63. Kliewer DV, Demers AA, Brisson M, et al. The Manitoba human papillomavirus vaccine surveillance and evaluation system. Health Rep 2010;21:37–42.
64. Hariri S, Unger ER, Powell SE, et al. The HPV vaccine impact monitoring project (HPV-IMPACT): assessing early evidence of vaccination impact on HPV-associated cervical cancer precursor lesions. Cancer Causes Control 2012;23:281–8.
65. Wheeler CM, Hunt WC, Cuzick J, et al. A population-based study of human papillomavirus genotype prevalence in the United States: baseline measures prior to mass human papillomavirus vaccination. Int J Cancer 2013;132:198–207.
66. Serrano B, Alemany L, Tous S, et al. Potential impact of a nine-valent vaccine in human papillomavirus related cervical disease. Infect Agent Cancer 2012;7:38.
67. Tumban E, Peabody J, Tyler M, et al. VLPs displaying a single L2 epitope induce broadly cross-neutralizing antibodies against human papillomavirus. PLoS One 2012;7:e49751. http://dx.doi.org/10.1371/journal.pone.0049751.

Cervical Cancer Screening in Pregnancy

Jody Stonehocker, MD

KEYWORDS

- Cervical cancer screening • Pregnancy • Pap smear
- Cervical intraepithelial neoplasia • Cervical cancer
- Management of abnormal Pap smear in pregnancy

KEY POINTS

- Pap smears should only be performed in pregnancy if indicated under current screening guidelines.
- Colposcopy may be deferred in pregnancy for atypical squamous cells undetermined significance and low-grade squamous intraepithelial lesion, but should be used to triage more serious abnormalities.
- Cervical biopsies should be performed to exclude invasive cervical cancer.
- Cervical dysplasia should never be treated during pregnancy.
- Treatment guidelines for advanced invasive cervical cancer are not well studied and controversial.

SCREENING AND CERVICAL CYTOLOGY IN PREGNANCY

The goal of cervical cancer screening programs is to reduce the incidence of and mortality from cervical cancer through the detection and treatment of preinvasive lesions and early-stage cervical cancer. With the introduction of cervical cancer screening in the United States, cervical cancer deaths have been successfully reduced from the leading cause to 14th of all cancer deaths. Nevertheless in 2012 it was estimated that 12,170 women will be diagnosed with invasive cervical cancer and 4220 will die of their disease.[1] In the past it has been recommended that all pregnant women undergo Papanicolaou test (Pap) screening at the time of their initial prenatal examination in an effort to increase detection.[2] It has become clear that such opportunistic screening, in an already well-screened population, is not effective.[3,4] Under current guidelines there is no role for annual or even more frequent than annual screening (ie, at initiation of prenatal care and postpartum). It is recommended to screen

Division of Gynecology, Department of Obstetrics and Gynecology, University of New Mexico, MSC 10 5580, 1 University of New Mexico, Albuquerque, NM 87131-0001, USA
E-mail address: jstonehocker@salud.unm.edu

Obstet Gynecol Clin N Am 40 (2013) 269–282
http://dx.doi.org/10.1016/j.ogc.2013.03.005
0889-8545/13/$ – see front matter © 2013 Elsevier Inc. All rights reserved.

Table 1		
Recommended cervical cancer screening under updated guidelines		
Population	**USPSTF**	**ACS/ASCCP/ASCP**
<21 y	Do not screen, regardless of the age of sexual initiation and other risk factors	
21–29 y	Screen with cytology every 3 y. No role for HPV screening.	
30–65 y	Screen with cytology every 3 y (preferred) or with a combination of cytology and HPV testing every 5 y	Screen with a combination of cytology and HPV testing every 5 y (preferred) or cytology alone every 3 y
HPV-vaccinated	Continue screening, according to age and clinical history	

Abbreviations: ACS, American Cancer Society; ASCCP, American Society for Colposcopy and Cervical Pathology; ASCP, American Society for Clinical Pathology; USPSTF, US Preventive Services Task Force.

pregnant women with a Pap test only if they would qualify for screening under current screening guidelines (**Table 1**).

Some practitioners may be concerned about placing an instrument into the endocervical canal such as a cytobrush. One randomized study compared the use of a cytobrush to the presumed gentler, Dacron swab. They reported improved yield of endocervical cells for the cytobrush (96% vs 70%) without any difference in complications, including bleeding and spontaneous abortion.[5] As such, it is recommended to use the cytobrush, or comparable combination broom, during the collection of a prenatal Pap test.

Cytologic specimens are more difficult to interpret in pregnancy because of hormonal changes in the squamous and glandular epithelial cells. The Arias-Stella reaction or decidual cells are large hypervacuolated cells with variably staining cytoplasm and large nuclei that can often be misinterpreted as dysplastic cells. Immature metaplastic cells are also present in large quantities, which may appear similar to high-grade intraepithelial lesions. There are more inflammatory cells present in cervical cytology obtained during pregnancy. In addition, cytotrophoblast and syncytiotrophoblast cells may be seen in cytologic specimens. Despite these challenges, the Pap test seems to demonstrate equivalent accuracy in pregnancy compared with the nonpregnant patient.[6] It is of utmost importance that the pathologist be notified of the patient's pregnant state to facilitate an accurate interpretation.

COLPOSCOPY IN PREGNANCY

Once an abnormal screening cervical cytology result is obtained, patients and some practitioners may question the safety of colposcopy in pregnancy. It has been well established that colposcopy with or without directed biopsies is safe in pregnancy without an increased incidence of hemorrhage, premature labor, abortion, or infection.[7] Although colposcopy does not cause abortion, if performed in the first trimester when the rate of spontaneous abortion is increased, colposcopy may be temporally related and blamed for the pregnancy loss. To avoid this confusion, it is most often recommended to perform colposcopy in the second trimester of pregnancy.

Colposcopy Technique

Practitioners who have performed colposcopy in pregnancy are aware that although it may be safe, it is a more difficult examination to perform. The hormonal changes of pregnancy cause laxity in the vaginal walls, increased mucous production of the cervix, and engorgement and enlargement of the cervix itself. There are techniques that can help overcome these obstacles. First, before 20 weeks' gestation patient positioning does not need to change. After 20 weeks' gestation, a rolled sheet should be placed behind the patient's right hip to avoid supine hypotension. It is important to use the longest and widest speculum that will be tolerated by the patient for your examination. If the vaginal walls still preclude visualization of the cervix, vaginal wall retractors may be used. A condom may also be placed over the speculum, removing the distal end, in place of vaginal wall retractors.

Cervical mucus in pregnancy is abundant and tenacious. A ring forceps may be used to gently remove mucous from the cervical os to allow for visualization. If this is not successful, the mucus may be wrapped around a dry sterile swab and moved from quadrant to quadrant during the examination. The enlarged and engorged pregnant cervix, especially later in pregnancy, may be too large to visualize in its entirety. If so, it is acceptable to manipulate the cervix with a large cotton swab, allowing for thorough visualization of one quadrant at a time. The hormonal changes of pregnancy cause eversion of the endocervical canal.[8] This enlargement of the transformation zone makes a satisfactory colposcopy more likely. If colposcopy is performed in early pregnancy and is unsatisfactory, the examination should be repeated in the second trimester when it will almost certainly be achievable.[9] The enlarged transformation zone also causes greater friability of the pregnant cervix, so acetic acid should be applied with care to avoid bleeding that can make the examination more difficult.

The same hormonal changes of pregnancy that render cervical cytology more difficult to interpret also make the colposcopic appearance of the cervix change dramatically during pregnancy. Active immature metaplasia often causes large areas of thin acetowhite changes, which may contain fine punctuation or mosaicism, making it difficult to distinguish from low-grade dysplasia. As pregnancy progresses, decidualization of the stroma may become prominent, appearing as dense acetowhite lesions with lacy superficial blood vessels that may be confused for a high-grade lesion. Normal capillaries may also have a thin ring of decidualized stroma around them, which will also appear acetowhite, causing the "starry-sky" appearance.[10]

Given these changes, it is recommended that an expert colposcopist perform the examination during pregnancy. Many studies have shown that when performed by an experienced colposcopist, the visual impression has a reliable correlation with histology.[11-13] Most recently the largest series in the literature (n = 1079) of pregnant women with abnormal cervical cytology and antepartum colposcopic assessment was published. Fader and colleagues[14] found that women who had a colposcopic impression of cervical intraepithelial neoplasia (CIN) 1 or less, biopsy histology correlated with clinical impression in 81.5% of cases. For those with a colposcopic impression of CIN2 or 3, histology correlated with clinical impression or lower grade dysplasia in 100% of cases.

Biopsy Technique

Because the purpose of colposcopy is to exclude malignancy, if colposcopic impression favors high-grade dysplasia and microinvasion cannot be excluded, or invasive cancer is suspected, directed biopsies should be performed. Anecdotally most practitioners note increased bleeding from the pregnant cervix when biopsied, but again there is no evidence to support the clinical significance of this bleeding, including poor pregnancy outcome. In preparation for a biopsy it is helpful to place an absorbent pad under the patient that extends under the speculum handle. A small, sharp biopsy forceps should be used and pressure should be applied immediately to the biopsy site with a large cotton swab held in the nondominant hand to prevent blood from welling up. Once the specimen has been handed off, pressure should only be released to apply a hemostatic substance such as Monsel's solution or silver nitrate, both of which are safe in pregnancy. If bleeding is excessive, cautery, fine suture, or vaginal packing may be used.

Endocervical Curettage

Although accumulated evidence supports the safety of colposcopic biopsy, there is no body of evidence to support the safety of endocervical curettage (ECC). One retrospective study described the use of ECC in the diagnosis of carcinoma in situ in 33 pregnant patients. They found that 97% delivered at term, with no significant difference in pregnancy outcome compared with the general population.[15] Despite this limited data, it is currently considered unacceptable to perform ECC in pregnancy.

MANAGEMENT OF ABNORMAL CYTOLOGY
Atypical Squamous Cells Undetermined Significance ± Human Papillomavirus

Despite the relative immunocompromised status of pregnancy, there is no current evidence to suggest that the natural history or prevalence of HPV infection differs in the pregnant patient.[16] Therefore, it is valid to use the high-risk human papillomavirus (HPV) DNA test to triage atypical squamous cells of undetermined significance (ASCUS) test results. Those women found to be HPV-negative should return to routine screening. When found to be HPV-positive, the likelihood of finding CIN2/3 on biopsy is low. Wetta and colleagues[17] determined 25.6% of women with either ASCUS or low-grade squamous intraepithelial lesion (LGSIL) had CIN2/3 on biopsy, whereas others have found rates as low as 10%.[18] The likelihood of finding invasive cervical cancer is even lower, estimated to be less than 1%. Given this information, it is acceptable to perform colposcopy in pregnancy, but preferable to defer evaluation to no sooner than 6 weeks' postpartum. At that time, repeat cytology or colposcopic evaluation may be performed. According to the American Society for Colposcopy and Cervical Pathology (ASCCP) 2013 guidelines, if the patient is between the ages of 21 and 24 years, HPV testing is not preferred, but repeat cytology in 12 months should be performed (**Fig. 1**).[19]

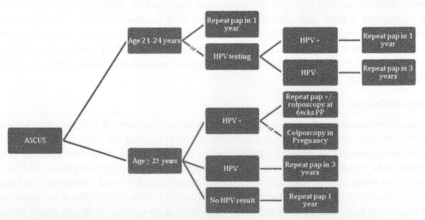

Fig. 1. Management of ASCUS Pap smear results in pregnancy. PP, postpartum.

Atypical Squamous Cells Favor High Grade

Because the risk of finding CIN2/3 on colposcopic biopsy approaches 50% for women with atypical squamous cells favor high grade Pap test results,[17] it is recommended that all of these patients have colposcopy performed in pregnancy.

LGSIL

As stated previously, patients with LGSIL cytology results are very unlikely to have a high-grade histologic lesion or invasive cancer. There is also evidence that CIN1 lesions have a high rate of regression postpartum. Serati and colleagues[20] found 69% of CIN1 lesions regressed at 8 weeks' postpartum, whereas 16.6% persisted as CIN1 and 14.3% progressed to CIN2/3. The rate of regression seems to be even higher for younger women. Cubo-Abert and colleagues[21] found an overall regression rate of 45% in their LGSIL population. When they stratified these patients by age, 50% of women less than 25 years old experienced regression, whereas those older than 25 years had a regression rate of 42.8%. ASCCP guidelines were updated in 2007 to reflect this information. Although colposcopy during pregnancy is still the preferred method to evaluate LGSIL, it is acceptable to defer evaluation until no sooner than 6 weeks' postpartum. Since 2007 evidence has continued to accumulate regarding the benign nature of LGSIL lesions and some authors have suggested that colposcopic evaluation is neither cost effective nor necessary and suggest performing repeat cervical cytology at 6 weeks' postpartum.[2,18] The current ASSCP guidelines from 2013 still recommend using colposcopy at 6 weeks' postpartum for evaluation, if not performed during pregnancy, which is still the preferred option for women aged 25 years or older. For women aged 21 to 24 years, repeat cytology in 1 year is preferred (**Fig. 2**).[19]

High-Grade Squamous Intraepithelial Lesion

All women with high-grade cytology should undergo colposcopic evaluation in pregnancy. Biopsies should be performed of all suspicious lesions, but an endocervical curettage should not be performed. The risk of finding an invasive cancer is estimated at 1%, but in a small retrospective study 3 of 19 patients (11%) followed in pregnancy for high-grade squamous intraepithelial lesion were found to have microinvasive cervical cancer (stage IA1) on postpartum conization.[22] If invasion cannot be excluded from the colpscopic impression performed by an expert colposcopist, some would suggest using an excisional procedure in addition to directed biopsies to confirm the diagnosis.

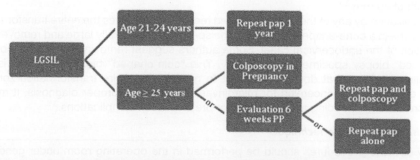

Fig. 2. Management of LGSIL Pap smear results in pregnancy. PP, postpartum.

Glandular Abnormalities

Adenocarncinoma in situ and primary adenocarcinoma of the cervix are uncommon, accounting for up to only 15% of all cervical neoplasms. Following a Pap test with atypical glandular cells, a patient would typically undergo colposcopy, endocervical curettage, and endometrial biopsy. Clearly this approach is problematic in pregnancy whereby endocervical curettage and endometrial biopsy are contraindicated. There is little evidence to direct the management of pregnant women with atypical glandular cells Pap test results, but it is clear they should have colposcopic evaluation. The most common lesion encountered at the time of colposcopy, just as in nonpregnant women, is a squamous neoplasia. In one study these patients were also examined by transrectal ultrasonography to exclude invasive endocervical cancer.[23] Others suggest consideration of diagnostic conization for all women with atypical glandular cells-favor neoplasia or adenocarncinoma in situ Pap test results.[24]

EXCISIONAL PROCEDURES

In the past the cold-knife cone (CKC) procedure was the only excisional procedure available for this purpose. It was associated with heavy vaginal bleeding (5%–15%), an increased rate of spontaneous abortion (up to 33%), and a high rate of postpartum recurrence of dysplasia.[25,26] It is currently not recommended in pregnancy.

Since the loop electrosurgical excision procedure (LEEP) has become commonplace in the treatment of cervical dysplasia, it has been increasingly studied in pregnancy. Most recently Schaefer and colleagues[27] published a series of 27 women who underwent LEEP in pregnancy as microinvasive disease could not be excluded by colposcopy. One pathologic specimen contained CIN2 and 22 specimens contained CIN3. Microinvasive cancer was found in 2 specimens and invasive cancer was found in 1 case (11% of procedures), emphasizing the importance of performing the procedure when the combination of cytology, histology from any colposcopically directed biopsies, and colposcopic impression leave concern for invasion. They also found that the procedure was relatively safe with no bleeding complications requiring transfusion or reoperation. It was associated with one spontaneous abortion (although the patient had had one previous spontaneous abortion), 3 premature deliveries before 37 weeks' gestation (2 in twin gestations), and 2 cases of incompetent cervix (one in twin gestation). Other studies have also found no correlation between LEEP during pregnancy and preterm delivery[28] or spontaneous abortion.[29]

Although less common, some prefer to use the carbon dioxide laser for excision of the transformation zone. Another retrospective study was published examining the safety and effectiveness of its use in pregnancy. The authors did not find laser conization–related obstetric complications and thought that it was safe in pregnancy up to a depth of 20 mm.[30]

Conization by any of the aforementioned techniques removes the entire transformation zone in a cone-shaped specimen. The specimen is generally large and removes a portion of the endocervical canal. Some authors suggest removing a smaller, "coin-shaped" biopsy specimen in pregnancy. This "coin-shaped" biopsy specimen is a shallow excision that does not attempt to remove the entire transformation zone, but only the area concerning for microinvasion to make a proper diagnosis. It may decrease both bleeding and concerns for preterm labor complications.[31]

Excisional Procedure Technique

Any of these procedures should be performed in the operating room under general anesthesia. It is best to perform them after the completion of the first trimester to avoid association with spontaneous abortion, but before the third trimester, because bleeding complications increase in later gestations. Blood products should be readily available and some advocate placing anywhere between 2 and 6 hemostatic sutures in the cervix, or even a prophylactic cerclage, before beginning the excision. The purpose of the procedure should always be diagnosis of invasive disease, not treatment of cervical dysplasia.

MANAGEMENT OF ABNORMAL HISTOLOGY
CIN1

Once a satisfactory colposcopy has been performed in pregnancy and directed biopsy has proven CIN1, no further evaluation or treatment during pregnancy should be completed. It has already been established that CIN1 does not progress to invasive cervical cancer during the course of pregnancy and that the rate of regression during the postpartum period is high. Given this, no further cytologic or colposcopic evaluation in pregnancy is warranted and treatment of CIN1 during pregnancy is unacceptable. **Fig. 3** shows specific follow-up recommendations.[19]

CIN2/CIN3

If CIN2, CIN3, or CIN2/3 are diagnosed at the time of colposcopy and invasive disease is not suspected, repeat cytology and colposcopy testing are acceptable during pregnancy but no more frequently than every 12 weeks. Repeat biopsy should be performed only if the lesion has a worsening colposcopic appearance or cytology is suggestive of invasive disease. The rate of progression from high-grade intraepithelial neoplasia to invasive carcinoma during pregnancy is estimated to be 0.4%.[10] Given such, it is also acceptable to defer any reevaluation until no sooner than 6 weeks' postpartum. At the postpartum evaluation, both cytology and colposcopy should be performed. Although the rate of regression for CIN2 or CIN3 is less than low-grade lesions, regression still does occur during the postpartum period and an excisional procedure should not be performed prior to reevaluation with cytology and colposcopy.

If invasive cancer is suspected during pregnancy even after directed biopsy returns CIN2 or CIN3, an excisional procedure is recommended as discussed previously. Treatment of CIN2 or CIN3 in pregnancy is never acceptable.

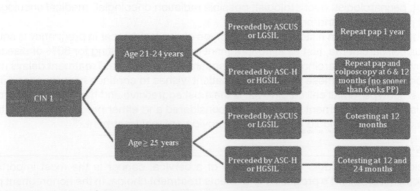

Fig. 3. Management of CIN 1 in pregnancy. PP, postpartum.

Mode of delivery
It has been hypothesized that the local inflammation and remodeling that occurs following cervical trauma at the time of a vaginal birth would improve the rate of regression of intraepithelial lesions. There have been studies performed that suggested this correlation,[32,33] but others that refute the relationship. A recent retrospective cohort study following 100 women with abnormal Pap tests found that the risk of progression, persistence, or regression had no significant association to the mode of delivery.[21] Although no clear benefit can be proven for vaginal delivery, it is clear that normal birth does not worsen the outcome for intraepithelial lesions. Given this, route of delivery for women with CIN1, CIN2, or CIN3 should be based on obstetric indications alone.

Risk of excisional procedures on future pregnancies
Information regarding the impact of treatment on future pregnancy is conflicting, although most studies indicate an increased preterm delivery risk. A recent meta-analysis indicates that cervical disease treatment increases risk for subsequent preterm delivery and other complications of pregnancy by approximately twofold.[34] The increased preterm delivery risk is presumed to result from deficient cervical stroma, and the risk does seem to increase with larger excisional procedures and the number of excisions performed. Some would argue that this increased risk seen in retrospective studies is no more than a casual relationship. Women with CIN may be at increased risk for preterm delivery even when untreated, potentially because of confounding factors that have not been controlled for in these studies or shared risk factors. Despite this, because any pregnancy complication, and especially preterm birth, can be devastating, the potential benefits of treatment of intraepithelial lesions should be balanced against the risk to future pregnancies. Special consideration should be given to any woman who has not completed child-bearing, but especially to those aged 21 to 24 years of age.[19]

MANAGEMENT OF INVASIVE CERVICAL CANCER

As previously discussed, the diagnosis of invasive cervical carcinoma in pregnancy is rare, occurring in 1 to 12 per 10,000 pregnancies.[35] Although pregnancy does not alter the prognosis of cervical cancer, as pregnant and nonpregnant women have the same outcomes,[36,37] it does alter treatment of the disease. Treatment planning depends on the patient's desires to continue or terminate the pregnancy, histopathologic subtype, clinical staging, and the gestational age at which the diagnosis is made. The patient must be managed by a multidisciplinary team that should include a gynecologic oncologist, perinatologist, neonatologist, possible radiation oncologist, medical oncologist, and psychological and/or pastoral care.

The most common histopathologic subtype of cervical cancer in pregnancy is squamous cell carcinoma, just as in nonpregnant patients, accounting for 80% of disease, followed by adenocarcinoma and adenosquamous carcinoma. Treatment delays may be considered with these cancers if the patient wishes to continue her pregnancy. The rarest subtype, small cell carcinoma, is the most aggressive and has a very poor prognosis. Delay of treatment should not be considered and either pregnancy termination or a delivery plan should be initiated to provide optimal treatment.[38]

Staging

Besides histopathologic subtype, stage of a cervical cancer is the most important indicator of a patient's prognosis and directs treatment choice. In the nonpregnant patient staging is based on the clinical examination and radiologic studies to determine distant spread (**Table 2**). The clinical examination may be more difficult in the pregnant patient and some are hesitant to offer pregnant women radiologic studies because of the risk of ionizing radiation. Patients with lesions greater than microinvasive disease should be offered accurate staging.

Computed tomography may be performed in the pregnant patient with minimal risk, delivering approximately 30 mGy to the fetus.[39] Because magnetic resonance imaging delivers no radiation to the fetus, it is currently considered the best imaging modality to determine the extent of both local spread and nodal metastases. Positron emission tomography-computed tomography use in pregnancy is still controversial as the used radionuclide (fluorodeoxyglucose) is not well studied and initial studies do suggest increased uptake and longer retention by the fetus that would exceed dosimetric standards.

The gold standard to determine nodal status is lymphadenectomy. The presence of positive lymph nodes changes the treatment plan and affects the outcome of the pregnancy particularly for early stage disease (IA2, IB1, and IIA). Laparoscopic lymphadenectomy is feasible at least up to 20 weeks' gestation, but has been reported up to 32 weeks' gestation. It may be performed by either the transperitoneal or the preperitoneal route. Thirty-one cases have been reported in the literature,[40,41] in which 25 patients had early-stage disease and 6 had bulky disease (>IB2). No conversions to laparotomy were required and no surgical complications, including negative pregnancy effects, were reported. In those with early-stage disease, positive lymph node metastases were found in 12%, compared with 50% in those with bulky disease. This rate of metastases is similar to the recorded rate for nonpregnant patients with

Table 2 FIGO staging of cervical cancer	
Stage	
I	Lesion is confined to cervix
IA	No visual lesion identifiable, but only by microscopic examination. Depth of invasion is no greater than 5 mm and lesion is no wider than 7 mm in diameter.
IA1	Stromal invasion is no greater than 3 mm in depth and no wider than 7 mm
IA2	Stromal invasion between 3 and 5 mm in depth and is no wider than 7 mm
IB	Lesion is visible and confined to the cervix or is preclinical but larger than the limits of stage IA
IB1	Lesion is no larger than 4 cm
IB2	Lesion is larger than 4 cm
II	Lesion extends into the vagina but no further than the upper two-thirds and or extends into the parametria but not to the pelvic side wall
IIA	Lesion extends into the upper two thirds of the vagina; no parametrial involvement
IIB	Obvious parametrial involvement: does not extend to pelvic sidewall
III	Lesion extends into lower one-third of the vagina or extends to pelvic sidewall; or there is evidence of hydronephrosis or a nonfunctioning kidney without a noncancerous cause
IIIA	Lesion extends into the lower one-third of the vagina but not to pelvic sidewall
IIIB	Lesion extends to pelvic sidewall or hydronephrosis or nonfunctioning kidney
IV	Tumor extends beyond true pelvis or clinically involves the mucosa of the bladder or rectum
IVA	Tumor has spread to adjacent organs
IVB	Tumor has spread to distant organs

disease of the same stage. As discussed with other histologic examinations in pregnancy, the examination of lymph nodes is also more complex. Decidual changes can mimic nodal metastases, especially in squamous cell carcinoma. An experienced pathologist should perform the examination and should clearly be notified of the patient's pregnant state.

Microinvasive carcinoma (stage IA1)

In the nonpregnant patient a CKC with negative margins or simple hysterectomy (if fertility is not desired) is considered adequate treatment in this earliest stage disease. If microinvasion is identified on an initial biopsy during early pregnancy, CKC or laser conization is recommended to exclude the possibility of more advanced stage disease. If cone margins are negative, the patient may be followed with colposcopy every 2 months until delivery and reevaluated 6 weeks' postpartum with cytology, colposcopy, and biopsies. If microinvasion is identified on an initial biopsy after 24 weeks' gestation, the risk of pregnancy complications from a CKC is increased (especially bleeding) and it may be reasonable to delay conization until the postpartum period as the likelihood of significant disease progression is small.[42] Patients with microinvasive cervical cancer that has been treated with negative CKC margins may deliver via the vaginal route without significant change in disease prognosis.

Early invasive carcinoma (stage IA2, IB1, IIA)

In the nonpregnant patient with early invasive disease, radical hysterectomy with pelvic lymphadenectomy is the treatment option of choice. Fertility-sparing surgery can be considered and would consist of pelvic lymphadenectomy and radical trachelectomy. When early invasive disease is diagnosed in a previable pregnancy and the patient does not wish to continue the pregnancy, radical hysterectomy can be performed with the fetus in situ. If the pregnancy is desired, radical trachelectomy is a treatment option but does have a high rate of complication including 33% fetal loss.[40,43–47] It should clearly only be performed in centers with experience in this procedure. If radical trachelectomy is not going to be performed, some would suggest neoadjuvant chemotherapy be considered while awaiting fetal lung maturity.[48] When early invasive disease is diagnosed in later gestation, expectant management can be considered. When fetal lung maturity is achieved, delivery should be undertaken by classical cesarean section (to avoid interrupting the lower uterine segment) and completion radical hysterectomy and pelvic lymphadenectomy performed immediately thereafter. After radical hysterectomy, the decision regarding adjuvant treatment should be based on the same factors as the nonpregnant patient, including depth of stromal invasion, parametrial involvement, and angiolymphatic invasion. Treatment delay in limited studies between 6 and 15 weeks does not seem to affect prognosis.[42]

The preferred route of delivery in early invasive carcinoma is by cesarean section. Vaginal delivery may increase the risk of lymphovascular dissemination of disease, lead to excessive bleeding, obstruction from tumor burden, and laceration of the diseased cervix. There have also been case reports of implantation of malignant cells at the episiotomy site.[49,50] Sood and colleagues[51] performed a matched case-control study of 56 pregnant women with invasive cervical cancer and showed a lower rate of recurrence in those who delivered by cesarean section (14% vs 56% vaginal delivery). Route of delivery was the most significant predictor of recurrence in multivariate analysis.

Advanced invasive carcinoma (stage IB2-IV)

In the nonpregnant patient, concominant chemotherapy and radiation would be the preferred treatment when bulky disease is diagnosed. If a patient in early pregnancy is diagnosed with advanced invasive carcinoma and opts for immediate treatment, the pregnancy should be terminated before beginning radiation therapy. In cases where pregnancy termination cannot be achieved because of tumor obstruction of the cervix, radiation therapy can be initiated with fetal demise and expulsion expected within 3 weeks.[52] Occasionally hysterotomy must be performed to complete evacuation of the uterus and stop excessive bleeding. If the patient wishes to continue the pregnancy, neoadjuvant chemotherapy may be the best alternative. This treatment is still controversial and not well studied, but would be followed by either surgical treatment postpartum (when tumor volume decreases to a surgically treatable size) or chemotherapy with radiation. Neoadjuvant chemotherapy should be platinum based and can be administered in the second or third trimesters of pregnancy without report of congenital malformations.[53] Long-term outcomes of exposed children have not been well studied, but no sequelae have been reported.[54] Neoadjuvant chemotherapy should not be administered within 4 weeks of delivery to avoid bone marrow suppression in the fetus at the time of delivery.

OUTCOMES

A recently published population-based cohort study including 8.8 million births over a period of 10 years looked at the maternal and fetal outcomes of pregnant women with CIN and cervical cancer.[55] They confirmed, as stated previously, that there was no observed increased risk of maternal mortality in this population. They also did not find any increased risk of pulmonary embolism or deep venous thrombosis. Women with cervical cancer were at greater risk for prematurity, cesarean delivery, and blood transfusion. These same risks were not present for women with CIN. Both groups were at higher risk for having a hysterectomy performed during the same admission as their delivery. Neither group had increased risk for intrauterine growth restriction, preterm premature rupture of membranes, or intrauterine fetal death.

SUMMARY

Pregnancy offers many young, healthy women an opportunity to seek care that otherwise may not be seen by a health care provider regularly or consistently. Cervical cancer screening guidelines are no different in the pregnant population than the nonpregnant population. If cervical cancer screening is performed and an abnormal Pap test is obtained, it should be triaged according to established guidelines. Colposcopy can often be deferred until postpartum with ASCUS or LGSIL results, but should performed for more serious abnormalities. The goal of colposcopy is to exclude invasive disease and biopsies should be performed as needed to meet this goal. Cervical dysplasia should never be treated in pregnancy. Once invasive disease has been identified, treatment protocols become controversial and are not well studied. Treatment recommendations should be flexible and addressed by multidisciplinary experts to accommodate this unique medical, ethical, and emotional dilemma.

REFERENCES

1. Siegel R, Naishadham D, Jemal A. Cancer statistics, 2012. CA Cancer J Clin 2012;62:10–29.
2. Hunter MI, Monk BJ, Tewari KS. Cervical neoplasia in pregnancy. Part 1: screening and management of preinvasive disease. Am J Obstet Gynecol 2008;199(1):3–9.

3. Saslow D, Castle P, Myers E, et al. American Cancer Society, American Society for Colposcopy and Cervical Pathology, and American Society for Clinical Pathology screening guidelines for the prevention and early detection of cervical cancer. CA Cancer J Clin 2012;62:147–72.

4. Saslow D, Herschel WL, Waldman J, et al. American Cancer Society, American Society for Colposcopy and Cervical Pathology, and American Society for Clinical Pathology screening guidelines for the prevention and early detection of cervical cancer. J Low Genit Tract Dis 2012;16(3):175–204.

5. Stillson T, Knight AL, Elswich RK Jr. The effectiveness and safety of two cervical cytology techniques during pregnancy. J Fam Pract 1997;45:159–63.

6. Morimura Y, Fujimori K, Soeda S. Cervical cytology during pregnancy–a comparison with non-pregnant women and management of women with abnormal cytology. Fukushima J Med Sci 2001;48:27–37.

7. Kohan S, Beckman EM, Bigelow B. The role of colposcopy in the managment of cervical intraepithelial neoplasia during pregnancy and postpartum. J Reprod Med 1980;25(5):279–84.

8. Nguyen C, Montz FJ, Bristow RE. Managment of stage I cervical cancer in pregnancy. Obstet Gynecol Surv 2000;55:633–43.

9. Economos K, Perez Veridiano N, Delke I, et al. Abnormal cervical cytology in pregnancy: a 17 year experience. Obstet Gynecol 1993;81:915–8.

10. McIntyre-Seltman K, Lesnock J. Cervical cancer screening in pregnancy. Obstet Gynecol Clin North Am 2008;35:645–58.

11. Broderick D, Matityahu D, Dudhbhai M, et al. Histologic and colposcopic correlates of ASCUS Pap smears in pregnancy. J Low Genit Tract Dis 2002;6(2):116–9.

12. Woodrow N, Permezel M, Butterfield L. Abnormal cervical cytology in pregnancy: experience of 811 cases. Aust N Z J Obstet Gynaecol 1998;38:161–5.

13. Benedet JL, Selke PA, Nickerson KG. Colposcopic evaluation of abnormal Papanicolaou smears in pregnancy. Am J Obstet Gynecol 1987;157:932–7.

14. Fader A, Alward E, Niederhauser A. Cervical dysplasia in pregnancy: a multi-institutional evaluation. Am J Obstet Gynecol 2010;203(2):113.e1–6.

15. El-Bastawissi AY, Becker TM, Daling JR. Effect of cervical carcinoma in situ and its managment on pregnancy outcome. Obstet Gynecol 1999;93:207–12.

16. Lu DW, Pirog EC, Zhu X. Prevalence and typing of HPV DNA in atypical squamous cells in pregnant women. Acta Cytol 2003;47:1008–16.

17. Wetta L, Matthews K, Kemper M. The managment of cervical intraepithelial neoplasia in pregnancy: is colposcopy necessary? J Low Genit Tract Dis 2009;13(3):182–5.

18. Jain AG, Higgins RV, Boyle MJ. Managment of low-grade squamous intraepithelial lesions during pregnancy. Am J Obstet Gynecol 1997;177:298–302.

19. Massad LS, Einstein MH, Huh WR, et al. 2012 updated consensus guidelines for the management of abnormal cervical cancer screening tests and cancer precursors. J Low Genit Tract Dis 2013;17(5 Suppl 1):S1–27.

20. Serati M, Uccella S, Laterza RM. Natural history of cervical intraepithelial neoplasia during pregnancy. Acta Obstet Gynecol Scand 2008;87(12):1296–300.

21. Cubo-Abert M, Centeno-Mediavilla C, Franco-Zabala P. Risk factors for progression or persistence of squamous intraepithelial lesions diagnosed during pregnancy. J Low Genit Tract Dis 2011;16(1):34–8.

22. Kaplan KJ. Prognosis and recurrence risk for patients with cervical squamous intraepithelial lesions diagnosed during pregnancy. Cancer 2004;102:22–232.

23. Slama J, Freitag P, Dundr P, et al. Outcomes of pregnant patients with Pap smears classified as atypical glandular cells. Cytopathology 2012;23(6):383–8.
24. Freeman-Wang T, Walker P. Colposcopy in special circumstances: pregnancy, immunocompromise, including HIV and transplants, adolescence and menopause. Clin Obstet Gynecol 2011;25(5):653–65.
25. Avarette HE, Nasser N, Yankow SL, et al. Cervical conization in pregnancy. Analysis of 180 operations. Am J Obstet Gynecol 1970;106:543–9.
26. Hannigan EV, Whitehouse HH, Atkinson WD, et al. Cone biopsy during pregnancy. Obstet Gynecol 1982;59:735–46.
27. Schaefer K, Peters D, Aulmann S, et al. Value and feasibility of LLETZ procedures for pregnant women with suspected high-grade squamous intraepithelial lesions and microinvasive cervical cancer. Int J Gynaecol Obstet 2012;118: 141–4.
28. Pena C, Fallani MG, Maggiorelli M, et al. High-grade cervical intraepithelial neoplasia (CIN) in pregnancy: clinicotherapeutic managment. Tumori 1998; 84(5):567–70.
29. Robova H, Rob L, Pluta M, et al. Squamous intraepithelial lesion-microinvasive carcinoma of the cervix during pregnancy. Eur J Gynaecol Oncol 2005;26(6): 611–4.
30. Tsuritani M, Watanabe Y, Kotani Y, et al. Retrospective evaluation of CO(2) laser conization in pregnant women with carcinoma in situ or mircoinvasive carcinoma. Gynecol Obstet Invest 2009;68:230–3.
31. DiSaia. Clinical gynecologic oncology. St Louis (MO): Mosby, Inc; 2002.
32. Siristatidis C, Vitoratos N, Michailidis E, et al. The role of the mode of delivery in the alteration of intrapartum pathological cervical cytologic findings during the postpartum period. Eur J Gynaecol Oncol 2002;23:358–60.
33. Ueda Y, Enomoto T, Miyatake T, et al. Postpartum outcome of cervical intraepithelial neoplasia in pregnant women determined by route of delivery. Reprod Sci 2009;16:1034–9.
34. Bruinsma FJ, Quinn MA. The risk of preterm birth following treatment for precancerous changes in the cervix: a systematic review and meta-analysis. BJOG 2011;118:1031–41.
35. Pavlidis N. Coexistence of pregnancy and malignancy. Oncologist 2002;7: 279–87.
36. Stensheim H, Moller B, van Dijk T, et al. Cause-specific survival for women diagnosed with cancer during pregnancy or lactation: a registry-based cohort study. J Clin Oncol 2009;27:45–51.
37. Zemlickis D, Lishner M, Degendorger P, et al. Maternal and fetal outcome after invasive cervical cancer in pregnancy. J Clin Oncol 1991;9:195–6.
38. Morice P, Uzan C, Gouy S, et al. Gynaecological cancers in pregnancy. Lancet 2012;379:558–69.
39. Hunter M, Tewari K, Monk B. Cervical neoplasia in pregnancy. Part 2: current treatment of invasive disease. Am J Obstet Gynecol 2008;199(1):10–8.
40. Alouini S, Rida K, Mathevet P. Cervical cancer complicating pregnancy: implications of laparoscopic lymphadenectomy. Gynecol Oncol 2008;108:472–7.
41. Sioutas A, Schedvins K, Larson B, et al. Three cases of vaginal radical trachelectomy in pregnancy. Gynecol Oncol 2010;121:420–1.
42. Takushi M, Moromizato H, Sakumoto K, et al. Managment of invasive carcinoma of the uterine cervix associated with pregnancy: outcome of intentional delay in treatment. Gynecol Oncol 2002;87:185–9.

43. Ungar L, Smith JR, Palfalvi L, et al. Abdominal radical trachelectomy during pregnancy to preserve pregnancy and fertility. Obstet Gynecol 2006;108:811–4.
44. Van de Nieuwenhof HP, van Ham MA, Lotgering FK, et al. First case of vaginal radical trachelectomy in a pregnant patient. Int J Gynecol Cancer 2008;18: 1381–5.
45. Mandic A, Novakovic P, Nincic D, et al. Radical abdominal trachelectomy in the 19th gestation week in patients with early invasive cervical carcinoma: case study and overview of literature. Am J Obstet Gynecol 2009;201:e6–8.
46. Abu-Rustum NR, Tal MN, DeLair D, et al. Radical abdominal trachelectomy for stage IB1 cervical cancer at 15-week gestation. Gynecol Oncol 2010;116: 151–2.
47. Karateke A, Cam C, Celik C, et al. Radical trachelectomy in late pregnancy: is it an option? Eur J Obstet Gynecol Reprod Biol 2010;152:112–3.
48. Manara H, de Andrade J, da Silva Mathes A, et al. Chemotherapy in the treatment of locally advanced cervical carcinoma. Gynecol Oncol 2001;80(2):272–4.
49. van der Vange N, Weverling GJ, Ketting BW, et al. The prognosis of cervical cancer associated with pregnancy: a matched cohort study. Obstet Gynecol 1995;85:1022–6.
50. Baloglu A, Uysal D, Aslan N, et al. Advanced stage of cervical carcinoma undiagnosed during antenatal period in term pregnancy and concominant metastasis on episiotomy scar during delivery: a case report and review of the literature. Int J Gynecol Cancer 2007;17:1155–9.
51. Sood AK, Sorosky JI, Mayr N, et al. Cervical cancer diagnosed shortly after pregnancy: prognostic variables and delivery routes. Obstet Gynecol 2009; 95(Pt 1):832–8.
52. Benhaim Y, Haie-Meder C, Lhomme C, et al. Chemoradiation therapy in pregnant patients treated for advanced-stage cervical carcinoma during the first trimester of pregnancy: report of two cases. Int J Gynecol Cancer 2007;17: 270–4.
53. Tewari K, Cappuccini F, Gambino A, et al. Neoadjuvant chemotherapy in the treatment of locally advanced cervical carcinoma in pregnancy: a report of two cases and review of issues specific to the management of cervical carcinoma in pregnancy including planned delay of therapy. Cancer 1998;82: 1529–34.
54. Bader A, Petru E, Winter R. Long-term follow-up after neoadjuvant chemotherapy for high-risk cervical cancer during pregnancy. Gynecol Oncol 2007; 105:269–72.
55. Al-Halal H, Kezouh A, Abenhaim H. Incidence and obstetrical outcomes of cervical intraepithelial neoplasia and cervical cancer in pregnancy. Arch Gynecol Obstet 2013;287(2):245–50.

LSIL: Definition and Management

Meggan Zsemlye, MD

KEYWORDS

- Cervical intraepithelial neoplasia • Human papilloma virus
- Cervical cancer screening • Cervical intraepithelial neoplasia, management

KEY POINTS

- Low-grade squamous intraepithelial lesion (LSIL) is a relatively common diagnosis on cervical cytology. Recent guidelines from the American Society for Colposcopy and Cervical Pathology (ASCCP) for the management of LSIL are reviewed.
- LSIL rarely leads to cervical cancer and is, therefore, best managed conservatively, especially in adolescents and young women.
- The use of p16 as part of the diagnostic tests on cervical histology should be encouraged.
- Cotesting with human papilloma virus (HPV) DNA tests should be encouraged because screening and HPV testing are utilized in the follow-up according to the ASCCP's 2012 guidelines.

LOW-GRADE SQUAMOUS INTRAEPITHELIAL LESION

The management of low-grade squamous intraepithelial lesions (LSIL) has changed greatly over the past 2 decades. The most recent recommendations propose avoiding treatment while continuing to monitor patients for clearance of disease or a change to a more severe diagnosis. Knowledge of the correct way to manage LSIL is important because LSIL is a relatively common diagnosis found on cervical cytology. Especially since the introduction of liquid-based cytology, the diagnosis of LSIL has become more frequent. The College of American Pathologists estimated in 2003 that the reporting rate for LSIL was 2.9%.[1] As we know from many studies of the pathophysiology of human papilloma virus (HPV)-related disease, most women with LSIL will be infected with HPV. Infection rates in women with LSIL range from 76.6% to more than 80.0%.[2] HPV infections in LSIL are most likely caused by high-risk HPV types, although a small percentage are caused by low-risk HPV types.

LSIL AND HPV

The conventional wisdom is that most women will be infected with HPV at some point in their life. Patients may be counseled that 80% of women show evidence of infection at some point. The likelihood of a woman having an HPV infection at a particular time

Department of Obstetrics and Gynecology, University of New Mexico School of Medicine, MSC 10 5580, 1 University of New Mexico, Albuquerque, NM 87131-0001, USA
E-mail address: mzsemlye@salud.unm.edu

Obstet Gynecol Clin N Am 40 (2013) 283–289
http://dx.doi.org/10.1016/j.ogc.2013.03.008
0889-8545/13/$ – see front matter © 2013 Elsevier Inc. All rights reserved.

is, to some extent, dependent on her age. Women in their early twenties have a high prevalence of HPV infection, approximately 20%.[3] Postmenopausal women have lower rates of HPV infection as well as lower rates of high-grade dysplasia.[4]

Most women with LSIL are infected with HPV. HPV infections that cause LSIL in the cervix are viral infections of the epithelium. In these cases, the HPV virus is expressed and viral particles are assembled and eventually shed, which allows for transmission. In higher-grade lesions, HPV is incorporated into the host genome and may eventually lead to a precancerous lesion.[5]

Most HPV infections are self-limited, and the data show that 90% of infections are cleared within a few years.[6] Clearance of the infection is brought about by cell-mediated immunity, although the details are not clear. Some women do not clear the infection and, thus, remain HPV positive. Persistent HPV infection is the underlying basis for the development of high-grade cervical dysplasia and eventually cervical cancer.[7] For this reason, women with persistent HPV infections, even those without obvious lesions, must be monitored.

TERMINOLOGY

The terminology used for the description of abnormal cervical cytology and dysplastic cervical intraepithelial lesions is complex. Recent recommendations for simplifying the terminology and incorporating the use of biomarkers may make treatment decisions easier for the clinician.

The 2001 Bethesda system organized the categorization of abnormal cervical cytology into categories including LSIL and high-grade squamous intraepithelial lesions (HSIL). Dysplastic cervical histology was divided into 3 categories: cervical intraepithelial neoplasia (CIN) I, CIN II, and CIN III.[8] CIN I is understood to represent an HPV infection in the cervical epithelium but not a precancerous process. CIN II and CIN III are considered potentially precancerous processes with HPV having incorporated into the host cell genome. The treatment of CIN II and III is generally similar, although CIN II is treated less aggressively in adolescents because of a high rate of regression seen with these lesions. Unfortunately, CIN II is often a difficult histologic diagnosis to make. The ALTS (ASC-US Low Grade Triage Study) trial showed that with blinded histologic examinations, the diagnosis of CIN II is not reproducible in a large number of patients. The same lack of reproducibility was noted in cytology specimens and in other grades of dysplasia.[9]

A consensus statement in 2012 produced by working groups from the College of American Pathologists and the American Society for Colposcopy and Cervical Pathology proposes a modified terminology that aims to bring the terms for histology of cervical dysplasia more in line with what we have now learned about the pathophysiology of HPV infection. The LAST project (Lower Anogenital Squamous Terminology Standardization Project for HPV Associated Lesions) proposes a unified nomenclature for cytologic and histologic diagnoses. The LAST terminology proposes the use of the term LSIL for CIN I and HSIL for CIN II, III. Also recommended is the use of p16 biomarkers in those cases when it is difficult to differentiate HPV infections from precancerous HPV lesions.[10] Using LAST terminology, a biopsy diagnosis of CIN I (confirmed, if necessary, by histochemical analysis) would be referred to as LSIL. A biopsy diagnosis of CIN II or CIN III (again, confirmed if necessary by histochemical analysis) would be referred to as HSIL.

MANAGEMENT GUIDELINES

Guidelines for the management of abnormal cervical cytology and abnormal cervical histology have recently been published[11] The American Society for Colposcopy and

Cervical Pathology (ASCCP) has published guidelines for this area 3 times since 2001, when a consensus conference was convened in response to the revised Bethesda system terminology. The consensus conferences are large gatherings of members of professional, governmental, and advocacy groups. Updates to the 2001 guidelines were agreed on and published in 2007 and 2013 because of new knowledge about the pathophysiology of HPV infection and the results of large studies of the natural history of infection and the results of treatment. Most recently, the guidelines were updated because of the evaluation of large-scale studies from the United States and other countries. Furthermore, the newest guidelines take into account the use of cotesting with HPV and cytology, which has been incorporated into screening. In addition, new techniques, such as HPV genotyping, are incorporated.

In 2012, data were published from a large-scale study of data from nearly 1.4 million women from the Northern California Kaiser group (KPNC) in collaboration with the National Institutes of Health scientists.[13] The information from this study allowed for comparison with the data from the ALTS trial from 2003, which was used extensively to generate guidelines for the management of women with low-grade abnormalities. The KPNC study is an observational study with a follow-up length of 8 years. Use of this large data set enabled the most recent consensus conference to modify and refine guidelines currently in use. Many of the trends we have seen in cervical cancer screening, treatment, and follow-up continue in the newest guidelines; time intervals between testing is increased, use of cotesting is encouraged, and the treatment of young women is not recommended. Of note, consensus conference participants agreed that the ASCCP's 2006 guidelines remain valid except for the specific areas modified by the new guidelines.[11]

The discussion of the ASCCP's new guidelines in this article is based on the article by Massad and colleagues,[12] which is in press at the time of this writing. From here on, these new guidelines are referred to as the ASCCP's 2012 guidelines. There are 2 important items to remember about the guidelines. First, for all of the ASCCP's guidelines, when the term *HPV testing* is used, it refers to the use of validated HPV tests. The results of HPV tests should only indicate whether high-risk HPV types are present; there is no clinical usefulness to knowing if low-risk HPV types are present. Laboratory-specific or nonvalidated HPV tests may provide inaccurate results. HPV genotyping is mentioned in the guidelines; again, only validated HPV genotyping tests should be used. Secondly, the ASCCP's guidelines use the terms *recommended*, *preferred*, *acceptable,* and *not recommended*. This terminology indicates the relative strength of evidence behind the guideline. Items that are designated as *recommended* and *preferred* have stronger evidence than those designated as *acceptable*. Items noted as *not recommended* are not supported by evidence.

ASCCP'S 2012 GUIDELINES FOR LSIL CYTOLOGY

New information included in the 2012 guidelines incorporate recommendations for patients who undergo cotesting with cytology and HPV testing. The previous guideline recommendation for a woman with a cytologic diagnosis of LSIL was direct referral for colposcopy in adult women (not pregnant, adolescent, or postmenopausal). The diagnosis of LSIL is an indirect indicator of HPV positivity; close to 80% of women with LSIL on cytology will be HPV positive.[14] There will, however, be some women who are HPV negative with an LSIL Papanicolaou test when they undergo cotesting. The ASCCP's 2012 guidelines state that for those women who have undergone cotesting, if the Papanicolaou test shows LSIL and HPV is negative, women preferably should have repeat cotesting in 1 year. If in 1 year the cytology is atypical squamous cells of uncertain significance (ASC-US) or greater or if HPV is positive, patients should have a colposcopy. If, however, both cytology and HPV testing are negative at this follow-up, repeat cotesting should occur in 3 years. Repeat cotesting in 1 year after a negative HPV, but LSIL cytology is the preferred follow-up according to the new guidelines; but it is still acceptable for patients to be sent directly to colposcopy.

Another new area in the ASCCP's 2012 guidelines includes the management of young women, aged 21 to 24 years. The ASCCP's previous guidelines have offered management recommendations for adolescent women. The most recent cervical cancer screening guidelines from multiple US groups (US Preventative Services Task Force, American Congress of Obstetricians and Gynecologists, and the ASCCP) recommend that screening start at 21 years of age. Therefore, most adolescents should not be having Papanicolaou testing performed. The risk of cervical cancer in women younger than 25 years is very low (1.4 per 100 000 women annually); but in the United States, this level of risk is considered high enough to justify routine screening for women aged 21 years and older.[15] Women in young age groups are frequently HPV positive; however, their HPV-related lesions are more likely to regress.[16] With this evidence in mind, the ASCCP's 2012 guidelines recommend that women aged 21 to 24 years who have LSIL on cytology should follow up with repeat cytology yearly for 2 years. If the first repeat cytology shows ASC-H or HSIL, colposcopy is recommended. Women who have ASC-US or worse at the second repeat cytology (2 years) should undergo colposcopy. If women aged 21 to 24 years have 2 negative cytology results after their initial LSIL cytology, they may return to routine screening. This new guideline allows young women the time for their lesion to regress while protecting them from tests and treatment that may cause distress or have an impact on future childbearing.

For pregnant women with LSIL cytology, the new guidelines do not suggest many changes to current practice. The ASCCP's 2006 guidelines recommend colposcopy for women who have LSIL on cytology in pregnancy, with the option of waiting to perform colposcopy at 6 weeks post partum considered acceptable. In the new guidelines, recommendations remain the same except that women aged 21 to 24 years with LSIL cytology during pregnancy should be followed with cytology at 12-month intervals as discussed earlier in the recommendations for nonpregnant women aged 21 to 24 years. Endocervical curettage is not recommended in pregnancy. For those women who do have colposcopy during pregnancy, the colposcopy should not be repeated unless CIN II or worse is suspected cytologically, histologically, or colposcopically. Follow-up post partum is recommended for those without suspicion of CIN II or worse.

The recommendations for postmenopausal women with LSIL cytology remain unchanged in the new guidelines. These women can be triaged to an HPV test, cytologic testing at 6 and 12 months, or direct referral to colposcopy. If HPV testing returns negative or no dysplasia is identified on colposcopically directed biopsy, retesting with cytology in 1 year is recommended. If patients choose the option of repeat cytologic testing at 6 and 12 months, they should be referred for colposcopy if either of those tests show ASC-US or greater. If not, she may return to routine screening.

ASCCP'S 2012 GUIDELINES FOR CIN I HISTOLOGY

Low-grade disease in the cervix indicates an HPV infection as opposed to high-grade disease, which is associated with the integration of HPV into the host genome. The term for low-grade HPV infection in histologic terms is CIN I (or LSIL according to the LAST guidelines). These terms refer to the fact that HPV has infected cervical epithelium but that the cellular changes associated with dysplasia are visible only in the lower one-third of the epithelium. Patients with CIN I have a high chance of disease regression and a generally low chance of high-grade or precancerous disease in the next 5 years. The risk of finding high-grade disease in patients who are diagnosed with CIN I on colposcopically directed biopsy is related to the relative degree of abnormality that was noted in the cytologic test leading to the colposcopy. In the KPNC study, investigators evaluated women who had CIN I on biopsy after an abnormal cytology result and looked at the risk of finding high-grade disease (CIN III or worse) within the next 5 years. For women with initial cytology showing LSIL or ASC-US with positive HPV, the risk was 3.8%. Those women whose initial cytology showed HSIL had a 5-year risk of CIN III or worse of 15%.[13] Therefore, management guidelines for women with a biopsy showing CIN I should take into consideration the severity of the Papanicolaou test preceding the colposcopy.

The ASCCP's new 2012 guidelines state that women with CIN I or no lesion on biopsy if preceded by a "lesser abnormality" (LSIL or ASC-US cytology) should be followed with cotesting in 1 year. If both are negative, patients may have age-appropriate routine screening in 3 years. If those tests are negative, patients should return to routine screening. If any of the tests results are abnormal, colposcopy is recommended. For those patients who have persistent CIN I on biopsy for 2 years, both treatment and continued follow-up is acceptable. CIN I should not be treated at the first biopsy, and hysterectomy as the primary treatment of CIN I on biopsy is not acceptable. Treatment can consist of ablation or excision depending on the practitioner's comfort level and the patients' characteristics. Ablation should not be used in cases when the colposcopy is unsatisfactory, if patients have CIN II or worse on endocervical sampling, or if patients have been previously treated for dysplasia.

If patients have CIN I on biopsy but the preceding cytology was ASC-H or HSIL, the follow-up is somewhat more intensive.

Similar to previous recommendations, the ASCCP's 2012 guidelines state that patients in this situation may have a diagnostic excisional procedure, follow-up, or a review of the findings. If excision is chosen, patients must have had a satisfactory colposcopy and negative endocervical sampling. The follow-up should be in the form of cotesting with cytology and HPV at 12 and 24 months. If both are normal, patients may wait for 3 years until the next cotest. If any of the cotesting results are abnormal at 12 or 24 months, patients should be referred for colposcopy. Cytology results showing HSIL at either the 12- or 24-month follow-up should cause patients to be sent for an excisional procedure.

A new area in the ASCCP's 2012 guidelines is a discussion of the management of the finding of CIN I on endocervical sampling. Previously, any dysplasia in an endocervical sample was cause for excisional treatment. More recent research shows that women with CIN I on endocervical sampling are at low risk for CIN II or worse.[17] The ASCCP's 2012 guidelines incorporate this evidence by recommending that women with CIN I found on endocervical sampling be treated as women with a biopsy diagnosis of CIN I. The treatment will depend on the severity of the preceding cytology. Women who have a follow-up should have endocervical sampling done as part of their follow-up at 1 year.

Women aged 21 to 24 years with CIN I on biopsy should be managed conservatively according to the ASCCP's 2012 guidelines. Those young women whose preceding cytology was ASC-US or LSIL should be followed with cytology only at 12-month intervals. Those with HSIL or ASC-H at 12 months or any continued abnormality at 24 months should have a colposcopy. Two consecutive negative tests should cause patients to return to routine screening. If the cytology before the diagnosis of CIN I on histology was HSIL or ASC-H, patients should have every-6-month cytology and colposcopy for 2 years. If CIN II or worse is diagnosed histologically, patient care should follow the ASCCP's relevant guideline. If CIN II or worse is suspected colposcopically or cytologically, a biopsy should be done. If cytology shows HSIL for 2 years but no CIN II or worse is found histologically, a diagnostic excisional procedure is recommended. It is important to note that CIN I should not be treated in women aged 21 to 24 years.

SUMMARY

The release of new guidelines for the management of abnormal cervical cytology and histology has occurred twice since the ASCCP's first guidelines were released in 2001. Continually updating guidelines ensures that clinicians practice at the cutting edge of science as the results of new studies become available. The ASCCP's new 2012 guidelines for the management of LSIL on cytology and CIN I histology were written after the analysis of data from large numbers of patients in the KPNC study. These guidelines help to clarify the appropriate uses of cervical cancer screening tests. The use of cotesting for the follow-up of patients with abnormal cytology results is addressed. In addition, cotesting is used as a follow-up method more frequently in the new guidelines. The trend toward avoiding the treatment of low-grade disease and unnecessary procedures for young women is continued in these guidelines. Clinicians should be aware that the ASCCP's 2012 guidelines offer specific and evidence-based recommendations for the care of women with abnormalities in cervical cancer screening.

REFERENCES

1. Davey DD, Neal MH, Wilbur DC, et al. Bethesda 2001implementation and reporting rate: 2003 practices of participants in the College of American Pathologists Interlaboratory Comparison Program in Cervicovaginal Cytology. Arch Pathol Lab Med 2004;128:1224–9.
2. Arbyn M, Sasieni P, Meijer CJ, et al. Chapter 9: clinical applications of HPV testing: a summary of meta-analyses. Vaccine 2005;24(Suppl 3):S78–9.
3. Tjaima WA, Van Waes TR, Van den Eeden LE, et al. Role of human papillomavirus in the carcinogenesis of squamous cell carcinoma and adenocarcinoma of the cervix. Best Pract Res Clin Obstet Gynaecol 2005;19:469–83.
4. Evans MF, Adamson CS, Papillo JL, et al. Distribution of human papillomavirus types in ThinPrep Papanicolaou tests classified according to the Bethesda 2001 terminology and correlations with patient age and biopsy outcomes. Cancer 2006;106:1054–64.
5. Doorbar J. Molecular biology of human papillomavirus infection and cervical caner. Clin Sci (Lond) 2006;110:525–41.
6. Rodriguez AC, Schiffman M, Herrero R, et al. Rapid clearance of human papillomavirus and implications for clinical focus on persistent infections. J Natl Cancer Inst 2008;100(7):513–7.
7. Stanley M. Pathology and epidemiology of HPV infection in females. Gynecol Oncol 2010;117(Suppl 2):S5–10. http://dx.doi.org/10.1016/j.ygyno.2010.01.024.
8. Soloman D, Davey D, Kurman R, et al. The 2001 Bethesda System: terminology for reporting results of cervical cytology. JAMA 2002;287:2114–9.
9. Stoler MH, Schiffman M. Interobserver reproducibility of cervical cytologic and histologic interpretations: realistic estimates from the ASCUS-LSIL triage study. JAMA 2001;285:1500–5.

10. Darragh TM, Colgan TJ, Cox JT, et al. The lower anogenital squamous terminology standardization project for HPV-associated lesions: background and consensus recommendations from the College of American Pathologists and the American Society for Colposcopy and Cervical Pathology. J Low Genit Tract Dis 2012; 16(3):205–42.
11. Saslow D, Solomon D, Lawson HW, et al. American Cancer Society, American Society for Clinical Pathology screening guidelines for the prevention and early detection of cervical cancer. CA Cancer J Clin 2012;62:147–72.
12. Massad LS, Einstein MH, Huh WK, et al. 2012 ASCCP Consensus Guidelines Conference. 2012 updated consensus guidelines for the management of abnormal cervical cancer screening tests and cancer precursors. Obstet Gynecol 2013;121(4):829–46.
13. Katki HA, Schiffman M, Castle PE, et al. Benchmarking CIN3+ risk as the basis for incorporating HPV and Pap contesting into cervical screening and management guidelines. J Lower Genit Tract Dis 2013;17(5 Suppl 1):S28–35.
14. Arbyn M, Sasieni P, Meijer CJ, et al. Chapter 9: clinical applications of HPV testing: a summary of meta-analyses. Vaccine 2006;24(Suppl 3):S78–89.
15. Benard VB, Watson M, Castle PE, et al. Cervical cancer rates among young females in the U.S. Obstet Gynecol 2012;120:1117–23.
16. Moscicki AB, Hills N, Shiboski S, et al. Risks for incident human papillomavirus infection and low grade squamous intraepithelial lesion development in young females. JAMA 2001;285:2995–3002.
17. Petersen S, Belnap C, Larsen WI, et al. Grading of squamous dysplasia in endocervical curettage specimens: the case for conservative management of mild endocervical dysplasia. J Reprod Med 2007;52:917–21.

Treatment Options for High-Grade Squamous Intraepithelial Lesions

Stephanie Long, MD, Lawrence Leeman, MD, MPH*

KEYWORDS

- Human papillomavirus • High-grade squamous intraepithelial lesion
- Cervical intraepithelial neoplasia • Cervical cancer • "See and treat" • Cryotherapy
- Loop electrosurgical excision procedure • Cold knife conization

KEY POINTS

- Treatment of young women with the human papilloma virus (HPV) vaccination is strongly recommended, ideally before sexual debut; however, vaccination does not change screening or treatment recommendations.
- Young women with grade 2 cervical intraepithelial neoplasia (CIN 2) can be managed conservatively with colposcopy and Papanicolaou smear every 6 months for up to two years.
- A "see and treat" diagnostic excisional procedure (eg, loop electrosurgical excision procedure [LEEP]) following high-grade cytology rather than colposcopy is an option for women who are neither pregnant nor "young" in absolute years (21–24 years), or reproductively young with plans for future conception.
- Risk for preterm labor in a subsequent pregnancy is moderately increased by diagnostic excisional procedures (ie, LEEP excision); however, there may be an increased risk in women with cervical dysplasia with or without treatment.
- Cotesting with Papanicolaou and high-risk HPV testing is recommended at 12 and 24 months after treatment for a high-grade squamous intraepithelial lesion (HSIL). If negative, perform cotesting at 3 years and if negative, return to routine screening.
- Women treated for HSIL are considered at higher risk for recurrent disease for 20 years after treatment, and surveillance should continue beyond age 65 years if indicated.

INTRODUCTION

Over the last few decades our understanding about the natural history of cervical dysplasia has advanced greatly. Initial human papilloma virus (HPV) infection is rapidly cleared in most immunocompetent women. With the introduction of testing for

No disclosures.
No conflicts of interest.
Department of Family & Community Medicine, University of New Mexico, MSC09 5040, 1 University of New Mexico, Albuquerque, NM 87131, USA
* Corresponding author. Departments of Family & Community Medicine; Obstetrics & Gynecology.
E-mail address: lleeman@salud.unm.edu

Obstet Gynecol Clin N Am 40 (2013) 291–316
http://dx.doi.org/10.1016/j.ogc.2013.03.004
0889-8545/13/$ – see front matter © 2013 Elsevier Inc. All rights reserved.

obgyn.theclinics.com

high-risk HPV types, including subtyping for HPV-16 and HPV-18, and the introduction of P16 immunostaining of grade 2 cervical intraepithelial neoplasia (CIN 2) histologic specimens, it is possible to more accurately characterize the risk of progression versus regression for a particular cytologic or histologic sample. Observation with serial cytology or colposcopic examinations over time is now considered appropriate for women with low-grade cytologic and histologic lesions, as well as for women during pregnancy or for young women with certain high-grade lesions.

This article identifies the criteria for treatment of high-grade squamous lesions, and discusses the advantages and disadvantages of each type of treatment modality with an emphasis on the loop electrosurgical excision procedure (LEEP), which has become the predominant technique for the treatment of cervical dysplasia. The short-term and long-term complications and current recommendations for posttreatment follow-up are presented. The management of high-grade lesions is first addressed, followed by the specific treatment options for CIN. Equally as important as knowing how to perform cryotherapy or LEEP is knowing when to perform these procedures.

Current controversies in the treatment of CIN 2 and CIN 3 are discussed, including:

1. Is CIN 2 a distinct category, or should these lesions be histologically classified as either low-grade or high-grade intraepithelial lesions?
2. How does the management of high-grade squamous intraepithelial lesion (HSIL) differ in young women?
3. How does treatment failure differ between excision and ablative methods?
4. What is the risk of preterm labor after treatment?
5. What are the recommendations for follow-up after treatment of high-grade squamous lesions?

The authors have incorporated the 2012 American Society for Colposcopy and Cervical Pathology (ASCCP) guidelines and The Lower Anogenital Squamous Terminology (LAST) project's 2012 report.[1]

EPIDEMIOLOGY OF HPV

The National Health and Nutrition Examination Survey (NHANES) data from 2003/2004 estimated the overall prevalence of HPV in women aged 14 to 59 years at 26.8% (95% confidence interval [CI] 23.3%–30.9%).[2] Review of the same samples in 2006 showed an increase in HPV prevalence to 46.8%, owing to improved detection techniques.[3] The highest prevalence is among women aged 20 to 24, increasing each year from age 14 to 20 and decreasing from age 24 through 59.[2] HPV genotypes are subdivided into low-risk or nononcogenic types and high-risk or oncogenic types. HPV-6, -11, -40, -42, -43, -44, -54, -61, -72, and -81 are low-risk or nononcogenic.[4] HPV-16, -18, -31, -33, -35, -39, -45, -51, -52, -56, -58, -59, -68, -69, and -82 are high-risk or oncogenic subtypes.[4] HPV-16 and HPV-18 are responsible for about 50% of HSIL pathology, with HPV -16 causing 45.3% and HPV-18 causing 6.9%. HPV-16 and HPV-18 are responsible for about 70% of invasive cervical cancer, irrespective of geographic locale.[5] Independent risk factors for HPV positivity include young age, single marital status, and increased number of sexual partners.

MANAGEMENT OF HIGH-GRADE LESIONS

HSIL cytology is relatively uncommon, representing 0.6% of specimens,[6] however, an HSIL Papanicolaou (Pap) smear result carries significant prognostic information. Patients with HSIL cytology who have either a colposcopically directed cervical biopsy or a specimen from an excisional procedure will have CIN grade 2 or 3 on 70% to 75% of these histologic specimens.[7] **Table 1** demonstrates the risk of persistent HPV, progression to CIN, and risk of cancer with each grade of CIN.

CIN 2 has traditionally been grouped with CIN 3 in management algorithms, and treated in a similar fashion. The 2006 ASCCP guidelines offered the option of surveillance rather than treatment for CIN 2 in young women. The LAST project was jointly sponsored by the College of American Pathologists (CAP) and the ASCCP, and included 5 working groups whose goal was to standardize the terminology for HPV-associated lesions of the cervix, vagina, vulva, and anus. As reported by Waxman and colleagues,[8] CIN 2 represents "a heterogeneous mix that includes some [biopsies] that could arguably by called CIN 1 and some that other pathologists would call CIN 3." As a result, the LAST project recommended the use of p16 immunostaining to better differentiate oncogenic lesions from benign look-alikes.[8] CIN 2 can be dichotomized by p16 into a low-grade squamous intraepithelial lesion (LSIL) category with a low risk of progression and a higher rate of regression, and an HSIL category with a high risk of persistence and progression toward invasive cancer. In recognition of the heterogeneity of histologic specimens currently labeled as CIN 2, the LAST project has recommended revision of the histologic classification terminology and management by eliminating CIN 2 as a discrete category, instead using the terms LSIL and HSIL for histologic specimens. In addition, LAST recommended standardization of the terminology for cervical, vulvar, vaginal, and anal histology.

The ASCCP released new consensus management guidelines for cervical pathology in March 2013, which delineate management recommendations after colposcopic examination. The guidelines as they pertain to high-grade dysplasia are outlined in **Table 2**. The management is based primarily on the histologic diagnosis; however, it is influenced by the index cytologic diagnosis, age and future fertility plans, pregnancy, and presence of a satisfactory colposcopic examination or evidence of endocervical dysplasia. Unless otherwise stated, the recommendations as outlined here are taken from the ASCCP 2012 Consensus guidelines for the management of cervical pathology.[9] General recommendations for HSIL cytology and CIN 2 or CIN 3 histology are presented in **Table 2**, and any modifications for young women and pregnant women are then addressed.[10] A colposcopy should be performed after receiving a Pap result with the following cytologic diagnoses: HPV-positive atypical squamous cells (ASC) of undetermined significance (ASCUS), LSIL, HSIL, ASC-H (ie, ASC and cannot rule out HSIL), or atypical glandular cells (AGC).

Table 1			
Grade of cervical intraepithelial neoplasia and risk of progression over lifetime			
Degree of Cervical Intraepithelial Neoplasia	Risk of Persistent HPV	Risk of Progression to CIN 3	Risk of Progression to Cervical Cancer
CIN 1	30%	10%	1%
CIN 2	40%	20%	5%
CIN 3	n/a	n/a	12%

Abbreviation: n/a, not applicable.

Data from Padilla-Paz LA, Carlson J, Twiggs LB, et al. Evidence supporting the current management guidelines for high-grade squamous intraepithelial lesion cytology. J Low Genit Tract Dis 2004;8(2):139–46.

Table 2
Summary of 2013 ASCCP recommendations for high-grade dysplasia

Group	Colposcopy Diagnosis[a]	Management Options	Follow-Up
Women >25 y old and nonpregnant	CIN 1 or no lesion in setting of prior HSIL or ASC-H Pap	1. Cotesting at 12 and 24 mo	If HPV (−) and cytology negative at both time points, may return to routine screening. If HPV (+) or any abnormal cytology at level of ASCUS/HPV or worse, proceed to colposcopy. If negative at 12 and 24 months, then patient may resume routine screening.
			If HPV (+) or any abnormal cytology at level of ASCUS/HPV or worse, proceed to colposcopy. If HSIL at any time, proceed to diagnostic excisional procedure.
		2. Diagnostic excisional procedure	Negative margins and ECC: cotesting at 12 and 24 mo; if negative results x 2, may repeat cotesting in 3 y; if normal, may return to routine screening. If CIN1, see above recommendations for follow up. If CIN2/3 identified at margins or ECC positive, repeat cytology and ECC preferred at 4–6 mo, but repeat excision is acceptable or hysterectomy is acceptable alternative if reexcision not possible. If any follow-up test is abnormal, proceed to colposcopy and endocervical sampling.
		3. Review of material	Leading to change in diagnosis. Follow-up as recommended in ASCCP 2012 guidelines
	CIN 2 or 3	Adequate colposcopy: Excision or Ablation of the T-zone	Follow up as outlined above for diagnostic excisional procedure
		Inadequate colposcopy or recurrent CIN2/3 or ECC (+): Diagnostic Excisional Procedure	
		Inadequate colposcopy, recurrent CIN 2/3 or ECC (1)	

Pregnant women	CIN 1 or no lesion after HSIL or ASC-H Pap	Observation with colposcopy and cytology in postpartum period	Follow-up per ASCCP guidelines with repeat cytology and colposcopy
	CIN 2 or 3	Observation with colposcopy and cytology at time of diagnosis and postpartum period	Follow-up per ASCCP guidelines with repeat cytology and colposcopy
	Inadequate colposcopy	Observation with colposcopy and cytology in postpartum period	Follow-up per ASCCP guidelines with repeat cytology and colposcopy
Young women (<25 y with anticipated future fertility)	CIN 1 or no lesion in setting of prior HSIL or ASC-H Pap	Observation with colposcopy and cytology at 6-mo intervals for up to 24 mo	If HSIL or high grade colposcopic lesion persists for 1 year, then biopsy. If biopsy is CIN2 or 3, manage per ASCCP guidelines young women with CIN2,3. If biopsy is CIN1, continue observation.
			If HSIL persists for 24 months without CIN2,3 identified, proceed to Diagnostic Excisional Procedure
			Other results, manage per ASCCP guidelines
			If two consecutive cytology negative results and no high grade lesion on colposcopy, then may resume routine screening
	CIN 2	*Preferred:* Observation with colposcopy and cytology at 6-mo intervals for 12 mo	If negative cytology × 2 and normal colposcopy, may repeat cotest in 1 y. If both negative at that time, may cotest in 3 y. If any test abnormal, colposcopy worsens, or high-grade cytology persist for 1 y, repeat colposcopy and biopsy recommended. After that if CIN 3 or CIN 2/3 persist for 24 mo, treatment recommended.
		Acceptable: treatment using excision or ablation of T-zone	Follow-up as for women ≥ 25 years undergoing diagnostic excisional procedure
	CIN 3 or inadequate colposcopy	*Preferred:* Treatment using excision or ablation of T-zone	Follow-up as for women ≥ 25 years undergoing diagnostic excisional procedure
		Acceptable: observation with colposcopy and cytology at 6-mo intervals for 12 mo	If negative cytology × 2 and normal colposcopy, may repeat cotest in 1 y. If both negative at that time, may cotest in 3 y. If any test abnormal, colposcopy worsens, or high-grade cytology persist for 1 y, repeat colposcopy and biopsy recommended. After that if CIN 3 or CIN 2/3 persist for 24 mo, treatment recommended.

[a] Colposcopic diagnosis based on cervical biopsy and endocervical curettage when done.
Data from Wright TC, Cox JT, Massad LS, et al. 2012 Consensus guidelines for the management of cervical intraepithelial neoplasia. J Low Genit Tract Dis 2013;17(5):S1-27.

HSIL or ASC-H Cytology with Biopsy-Confirmed CIN 1 or Without a Lesion

If CIN 1 is identified on cervical biopsy after an HSIL or ASC-H cytology with a satisfactory colposcopy, three management approaches are acceptable: (1) observation with cytology and HPV ("cotesting") at 12 and 24 months, (2) diagnostic excisional procedure, or (3) a second review of the histology that may result in a change in the diagnosis. If cotesting results at 12 and 24 months are cytology and HPV negative, the patient should have a repeat Pap in 3 years. If at 12 or 24 months either the HPV is positive or there is any abnormality other than HSIL, colposcopy is recommended. If HSIL is subsequently identified at either time point, a diagnostic excision procedure is recommended.

After an HSIL Pap with inadequate colposcopy or positive endocervical curettage (ECC), an excisional procedure is recommended to simultaneously obtain a specimen for diagnosis and treat any potential dysplasia. The colposcopic examination is only considered "satisfactory" if the entire squamocolumnar junction can be visualized. If the entire squamocolumnar junction is not visualized the colposcopy is "unsatisfactory." Areas with a colposcopic impression of dysplasia are biopsied.

Biopsy-Confirmed CIN 2 or CIN 3

If CIN 2 or CIN2/3 is the histologic diagnosis from a cervical biopsy with an adequate colposcopy then either excision or ablation of the transformation zone is recommended unless the woman is pregnant, or if she is either young in absolute years (21–24 years) or reproductively young in that pregnancy is desired in the future. If the biopsy shows CIN 3, treatment is recommended regardless of the woman's age or future desire for fertility. If a biopsy from an unsatisfactory colposcopy returns with CIN 2 or CIN 3, if the CIN 2 or CIN 3 is recurrent, or if endocervical sampling reveals CIN 2 or CIN 3, a diagnostic excisional procedure is the next step. An ablative procedure is not appropriate in these situations because of the potential for missing endocervical dysplasia.

Option for immediate LEEP or "see and treat"

"See and treat" refers to the option to perform an excisional procedure with a LEEP after HSIL cytology without prior colposcopy. Most women with HSIL cytology will ultimately have a treatment procedure either because histology confirms CIN 2/3 or there is lack of concordance between the HSIL Pap and histology. Proceeding directly to an excisional LEEP has the advantage of decreasing the number of visits, minimizing the risk of loss to follow-up, and providing specimens for histology diagnosis to rule out undetected invasive cancer. See and treat is particularly advantageous in groups at risk for loss to follow-up owing to geographic or financial barriers or a history of poor adherence, as well as risk factors for persistence. Despite the advantages, see and treat is not appropriate for all patients.

Special treatment groups: young women and pregnancy

Pregnant patients are not candidates for a LEEP, given the risk to the pregnancy and blood loss.[11] Dysplasia has a high rate of regression after pregnancy, as demonstrated by Cubo-Abert and colleagues[12] in their study that followed 40 pregnant women with LSIL and 40 women with HSIL. Overall regression rates were 32.5% (45% for LSIL and 20% HSIL) between first screening in pregnancy and 6 to 8 weeks postpartum, with the highest rates observed in patients younger than 25 years. In patients older than 25 years, the HSIL regression rate was 20% with a 2-fold increased risk of progression/persistence, compared with younger women up to the age of 25, although there was no progression to invasive disease.[12] HPV subtyping of these lesions revealed that samples positive for HPV-16 had a rate of regression of 9.5% compared with 52.2% for HPV-16 negative lesions,[12] underscoring the oncogenic potential of some HPV subtypes. These results highlight that follow-up for LSIL and HSIL lesions in pregnancy can be safely delayed until the postpartum period.

Young women represent another special treatment group. Current ASCCP guidelines set the minimum age for cervical cancer screening at 21 years,[11] hence the category of "adolescent and young women" has been changed to simply "young women." Although some have proposed that young women should be defined as those 21 to 24 years of age, desired future fertility must also be considered when determining treatment plans.

CIN 2 in young women is associated with a high rate of regression. Moscicki and colleagues[13] looked at 95 patients with CIN 2 with a mean age of 20.4 ± 2.3 years over a 3-year time frame to assess progression and regression in younger women. Rates of regression were 38% by year 1, 63% by year 2, and 68% by year 3.[13] Only 15% of patients had progression of disease by year 3, and HPV-16 or HPV-18 positivity was associated with progression.[13] This finding fits with our current understanding about the nature of CIN 2, which can behave like CIN 1 or CIN 3 depending on the presence of certain biomarkers. Given the high rates of regression over time, the low risk for progression to invasive disease, and concerns for the effect of treatment on future pregnancies, it is not recommended to proceed directly to a see-and-treat excisional procedure in young women.[11]

After ASC-H or HSIL cytology in a young woman leads to an adequate colposcopy with no lesion identified or CIN 1, then observation with colposcopy and cytology are recommended at 6 month intervals for up to two years. If observation is pursued and both time points yield negative results, the patient may return to routine screening after 1 year. If the colposcopy is not satisfactory, a diagnostic excisional procedure is recommended.

After ASC-H or HSIL in young women with subsequent CIN 2 or CIN 3 histology and a satisfactory colposcopy, the options are either excision or ablation of the transformation zone or observation with colposcopy and cytology at 6 and 12 months. If the histologic diagnosis specifically states CIN 2 then observation is preferred, and if it specifies CIN 3 then excision is preferred. If observation is chosen, and at any point in the first year colposcopy has worsened or if HSIL persists, repeat colposcopy and biopsy are recommended. If these colposcopic examinations and cytology samples are negative, the patient may undergo a cotest in 1 year (or at the 24-month mark from index colposcopy). If the cotest results are normal then the patient may have a follow-up cotest in 3 years, and only then return to routine age-appropriate screening. However, if either cytology or HPV testing is abnormal at 1 year, repeat colposcopy and biopsy is recommended. If there is subsequent development of CIN 3, or CIN 2/3 persists for the 24 months of follow-up, excisional or ablative treatment is recommended.[9]

Women seropositive for human immunodeficiency virus

Women who are seropositive for human immunodeficiency virus (HIV) are at increased risk for CIN[14] in comparison with HIV-seronegative women. Resolution of CIN is also slower in HIV-seropositive women. However, despite their increased risk the overall progression to a high-grade lesion in HIV-seropositive women is still low, with only 5.9% of seropositive women developing a high-grade lesion in a study of 1639 women by Massad and colleagues.[14]

Young women with HIV disease also have low rates of progression to cervical cancer despite abnormal cytology. A prospective multicenter study of 132 adolescent HIV-seropositive women with normal cervical cytology at enrollment found that only

7% of women developed HSIL or CIN 2/3, with none developing invasive cervical cancer over a median of 2.6 years of observation.[15] This study supports the recommendation that young women with HIV be followed with the observational algorithms outlined in this article, rather than prophylactically treated with an ablative or excisional method.[15]

TREATMENT OPTIONS

Treatment options for high-grade lesions fall into two general categories: excisional (LEEP, cone knife biopsy) and ablative (cryotherapy, laser ablation). A 2010 Cochrane meta-analysis of 29 randomized controlled trials included 5441 women with CIN, and found no evidence to support one surgical method over another.[16] However, other studies such as the British Columbia Cancer cohort found greater failure rates for cryotherapy versus LEEP (see the section on outcomes after treatment).[17] In practice, there are histologic and patient factors that need to be considered when deciding on treatment modalities. As with any procedure, physicians should use methods for which they have received adequate training.

Cryotherapy

Cryotherapy uses a refrigerant under pressure, either carbon dioxide or nitrogen oxide, which provides cellular destruction through rapid freeze-thaw cycles.[18] The area of destruction depends on the size of the probe used and the lateral spread of the freeze zone evidenced by the ice crystals that form on the cryoprobe.[18] For example, 5 mm of spread beyond the probe tip ensures 5 mm depth of freeze.[18] In general, cryotherapy is recommended for smaller lesions that can be covered completely by the cryoprobe, are located in 1 or 2 quadrants, and do not extend into the endocervical canal.[18] The cryotherapy triage rules listed in **Box 1** are followed to determine when cryotherapy is an appropriate treatment.

Preprocedure counseling and consent forms should address the steps of the procedure, benefits, alternatives, and risks such as bleeding, infection, recurrence of disease, cervical stenosis, and injury to vaginal tissue (**Fig. 1**). Patients should be offered 600 to 800 mg of ibuprofen before the procedure. Patient consent forms must be signed, and all equipment must be readily available before performing cryotherapy. Recommended equipment should include, but is not limited to, the items listed in **Box 2**.

Patients are placed in the dorsal lithotomy position and a vaginal speculum is inserted. A vaginal side-wall retractor can be used if needed for visualization and to protect redundant vaginal tissue. The refrigerant should be turned on and checked

---

Box 1
Cryotherapy triage rules

Entire squamocolumnar junction must be visualized

Entire extent of lesion must be seen

CIN diagnosed by biopsy

Endocervical canal disease has been ruled out

Colposcopic impression, cytology, and histology correlate

Invasive disease is not present

Cryotherapy probe must cover lesion

CONSENT FOR COLPOSCOPY, CRYOTHERAPY AND / OR LEEP

Colposcopy: Colposcopy is recommended after an abnormal Pap smear. A microscope is used to take a look at the surface of the cervix, vulva or vagina after a small amount of vinegar solution is applied. If an area is abnormal, and you are not pregnant, then your provided will take a small biopsy, or pinch of tissue, at the abnormal spot to receive a more accurate diagnosis about the kind of cervical dysplasia, or change, that is present.

Cryotherapy: Cryotherapy is one method of treatment for precancerous lesions of the cervix. The abnormal tissue is visualized by colposcopy and frozen. It is a mildly uncomfortable procedure which produces menstrual like cramping. Very rarely is it described as very painful although each woman's response is unique. We recommend that all women take ibuprofen 600-800 mg prior to the procedure to help with cramping.

LEEP: Loop electrocautery excision procedure, or a LEEP, is an in office procedure that can be used to diagnose and / or treatment abnormalities of the cervix, vulva, and vaginal tissue. A local anesthetic is injected into the cervix to numb the cervix. Electric current is used to remove the abnormal tissue which is then sent to the pathologist for examination. LEEP aims to remove the entire transformation zone, or area of potential abnormal tissue, so that follow up biopsies and procedures can be lessened.

Risks of the above procedures include:
-**Bleeding:** since these procedures involve removing tissue, there may be some bleeding. Normally, this can be controlled using topical medication or a stitch if needed. Bleeding can show up as a late complication at 5 to 10 days. If bleeding heavier than a menstrual period occurs and persists, please contact our office.

-**Infection:** The cervix and vaginal rarely develop infections after colposcopy, cryotherapy or LEEP. If you develop unusual pain, discharge, heavy or excess bleeding, fever or foul smelling odor, please contact the office. To decrease the risk of infection, it is recommended that you do not use tampons, douche or have sexual intercourse for 1 week after a colposcopy and 3-4 weeks after LEEP or cryotherapy.

-**Cervical incompetence:** During a LEEP procedure, part of the cervix is removed. This has the potential to weaken the cervix and result in early dilation of the cervix during pregnancy. This risk increases with the number of LEEP procedures you have. Please discuss your plans for future pregnancies with your provider prior to undergoing a LEEP.

-**Residual disease:** Cryotherapy and LEEP cure rates are 90-95% but not 100%. Our goal is to destroy or remove all abnormal tissue. However, regular follow up is needed to ensure there is no recurrence of disease.

-**Cervical stenosis:** Although uncommon, the cervix can potentially narrow months after the procedure is performed which puts you at risk for retained blood in the uterus. This can be fixed by dilating the cervix. Please contact your provider if your periods are absent after your procedure.

-**Vaginal laceration or bowel / bladder injury:** There is a small risk of injury to the vaginal, bowel or bladder during your procedure. If it occurs, this would need to be fixed with a suture or additional procedures.

Regardless of the procedure you have today, it is vital that you follow up with your provider as she / he recommends. It is important that you notify us if your telephone number or address changes so we can keep in contact with you. Failure to comply with recommended treatment could place you at risk for progressive disease the possibility of developing cervical cancer.

Patient signature: _____   Date: _____

Witness signature: _____   Date: _____

Physician signature: _____   Date: _____

Fig. 1. Sample consent form for Colposcopy, Cryotherapy and LEEP.

Box 2
Cryotherapy equipment

Cryogun

Large nitrogen oxide or carbon dioxide tank with a pressure gauge and at least 20 psi pressure in the tank

Vaginal speculum

Vaginal wall retractors

Various sizes and shapes of cryotips (**Fig. 2**)

Water-soluble lubricating gel

Colposcope

Acetic acid or vinegar (3% or 5%)

Disinfectant for cryoprobes

---

to ensure that there is at least 20 pounds per square inch of pressure before starting the procedure, and all other instructions are followed according to the manufacturer's guidelines. An appropriately sized and shaped probe tip is selected and tightly secured in place, as shown in **Fig. 2**. However, the use of a probe tip that extends into the endocervix is not recommended because of an increased risk of cervical stenosis. Cryotherapy is completed using cycles of freeze-thaw-freeze. It is important to ensure that contact is maintained between the cryoprobe and the cervical tissue. The World Health Organization recommends a cycle of 3-minute freeze, 5-minute thaw, and 3-minute freeze (**Fig. 3**).[18] The probe must have thawed completely before removal, as the softer, central part of the freeze zone is friable and is a source of bleeding if disturbed.

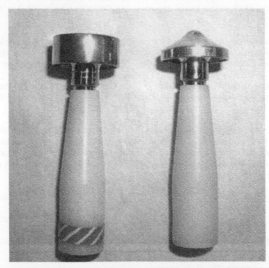

Fig. 2. Cryotherapy probes with various size tips. *From* Spitzer S, Brotzman GL, Apgar BS. Practical therapeutic options for treatment of cervical intraepithelial neoplasia. In: Apgar BS, Spitzer S, Brotzman GL, editors. Colposcopy, principles and practice. 2nd edition. Philadelphia: Saunders Elsevier; 2008; with permission.

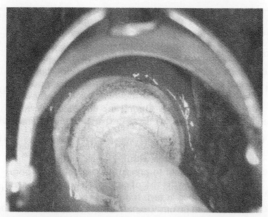

Fig. 3. Cryotherapy freeze cycle, showing extension of the freeze zone beyond the probe boundary. *From* Spitzer S, Brotzman GL, Apgar BS. Practical therapeutic options for treatment of cervical intraepithelial neoplasia. In: Apgar BS, Spitzer S, Brotzman GL, editors. Colposcopy, principles and practice. 2nd edition. Philadelphia: Saunders Elsevier; 2008; with permission.

Side effects from cryotherapy vary. Patients should be counseled to anticipate menstrual-like cramps, and some patients experience vasomotor symptoms such as flushing and light-headedness, with vasovagal syncope being rarer.[19] Aftercare instructions should be given to the patient. Many women experience vaginal bleeding (less than a menstrual flow), mild cramping, and brownish-black discharge at first and then a watery discharge that may last for 3 to 4 weeks.[19] Tampons, douching, and sexual intercourse should be avoided for up to 4 weeks after the procedure to avoid dislodging the eschar. Nahhas and colleagues[20] followed 36 women after cryotherapy in an attempt to evaluate removal of the eschar, with the aim of decreasing discharge after cryotherapy. Eighteen women were brought back at 72 hours for eschar removal. They found no statistical difference between discharge amounts or duration between the removal and standard follow-up group. The cervix heals by reepithelialization, which occurs in 47% of patients by 6 weeks and in all patients by 3 months.[21]

Loop Electrosurgical Excision Procedure

LEEP uses electric current to excise the entire transformation zone. It can be used for any degree of cervical dysplasia. LEEP has the advantages presented by Prendiville in 1995 and outlined in **Box 3**. Given the triage requirements and recommendations for the use of cryotherapy, LEEP may be the preferred modality for high-grade lesions in more than 2 quadrants, for lesions larger than the cryoprobe, lesions having an irregular ectocervical surface such that contact with the cryoprobe cannot be maintained, when there is endocervical disease, or if the dysplasia represents recurrence after previous treatment. Suspected invasive cancer, cervicitis, pregnancy, concurrent anticoagulation or hemorrhagic disorder, and presence of an implanted cardioverter-defibrillator and implantable loop recorder are contraindications to LEEP.

LEEP may be performed as an outpatient office procedure or in the operating room. The choice of setting may depend on where the physician has access to the appropriate equipment, the patient's preference for analgesia or anesthesia, and the anticipated technical difficulty of the procedure. A retrospective cohort study of 233 women compared 181 outpatient LEEPs with 52 inpatient LEEPs, looking at efficacy in the

> **Box 3**
> **LEEP advantages as published by Prendiville in 1995**
>
> It allows for histologic audit of the colposcopic diagnosis
>
> It allows histopathologic examination to rule out microinvasion
>
> It allows excision of the dysplastic lesion and the transformation zone, which may be confirmed histologically
>
> It may be performed at the first (assessment) colposcopic examination in selected patients
>
> It may be adapted to treat all cased of CIN, irrespective of the size and site of the transformation zone
>
> It is an easily learned technique
>
> It uses inexpensive, readily available equipment and has low operating costs
>
> It is usually an office or outpatient procedure performed using local anesthesia
>
> *Data from* Prendiville W. Large loop excision of the transformation zone. Clin Obstet Gynecol 1995;38:622–39.

sample obtained and complications such as hemorrhage and cervical stenosis.[22] Complications were comparable between groups, with the conclusion that inpatient and outpatient LEEPs were equally efficacious and safe.[22]

Although most women will do well with an outpatient LEEP procedure after oral analgesia and an intracervical block, those with a history of anxiety or panic attacks, substance abuse disorders, or difficult pelvic examinations consequent to a history of sexual abuse, may be best served by having the procedure in a setting where they can have conscious sedation with intravenous medications or general anesthesia. Women who may have a more difficult procedure owing to factors such as having had prior LEEP procedures resulting in the cervix now being almost flush with the vaginal mucosa, or morbid obesity requiring extensive retraction of the vaginal mucosa to visualize the cervix, may also be best served by an operating room setting.

Preprocedure counseling and consent forms should address the steps of the procedure, benefits, alternatives, and risks such as bleeding, infection, recurrence of disease, preterm delivery in future pregnancies, and injury to vaginal tissue or surrounding organs. Patients should be offered 600 to 800 mg of ibuprofen or another nonsteroidal anti-inflammatory medication before the procedure. In selected cases additional oral or intravenous medications may be used in the outpatient setting with appropriate monitoring, including opioids and benzodiazepines. Recommended equipment includes, but is not limited to, items listed in **Box 4** and shown in **Figs. 4–10**.

To perform a LEEP, the patient is placed in the dorsal lithotomy position, and a nonconductive speculum is placed in the vagina and connected to smoke evacuation tubing. A vaginal side-wall retractor may be needed if vaginal mucosa obscures visualization or access to the cervix. Lugol solution is used to both delineate the transformation zone and provide antisepsis. The transformation zone is visualized with a colposcope and the appropriately sized loop is chosen. There are various loop sizes and shapes available. A 20- by 8-mm loop is the most common choice in the United States; however, on occasion a smaller cervical transformation zone may be completely removed in a single pass with a 15- by 8-mm loop. An intracervical block is performed using a local anesthetic agent such as 1% lidocaine mixed with epinephrine or vasopressin, to provide vasoconstriction to decrease bleeding and extend the

Box 4
LEEP equipment
Electrosurgical generator (see **Fig. 4**)
Patient grounding (dispersive) pad
Insulated electrode handle
Nonconductive speculum with smoke-evacuator port (see **Fig. 5**)
Nonconductive vaginal side-wall reactor (see **Figs. 6** and **7**)
Smoke evacuator and filter system (see **Fig. 8**),
Insulated ring forceps
Insulated tenaculum
Various sizes and shapes of loop electrodes (see **Fig. 9**)
Ball electrode (3 mm, 5 mm sizes) (see **Fig. 10**)
Colposcope
Acetic acid or vinegar (3% or 5%)
Lugol solution
Monsel paste or gel
Large cotton swabs
Local anesthetic with vasopressin or epinephrine for intracervical block
Syringe with 27-gauge needle
Needle extender
Specimen bottles with 10% buffered formalin
Suturing equipment (if needed): long needle holder, forceps, and absorbable suture

length of analgesia. One technique is to inject one mL at 12, 3, 6, and 9 o'clock with 0.5 mL placed between these injection sites. The injection should be superficial with a depth of 3 to 4 mm. The use of vasopressin rather than epinephrine for vasoconstriction may avoid the anxiety that often occurs after epinephrine injection. Under direct colposcopic guidance and in a smooth motion moving from top to bottom, the entire transformation zone is removed in a single pass if possible (**Fig. 11**). If the transformation zone is too wide to be completely removed on a single pass with a 20- by 8-mm loop, the central transformation zone can be removed in the first pass, followed by removal of the remaining lateral margins of the transformation zone in separate passes on each lateral margin.

In the case of a lesion that is suspected to extend into the endocervix based on a prior positive endocervical curettage or colposcopic visualization, or in the instance where the entire transformation zone cannot be seen, a "top-hat" or "cowboy-hat" LEEP technique may be indicated.[23] In this situation the cervical transformation zone is removed as described with a 20- by 8-mm loop. Next, the cervical os is visualized and a 10- by 10-mm loop used to remove the endocervical canal as a separate specimen. The cervical os must be carefully identified after the initial removal of the cervical transformation zone, to assure a symmetric specimen that includes 360° removal of the endocervical canal. In general, less cervical tissue is removed with the top hat than with a cold knife conization.[24] Previously, a second pass has been recommended for a lack of concordance between cervical biopsy from colposcopy

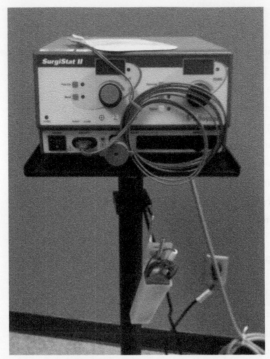

Fig. 4. Electrocautery unit. University of New Mexico, Family Medicine Center, Fall 2012.

and cytology. Lanneau and colleagues[25] undertook a study to determine the need for a 2-step (also known as a top-hat) procedure in this setting. The cohort included 59 patients with an HSIL diagnosis from a Pap smear, subsequently found to have no lesion or CIN 1 in their LEEP specimens. In this study, a second pass did not decrease

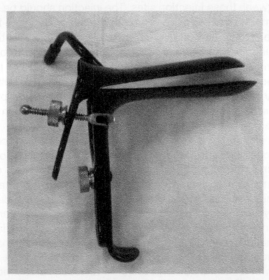

Fig. 5. Insulated speculum. University of New Mexico, Family Medicine Center, Fall 2012.

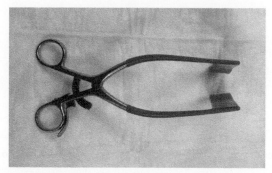

Fig. 6. Insulated side wall rectractor. University of New Mexico, Family Medicine Center, Fall 2012.

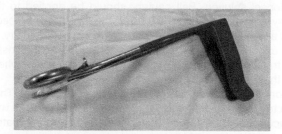

Fig. 7. Insulated side wall retractor (side view). University of New Mexico, Family Medicine Center. Fall 2012.

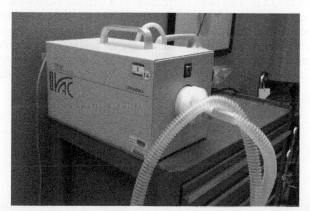

Fig. 8. Smoke evacuator unit. University of New Mexico, Family Medicine Center.

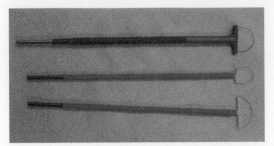

Fig. 9. Electrocautery loop tips, various sizes. University of New Mexico, Family Medicine Center, Fall 2012.

the discrepancy between a Pap and LEEP specimen, with 96% of second-pass LEEP specimens (*P*<.0001) having no lesion or only CIN 1 identified.

After the removal of the transformation zone and the endocervical canal when indicated, endocervical sampling curettage should be performed with a cytobrush or a metal endocervical curette. This is of particular importance when endocervical disease has been previously identified or suspected. After endocervical sampling, hemostasis of the cervix is typically achieved using ball electrocautery followed by the application of Monsel solution. Ball cautery should be applied to the ectocervical edge of the biopsy site while sparing the "crater" caused by the procedure. The crater area immediately around the cervical os is spared from electrocautery, as described in a study demonstrating a higher incidence of cervical stenosis and unsatisfactory visualization of the transformation zone on follow-up colposcopy when cautery was applied close to the cervical os.[26]

LEEP can be completed with an intrauterine device (IUD) in place. The strings can be moved from side to side or tucked into the canal and then retrieved with a cytobrush. Bailey and Darracott[27] also described a technique involving a sheath to protect the IUD strings in their article from 2010. In this study, a suture tie is placed on the IUD strings and is then threaded through the sheath (the hollow handle of a sterile absorbent-tipped applicator after removing the cotton tip), which is then passed into the cervix to a recommended depth of 2.5 cm. The loop excision is then performed, beginning at the 12 o'clock position and rotating clockwise around the sheath to the 6 o'clock position. The tube and electrocautery then switch hands and the excision continues in a clockwise fashion from 6 o'clock to 12 o'clock, still rotating around the sheath, until the LEEP has been completed in a circular clockwise fashion.[27] The plastic sheath of a spinal needle may also make an appropriate shield for IUD strings.

Immediate complications of LEEP such as bleeding and infection can occur in 1% to 2% of patients.[28] Bleeding at the post-LEEP cervical crater that is not controlled by the use of electrocautery and Monsel solution may require suture closure, although this is rarely needed. If the crater has continued oozing heavily despite the aforementioned

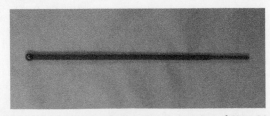

Fig. 10. Electrocautery roller ball coagulation tip. University of New Mexico, Family Medicine Center, Fall 2012.

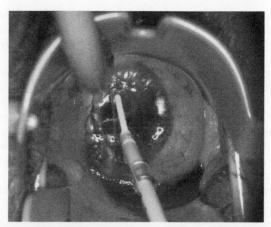

Fig. 11. LEEP probe in position. *From* Spitzer S, Brotzman GL, Apgar BS. Practical therapeutic options for treatment of cervical intraepithelial neoplasia. In: Apgar BS, Spitzer S, Brotzman GL, editors. Colposcopy, principles and practice. 2nd edition. Philadelphia: Saunders Elsevier; 2008; with permission.

treatments, the surgeon can attempt to achieve hemostasis by packing the crater with Monsel-soaked gauze or a hemostatic agent such as Surgicel™. In this scenario the speculum is then removed, leaving the gauze in place for 30 to 60 minutes before the speculum is replaced and the crater reexamined after gauze removal. A vaginal laceration can occur if the loop contacts the vaginal mucosa, as a result of either minimal clearance between the transformation zone and the vaginal mucosa or patient movement during the procedure. The vaginal laceration may become hemostatic with pressure and Monsel solution; however, a suture may be needed in this scenario. The LEEP surgeon should have ready access to the equipment needed to suture the vaginal mucosa or cervix, including a long needle holder, tissue forceps, and an absorbable suture on a large needle (such as 2-0 polyglactin on a CT-1 needle). Although it is possible to inadvertently enter the bladder or rectum through the vaginal mucosa, these injuries are fortunately extremely rare, with a single bowel injury documented in the authors' review of the literature.[29]

Patients should be instructed that a heavy, brown, and sometimes malodorous discharge can occur for up to 2 to 3 weeks. Tampons, douching, and sexual intercourse should be avoided for up to 4 weeks after the procedure to avoid dislodging the eschar. Complications in the weeks after LEEP include late bleeding and infection. Excess bleeding may also occur days to weeks after the LEEP procedure is completed, if the eschar detaches at the site of a cervical vessel. Late bleeding is described in 2% to 4% of women.[30–32] In the authors' experience it is not uncommon for women to present with a concern for infection in the days and weeks after a LEEP procedure because of a persistent, sometimes malodorous discharge. However, actual infection appears to be uncommon, although the incidence is not well described in the literature. Prophylactic antibiotics are not indicated before LEEP; nevertheless, screening for sexually transmitted infections, based on age and risk, is appropriate. Patients should be given clear instructions on when to seek urgent care and/or contact the surgeon performing the LEEP. Soaking a pad per hour for 2 hours would be an indication for seeking urgent evaluation, and bleeding continuing beyond 3 to 4 weeks should lead to an office examination.

Delayed complications include cervical stenosis, leading to difficultly performing future Pap smears and obtaining adequate colposcopic examinations. Cervical stenosis is seen in 3% to 4% of patients after LEEP.[33,34] A retrospective study demonstrated a higher incidence of cervical stenosis in women receiving depot medroxyprogesterone (DMPA).[35] A retrospective study of 257 patients showed that of those using DMPA, 41% developed stenosis versus 15.2% of those not on DMPA (odds ratio = 3.85, 95% CI = 1.41–10.50), although it is notable that the control group had a higher rate of stenosis than was reported in other case series.[35] Based on this study, consideration may be given to adding an estrogen-containing contraceptive (combined oral contraceptive, patch, or vaginal ring) for several months after LEEP, though this intervention has not been studied. On rare occasions the stenosis can lead to a hematometria if menstrual bleeding is unable to pass. The risk of preterm birth after LEEP, treatment failure, and recurrence of dysplasia are addressed in subsequent sections.

Cold Knife Conization

Cold knife conization (CKC) was the mainstay of treatment for cervical dysplasia before the availability of cryotherapy and LEEP. It has higher complication rates, including bleeding, infection, cervical stenosis, and cervical incompetency in pregnancy. For this reason, CKC is generally performed in the operating room and is reserved for clinical scenarios whereby LEEP would be technically difficult or whereby CKC is preferred owing to concern about the potential for thermal artifact obscuring evaluation of the margin of a LEEP excision. Two situations where having interpretable margins would be beneficial are when treating a woman who has had cytology has atypical glandular cells that "favor neoplasia," adenocarcinoma in situ (AIS) with a colposcopic examination negative for invasive disease, or suspected microinvasive carcinoma.[9] Given the success rates, and lower complication rates associated with LEEP and cryotherapy, the technique of CKC is only briefly described here, as a full discussion is beyond the scope of this article.

Preprocedure counseling and consent forms should address the steps of the procedure, benefits, alternatives, and risks such as bleeding, infection, recurrence of disease, cervical incompetence, or stenosis, and injury to vaginal tissue.

The patient is taken to the operating room and is placed in the dorsal lithotomy position; a speculum is inserted into the vagina. The transformation zone is delineated with either colposcopy or Lugol solution. Sutures can be placed at 3 and 9 o'clock at the approximate level of the descending cervical branches of the uterine arteries for hemostasis and traction prior to cervical incision.[36] A scalpel is then used to make a circumferential incision around the transformation zone that is tapered as it is carried to the deeper levels to remove a cone-shaped specimen. The final specimen is typically removed with scissors. Bleeding at the base of the biopsy site can be controlled through electrocautery, simple sutures, or Monsel solution, with no clearly superior method.[37] Vasopressin can be added to a local anesthetic block to provide vasoconstriction and decrease bleeding during and after a CKC as with a LEEP.[36] Electrocautery is favored over simple sutures with respect to blood loss, operative time, and rates of cervical stenosis.[38] Additionally, the cone bed may be packed with Surgicell™ and held in place by loosely tying together the stay sutures initially placed at 3 and 9 o'clock.

CKC appears to carry a higher complication rate than LEEP or cryotherapy. Significant bleeding occurs 5% to 10% of the time with CKC, although the need for transfusion is rare.[39] Rates of cervical stenosis are 2% to 3% according to most sources. The transformation zone may also be difficult to visualize after CKC.[36] However, the incidence of complications between LEEP and CKC was not statistically significantly different in a study by Zeng and colleagues,[40] 8.1% (6 of 74) for LEEP and 6.2% (54 of 869) for CKC.

FUTURE PREGNANCY AND TREATMENT OF DYSPLASIA

Women will commonly be concerned about the effect of CIN treatment on their future fertility, sexuality, and pregnancy complications and providers should preemptively address these concerns during their counseling. There are no known effects of CIN treatment on fertility. Nor are there any concerning changes in sexual function after the initial recommendations to avoid intercourse, tampons, and vaginal douching immediately after a treatment.[41,42] Concern for preterm birth after treatment for cervical dysplasia has lead to numerous research efforts to assess the effect of the treatment of CIN on future pregnancies, specifically the risk of the preterm birth.

Risk of Preterm Birth

Concern for the increase of preterm birth after the treatment of CIN has been a factor in changing the treatment guidelines for young women with high-grade dysplasia to favor a period of observation over immediate treatment.[9] A 2011 meta-analysis of thirty studies examined the association between cervical dysplasia and preterm delivery.[43] Excisional therapy carried an increased odds of preterm birth of 2.19 (95% CI 1.93–2.49) with an external comparison group of women who gave birth at the same center without a diagnosis of CIN, and 1.96 (95% CI 1.46–2.64) with an internal comparison group for whom the outcomes of births pretreatment were compared with outcomes of births after treatment in the same women.[43] Of note, untreated cervical dysplasia also carried a more modest but increased risk for preterm delivery with a relative risk (RR) of 1.25 (95% CI 0.98–1.58).[43] Interpreting these results together, while the treatment of cervical dysplasia raised the risk of preterm birth by a small measure. There may be factors related to the pathology of cervical dysplasia or confounding variables that raise the risk of preterm labor in patients with untreated lesions.[43] In the meta-analysis, ablative therapy minimally increased the risk of preterm delivery, but less so than having untreated cervical dysplasia or an excision procedure with an increased RR of 1.47 (95% CI 1.24-1.74) in comparison with women from the same centers that did not have dysplasia. Women having ablative therapy did not have an increased risk for preterm delivery in births after their procedure when compared to the gestational age of their own previous birth prior to ablative therapy (RR 1.24, 95% CI 0.73-2.10) or to women with dysplasia who had not been treated (RR 1.03, 95% CI 0.90 - 1.18).[43]

While there is conflicting evidence about the overall risk of preterm labor; however, it does seem clear that an increased risk of preterm labor correlates with increasing depth of transformation zone that is removed. Noehr and colleagues[44] demonstrated that each additional millimeter of tissue over 1.5 cm raised the risk of preterm delivery by 6%, with an odds ratio of 1.06 (95% CI 1.03–1.09). Data from Khalid and colleagues[45] suggested that there was 3 times the risk of preterm labor with excisions "thicker than 1.2 cm and larger than 6 cm^3 in volume." Increased risk after repeat procedures was also shown by Jakobsson and colleagues.[46] In the study of 1808 women in Ireland by Khalid and colleagues,[45] there was no association between time interval from LEEP and pregnancy, nor was there an association between CIN grade and risk of preterm labor.[45] Sadler and colleagues[47] arrived at similar results when controlling for known risk factors associated with preterm delivery and preterm premature rupture of membranes (PPROM) (age, socioeconomic factors, smoking, prior obstetric history). Regarding the type of procedure used to treat cervical dysplasia and its potential effect on the risk of preterm delivery, Sadler and colleagues[47] examined the differences between cone biopsy, ablation, and LEEP, and showed a significant association with both prior conization and LEEP with PPROM and preterm delivery, with an incidence of 15% for conization (RR 3.9, 95% CI 2.0–7.7) and incidence of 8.6% with LEEP (RR 2.2, 95% CI 1.2–4.2). Increased depth of the cone biopsy was associated with the greatest increased risk of preterm delivery, although LEEP also increased the risk of preterm delivery. The mean depth of the specimen removed was 1.40 cm on average (standard deviation [SD] 0.46 cm) for conization and 1.36 cm (SD 0.61 cm) for LEEP. The risk of preterm delivery increased with each increasing depth of cervix removed, with a 3-fold higher risk in women with a biopsy depth of 1.7 cm or more (RR 3.6, 95% CI 1.8–7.5).[47]

As previously mentioned, untreated CIN may also carry risks for PPROM and preterm labor distinct from any effect of treatment. A retrospective cohort study from Scottish national data showed an association of CIN 3, in comparison with the unexposed population, with increased spontaneous preterm delivery (11% vs 6%; OR 1.52, 95% CI 1.29–1.80, P<.001) and PPROM (8% vs 6%; OR 1.27, 95% CI 1.09–1.48, P = .001). By contrast, the CIN 3 group treated with excision had a lower incidence of PPROM and spontaneous preterm delivery compared with the unexposed population.

The use of cervical length screening by transvaginal ultrasonography (TVUS) in pregnant women with a history of a LEEP is controversial given conflicting evidence. Parikh and colleagues[48] conducted a retrospective chart review of 97 pregnant women who had previously undergone LEEP procedures. The 3 women in the study who delivered at less than 37 weeks reported no history of cervical shortening on TVUS, whereas other women noted to have cervical shortening on TVUS delivered at term.[48] However, Crane and colleagues[49] published a prospective study of cervical length screening in 75 women who had undergone LEEP, 21 who had CKC, and 36 who had cryotherapy. All had shorter cervical lengths (3.54 cm for LEEP, 3.69 cm for conization, 3.75 cm cryotherapy) when compared with a low-risk control group of 81 women without prior procedures or cervical dysplasia (4.21 cm). The treated group had cervical lengths similar to those of a group of 63 women with previous preterm birth (3.78 cm). In the Crane study, a cervical length of 3.0 cm or less was associated with a positive predictive value of 53.8% for preterm delivery, and a cervical length above 3.0 cm had a "negative predictive value of 95.2% for spontaneous preterm birth less than 37 weeks in women with a prior LEEP."[49] There is debate over the role of universal screening for cervical shortening versus selective screening for patients experiencing uterine contractions or with risk factors for preterm delivery. The benefit of progesterone for prevention of preterm labor in women with a short cervix has been well described[50]; however, data specific to women with a prior history of LEEP or cold knife cone biopsy are lacking.

Regarding the effect of a history of a prior excisional or ablative procedure on the course of labor, the increased incidence of preterm labor may be due to cervical incompetence caused by reduced cervical stroma, which could potentially result in more rapid labor or decreased incidence of labor dystocia. Although uncommon, most obstetricians can recall the anecdotal case of a woman with tight cervical stenosis after a prior cervical procedure that would not dilate or needed manual digital dilation to stretch past scar tissue. A retrospective cohort study of 598 women who had LEEP procedures did not show any difference in the overall incidence of cesarean delivery or in the incidence of cesarean for labor dystocia when compared with women who had only prior screening cytology or had a prior cervical punch biopsy.[51]

TREATMENT FAILURE AND RECURRENCE OF DYSPLASIA AFTER TREATMENT OF HIGH-GRADE SQUAMOUS DYSPLASIA

Treatment failure after excisional or ablative procedures for dysplasia may represent treatment failure or recurrence of disease. One study defined residual disease as dysplasia on cytology within 12 months of loop excision and recurrence as dysplasia at 12 months or longer after excision; however, this terminology has not been standardized.[52] The risk of recurrence after treatment for CIN depends on the original degree of dysplasia, the type of treatment, and the age of the woman (**Table 3**). Cryotherapy has demonstrated a 95% cure rate for CIN 1 or CIN 2 and 85% to 90% for CIN 3.[53] With cryotherapy the likelihood of cure decreases as the size of the lesion increases. Cryotherapy is successful in 90% of cases with only 1 involved quadrant, but treatment cure falls to 75% for lesions involving 3 to 4 quadrants.[53] A study of 1600 women treated with loop excision for CIN 2 or CIN 3 revealed 93.7% free of any dysplasia at cytologic follow-up if margins from the excision were clear, and 83% free of dysplasia if margins were positive.[52] The meta-analysis by Ghaem-Maghami and colleagues[53] of 35,109 women treated for CIN in England between 1960 and 1997 demonstrated that 23% had an "incomplete excision," defined as at least 1 positive margin on the excisional biopsy. In this analysis high-grade disease reoccurred in 18% of patients after an incomplete excision, versus a 3% recurrence in women with complete excision. After an incomplete excision the RR of recurrence of any dysplasia was 5.47 (95% CI 4.37–6.83) and for high-grade dysplasia (CIN 2, CIN 3, or HSIL) 6.09 (95% CI 3.87–9.60). The risk of recurrence of higher-grade lesions after LEEP was lower than after cryotherapy, but positive margins on LEEP specimens or endocervical lesions are associated with increased risk of recurrence.[53]

In regards to testing that should be done at follow-up after treatment of a high-grade lesion, if the biopsy margins were negative at the time of the procedure, traditional follow-up has consisted of serial cytologic or colposcopic examinations. Two recent publications demonstrate that HPV testing may have more sensitivity and specificity in follow-up. A meta-analysis included 1513 treated women and analyzed samples 6 months after treatment, and showed HPV testing to be more sensitive than cytology in the detection of posttreatment CIN 2/3.[54] This analysis demonstrated that cotesting was more sensitive at identifying recurrence, at 0.95 (95% CI 0.91–0.98), than HPV testing alone at 0.92 (95% CI 0.87–0.96) and far more sensitive than the 0.79 (95% CI 0.72–0.85) sensitivity of cytology alone.[54] In the meta-analysis by Paraskevaidis and colleagues,[55] a positive HPV test, even with normal cytology, described treatment failure earlier and more reliably than cytology. Cotesting with cytology and HPV at 12 and 24 months is recommended after either an excisional or ablative therapy. If results are

Table 3	
Association between risk factors and risk of invasive cancer after treatment for CIN over the first 10 years of follow-up	
Factor vs Comparison	**Adjusted OR (95% CI)**
Initial treatment with cryotherapy vs other	2.98 (2.09–4.26)
Initial diagnosis with CIN 3 vs CIN 1/2	4.10 (2.70–6.22)
Age ≥40 y vs <40 y	1.75 (1.12–2.74)

Abbreviations: CI, confidence interval; OR, odds ratio.

Data from Melnikow J, McGahan C, Sawaya GF, et al. Cervical intraepithelial neoplasia outcomes after treatment: long term follow up from the British Columbia Cohort Study. J Natl Cancer Inst 2009;101:721–8.

Table 4	
Rates of CIN 2 or CIN 3 in the first 6 years after treatment	
Initial Histology	Cumulative Rate of Recurrence of CIN 2/3 (95% CI) (%)
CIN 1	5.6 (4.91–5.21)
CIN 2	9.3 (9.09–9.42)
CIN 3	14.0 (13.84–14.15)

Data from Melnikow J, McGahan C, Sawaya GF, et al. Cervical intraepithelial neoplasia outcomes after treatment: long term follow up from the British Columbia Cohort Study. J Natl Cancer Inst 2009;101:721–8.

negative at both time points, repeat cotesting can occur in 3 years with a return to routine screening after that time if results remain normal. If any test is abnormal at 12 or 24 months, repeat colposcopy with ECC sampling is recommended. If positive margins are present with excisional therapy or an immediate post-procedure endocervical specimen is positive for dysplasia then repeat cytology and ECC should be performed within 4 to 6 months.

Regarding how long follow-up should last after treatment of high-grade cervical disease, the largest cohort for short-term[56] and long-term follow-up is the British Columbia Cancer Agency, which retrospectively identified 37,142 women from January 1986 through December 2000 who met study criteria and had continued follow-up through 2004.[17] Women older than 40 years with advanced dysplasia initially had higher recurrences of CIN 2/3 after treatment, with recurrences highest for cryo-therapy and lowest for cone biopsy.[17] **Table 4** outlines recurrence of CIN 2 and CIN 3 in the first 6 years after treatment. Overall, risk of recurrence of high-grade dysplasia, CIN 2, or CIN 3 after treatment was low, on the order of 1%, after 6 years.[17] There is a rapid decline in CIN 2 or CIN 3 in the first 2 years after follow-up, but there remains an ongoing elevated risk of cervical cancer for 10 to 20 years based on these data.[17]

These results support the ASCCP's 2012 recommendations regarding resuming routine screening after the period of cotesting at 12 and 24 months, and emphasize the importance of continued follow-up with a history of an HSIL cytology carrying an increased risk of cervical cancer for at least 20 years after treatment, even when that extends past age 65 years.[10]

SUMMARY

Treatment of high-grade cervical dysplasia has changed in significant ways in the past few decades. The ASCCP revised its consensus guidelines in 2012 to reflect the information regarding the natural history of HPV and increased use of testing for HPV. The data from the almost 1.4 million women in the Kaiser Permanente Northern California Medical (KPNC) plan, which includes follow-up for up to 8 years, has improved our ability to stratify risk based on age and specific cytologic or histologic abnormalities.[56] Using KPNC data, the ASCCP was able to develop standardized, evidence-based guidelines for the consistent follow-up of women with CIN and cancer. The standardization goals of the LAST project, with the use of a 2-tier SIL terminology, offers the promise of being able to dichotomize CIN 2 into lower-risk and higher-risk groups; however, outcomes data from this new classification system are still awaited.

Vaccines against the most common oncogenic subtypes of HPV that lead to invasive cervical cancer are widely available and effective. Current guidelines and studies do not differentiate management based on whether a woman has been vaccinated, as evidence is lacking in regard of the effect of vaccination on the natural history of HPV infection. This situation is expected to change as the girls and women who have been vaccinated since 2006 enter the age when women are at highest risk for CIN and cervical cancer.

Treatment of high-grade squamous lesions is essential in preventing cervical cancer. Although there remains some conflict in the literature, the presence of cervical dysplasia and the treatment of dysplasia both appear to be implicated in increasing the rates of preterm delivery. The concern for increasing the likelihood of preterm delivery, as well as the natural history of HPV infection, has informed our discussion of the risks and benefits of treatment versus observation in reproductive-age women with CIN 2 and CIN 3. With many women having been treated for cervical dysplasia during their reproductive years, the question arises as to whether there is any method to decrease the risk of preterm delivery after a LEEP has occurred. Studies on the use of cervical-length ultrasonography and progesterone are needed to determine whether women with a history of LEEP can benefit from this approach to screening and pharmacologic intervention.

Our understanding of HPV infection and cervical cancer has improved immensely in the past 20 years. This understanding has led to the creation of evidence-based guidelines for cervical cancer screening, management, and treatment to minimize the likelihood of progression to cervical cancer, while balancing the risks associated with treatment. To maximize the effect on morbidity and mortality from cervical cancer, the next step will be to strategize methods to have these guidelines widely implemented by all health care providers. This action will lead to a decrease in unnecessary tests and treatments, reduce the incidence of cervical cancer, and decrease morbidity associated with cervical dysplasia and treatment.

REFERENCES

1. Darragh TM, Colgan TJ, Cox JT, et al. The lower anogenital squamous terminology standardization project for HPV-associated lesions: background and consensus recommendations from the College of American Pathologists and the American Society for Colposcopy and Cervical Pathology. J Low Genit Tract Dis 2012;16(3):205–42.
2. Dunne EF, Unger ER, Sternberg M, et al. Prevalence of HPV infection among females in the United States. JAMA 2007;297(8):813–9.
3. Hariri S, Unger ER, Sternberg M, et al. Prevalence of genital human papillomavirus among females in the United States, the National Health and Nutrition Examination Survey, 2003-2006. J Infect Dis 2011;204(4):566–73.
4. Munoz N, Bosch FX, de Sanjose S, et al. Epidemiologic classification of human papillomavirus types associated with cervical cancer. N Engl J Med 2003; 348(6):518–27.
5. Stanley M. Pathology and epidemiology of HPV infection in females. Gynecol Oncol 2010;117(Suppl 2):S5–10.
6. Datta SD, Koutsky LA, Ratelle S, et al. Human papillomavirus infection and cervical cytology in women screened for cervical cancer in the United States, 2003-2005. Ann Intern Med 2008;148(7):493–500.
7. Padilla-Paz LA, Carlson J, Twiggs LB, et al. Evidence supporting the current management guidelines for high-grade squamous intraepithelial lesion cytology. J Low Genit Tract Dis 2004;8(2):139–46.
8. Waxman AG, Chelmow D, Darragh TM, et al. Revised terminology for cervical histopathology and its implications for management of high-grade

squamous intraepithelial lesions of the cervix. Obstet Gynecol 2012;120(6): 1465–71.

9. Wright TC, Cox JT, Massad LS, et al. 2012 Consensus guidelines for the management of cervical intraepithelial neoplasia. J Low Genit Tract Dis 2013; 17(5):S1–27.

10. American Society for Colposcopy and Cervical Pathology. Histology of the normal cervix. 2012. Available at: http://www.asccp.org/practicemanagement/cervix/histologyofthenormalcervix/tabid/5842/default.aspx. Accessed November 26, 2012.

11. Wright TC Jr, Massad LS, Dunton CJ, et al. 2006 consensus guidelines for the management of women with cervical intraepithelial neoplasia or adenocarcinoma in situ. J Low Genit Tract Dis 2007;11(4):223–39.

12. Cubo-Abert M, Centeno-Mediavilla C, Franco-Zabala P, et al. Risk factors for progression or persistence of squamous intraepithelial lesions diagnosed during pregnancy. J Low Genit Tract Dis 2012;16(1):34–8.

13. Moscicki AB, Ma Y, Wibbelsman C, et al. Rate of and risks for regression of cervical intraepithelial neoplasia 2 in adolescents and young women. Obstet Gynecol 2010;116(6):1373–80.

14. Massad LS, Ahdieh L, Benning L, et al. Evolution of cervical abnormalities among women with HIV-1: evidence from surveillance cytology in the women's interagency HIV study. J Acquir Immune Defic Syndr 2001;27(5):432–42.

15. Massad LS, Evans CT, D'Souza G, et al. High-grade cervical disease in adolescents with HIV. J Low Genit Tract Dis 2008;12(3):199–203.

16. Martin-Hirsch PP, Paraskevaidis E, Bryant A, et al. Interventions for preventing blood loss during the treatment of cervical intraepithelial neoplasia. Cochrane Database Syst Rev 2010;(6):CD001318.

17. Melnikow J, McGahan C, Sawaya GF, et al. Cervical intraepithelial neoplasia outcomes after treatment: long-term follow-up from the British Columbia Cohort Study. J Natl Cancer Inst 2009;101(10):721–8.

18. Santesso N, Schunemann H, Blumenthal P, et al. World Health Organization Guidelines: use of cryotherapy for cervical intraepithelial neoplasia. Int J Gynaecol Obstet 2012;118(2):97–102.

19. McClung EC, Blumenthal PD. Efficacy, safety, acceptability and affordability of cryotherapy: a review of current literature. Minerva Ginecol 2012;64(2): 149–71.

20. Nahhas WA, Whitney CW, Rine J. Evaluation of removing devitalized cervical tissue in the reduction of vaginal discharge after cervical cryotherapy: a prospective study. J Reprod Med 1981;26(5):263–4.

21. Townsend DE, Richart RM. Cryotherapy and carbon dioxide laser management of cervical intraepithelial neoplasia: a controlled comparison. Obstet Gynecol 1983;61(1):75–8.

22. Leimbacher B, Samartzis N, Imesch P, et al. Inpatient and outpatient loop electrosurgery excision procedure for cervical intraepithelial neoplasia: a retrospective analysis. Arch Gynecol Obstet 2012;285(5):1441–5.

23. Tillmanns TD, Falkner CA, Engle DB, et al. Preoperative predictors of positive margins after loop electrosurgical excisional procedure—Cone. Gynecol Oncol 2006;100(2):379–84.

24. Bruinsma F, Lumley J, Tan J, et al. Precancerous changes in the cervix and risk of subsequent preterm birth. BJOG 2007;114(1):70–80.

25. Lanneau GS, Skaggs V, Moore K, et al. A LEEP cervical conization is rarely indicated for a two-step discrepancy. J Low Genit Tract Dis 2007;11(3):134–7.

26. Paraskevaidis E, Koliopoulos G, Paschopoulos M, et al. Effects of ball cauterization following loop excision and follow-up colposcopy. Obstet Gynecol 2001; 97(4):617–20.
27. Bailey AP, Darracott MM. Loop electrosurgical excision procedure with an intrauterine device in place. Am J Obstet Gynecol 2010;203(3):291.e1–3.
28. Spitzer M, Chernys AE, Seltzer VL. The use of large-loop excision of the transformation zone in an inner-city population. Obstet Gynecol 1993;82(5): 731–5.
29. Dunn TS, Woods J, Burch J. Bowel injury occurring during an outpatient LLETZ procedure. A case report. J Reprod Med 2003;48(1):49–51.
30. Kietpeerakool C, Srisomboon J, Khobjai A, et al. Complications of loop electrosurgical excision procedure for cervical neoplasia: a prospective study. J Med Assoc Thai 2006;89(5):583–7.
31. Siegler E, Bornstein J. Loop electrosurgical excision procedures in Israel. Gynecol Obstet Invest 2011;72(2):85–9.
32. Sutthichon P, Kietpeerakool C. Perioperative complications of an outpatient loop electrosurgical excision procedure: a review of 857 consecutive cases. Asian Pac J Cancer Prev 2009;10(3):351–4.
33. Baldauf JJ, Dreyfus M, Wertz JP, et al. Consequences and treatment of cervical stenoses after laser conization or loop electrosurgical excision. J Gynecol Obstet Biol Reprod (Paris) 1997;26(1):64–70 [in French].
34. Mathevet P, Chemali E, Roy M, et al. Long-term outcome of a randomized study comparing three techniques of conization: cold knife, laser, and LEEP. Eur J Obstet Gynecol Reprod Biol 2003;106(2):214–8.
35. Martirosian TE, Smith SC, Baras AS, et al. Depot medroxyprogesterone acetate: a risk factor for cervical stenosis after loop electrosurgical excisional procedure management of cervical intraepithelial neoplasia? J Low Genit Tract Dis 2010; 14(1):37–42.
36. Toglia M. Cone biopsy: perfecting the procedure. J Fam Pract 2002;14(1):75–83.
37. Gilbert L, Saunders NJ, Stringer R, et al. Hemostasis and cold knife cone biopsy: a prospective randomized trial comparing a suture versus non-suture technique. Obstet Gynecol 1989;74(4):640–3.
38. Kamat AA, Kramer P, Soisson AP. Superiority of electrocautery over the suture method for achieving cervical cone bed hemostasis. Obstet Gynecol 2003; 102(4):726–30.
39. Jones HW 3rd. Cone biopsy and hysterectomy in the management of cervical intraepithelial neoplasia. Baillieres Clin Obstet Gynaecol 1995;9(1):221–36.
40. Zeng SY, Liang MR, Li LY, et al. Comparison of the efficacy and complications of different surgical methods for cervical intraepithelial neoplasia. Eur J Gynaecol Oncol 2012;33(3):257–60.
41. Inna N, Phianmongkhol Y, Charoenkwan K. Sexual function after loop electrosurgical excision procedure for cervical dysplasia. J Sex Med 2010;7(3):1291–7.
42. Serati M, Salvatore S, Cattoni E, et al. The impact of the loop electrosurgical excisional procedure for cervical intraepithelial lesions on female sexual function. J Sex Med 2010;7(6):2267–72.
43. Bruinsma FJ, Quinn MA. The risk of preterm birth following treatment for precancerous changes in the cervix: a systematic review and meta-analysis. BJOG 2011;118(9):1031–41.
44. Noehr B, Jensen A, Frederiksen K, et al. Depth of cervical cone removed by loop electrosurgical excision procedure and subsequent risk of spontaneous preterm delivery. Obstet Gynecol 2009;114(6):1232–8.

45. Khalid S, Dimitriou E, Conroy R, et al. The thickness and volume of LLETZ specimens can predict the relative risk of pregnancy-related morbidity. BJOG 2012; 119(6):685–91.
46. Jakobsson M, Gissler M, Paavonen J, et al. Loop electrosurgical excision procedure and the risk for preterm birth. Obstet Gynecol 2009;114(3):504–10.
47. Sadler L, Saftlas A, Wang W, et al. Treatment for cervical intraepithelial neoplasia and risk of preterm delivery. JAMA 2004;291(17):2100–6.
48. Parikh R, Horne H, Feinstein SJ, et al. Cervical length screening in patients who have undergone loop electrosurgical excision procedure. J Reprod Med 2008; 53(12):909–13.
49. Crane JM, Delaney T, Hutchens D. Transvaginal ultrasonography in the prediction of preterm birth after treatment for cervical intraepithelial neoplasia. Obstet Gynecol 2006;107(1):37–44.
50. Romero R, Nicolaides K, Conde-Agudelo A, et al. Vaginal progesterone in women with an asymptomatic sonographic short cervix in the midtrimester decreases preterm delivery and neonatal morbidity: a systematic review and metaanalysis of individual patient data. Am J Obstet Gynecol 2012;206(2):124.e1–19.
51. Frey HA, Stout MJ, Odibo AO, et al. Risk of cesarean delivery after loop electrosurgical excision procedure. Obstet Gynecol 2013;121(1):39–45.
52. Zaitoun AM, McKee G, Coppen MJ, et al. Completeness of excision and follow up cytology in patients treated with loop excision biopsy. J Clin Pathol 2000; 53(3):191–6.
53. Ghaem-Maghami S, Sagi S, Majeed G, et al. Incomplete excision of cervical intraepithelial neoplasia and risk of treatment failure: a meta-analysis. Lancet Oncol 2007;8(11):985–93.
54. Kocken M, Uijterwaal MH, de Vries AL, et al. High-risk human papillomavirus testing versus cytology in predicting post-treatment disease in women treated for high-grade cervical disease: a systematic review and meta-analysis. Gynecol Oncol 2012;125(2):500–7.
55. Paraskevaidis E, Arbyn M, Sotiriadis A, et al. The role of HPV DNA testing in the follow-up period after treatment for CIN: a systematic review of the literature. Cancer Treat Rev 2004;30(2):205–11.
56. Katki H, Schiffman M, Castle P, et al. Benchmarking CIN3+ Risk as the Basis for Incorporating HPV and Pap Cotesting into Cervical Screening and Management Guidelines. J Low Genit Tract Dis 2013;17(5):S28–35.

Nongenital Human Papillomavirus Disease

E.J. Mayeaux Jr, MD[a],*, Michelle J. Khan, MD, MPH[b]

KEYWORDS

- Human papillomavirus • Anal cancer • Head and neck cancer
- Respiratory papillomatosis

KEY POINTS

- Human papillomavirus (HPV) has been shown to be associated with several anogenital malignancies and with oral pharyngeal cancers.
- Primary prevention of anal cancer may be possible through widespread HPV vaccination.
- Recurrent respiratory papillomatosis is characterized by nonmalignant, yet aggressive neoplasms, and is caused by HPV.
- Many oropharyngeal squamous cell carcinomas, especially those found in the tonsils and on the base of the tongue, are associated with HPV.
- Prophylactic quadrivalent HPV vaccination should prevent respiratory papillomatosis, and both the quadrivalent and bivalent HPV vaccines could prevent HPV-related head and neck cancers.
- Secondary prevention of anal cancer may be possible through screening and treatment of precancerous anal lesions.

INTRODUCTION

Over the last several decades, the incidence of cervical cancer has decreased in industrialized countries since the introduction of the Papanicolaou (Pap) test, colposcopy, and treatments for cervical dysplasia. During this time, however, there have been increases in the incidence of oral and anal squamous cell carcinomas (SCCs).[1,2] Although the link with lower female genital tract cancers and infection with high-risk human papillomavirus (HPV) types has been well established, it has been more recently learned that both anal[3] and oral pharyngeal[2] cancers are associated with these high-risk HPV infections.

Disclosure: E.J.M. has served on advisory boards and as a speaker for Merck vaccine division, Pharmaderm, and Roche Diagnostics, but has resigned from all potential conflict activities.
^a Departments of Family Medicine and Obstetrics and Gynecology, Louisiana State University Health Sciences Center, 1501 Kings Highway, Shreveport, LA 71130, USA; ^b Department of Ob/Gyn and Reproductive Sciences, University of California, San Francisco, San Francisco, CA, USA
* Corresponding author.
E-mail address: emayea@lsuhsc.edu

Obstet Gynecol Clin N Am 40 (2013) 317–337
http://dx.doi.org/10.1016/j.ogc.2013.02.006
0889-8545/13/$ – see front matter © 2013 Elsevier Inc. All rights reserved.

obgyn.theclinics.com

HPV AND ANAL CANCER

Anal cancer is uncommon, with an estimated total in the United States of 6230 cancers in 2012.[4] However, its incidence has been rising in both men and women over the last 3 decades, doubling from 0.8 per 100,000 in 1975 to 1.7 per 100,000 in 2009. It remains more common in women (**Fig. 1**).[5] Biologically, anal cancer is very similar to cervical cancer in its causal relationship with high-risk HPV infection and the presumed progression from high-grade anal intraepithelial neoplasia (AIN) to invasive anal cancer.[6] A high prevalence of high-risk HPV in the anus has been reported in both human immunodeficiency virus (HIV)-positive and HIV-negative men and women.[1] Infection with high-risk types of HPV causes more than 80% of cases of anal cancer.[1,7] Populations at increased risk for anal cancer include men who have sex with men (MSM), women with previous high-grade lower genital tract dysplasia, immunosuppressed transplant recipients, and HIV-positive individuals.[8,9] MSM are about 20 times more likely than men who have sex with women (MSW) to develop anal cancer, with incidence rates as high as 128 per 100,000.[10,11]

It is also well established that individuals with active HIV disease have higher rates of anal HPV infection, especially HPV-16 and HPV-18, and higher rates of HPV-associated AIN.[1,12] Studies of anal HPV prevalence show rates ranging from 27% to 43% and 79% to 90% in HIV-negative and HIV-positive women, respectively,[13–15] from 50% to 60% and more than 90% in HIV-negative and HIV-positive MSM, respectively,[15–19] and from 25% to 59% among MSW.[15,20] Comparison of studies from the early 1990s to more recent years has shown that highly active antiretroviral therapy (HAART) does not appear to reduce the incidence of anal dysplasia, or clearance of high-risk HPV infection, although data are conflicting.[21] As HIV-positive patients survive longer with the widespread use of HAART, more cases of invasive anal intraepithelial neoplasia are being detected.[22] Recent studies demonstrated that the degree of immunosuppression in a person's lifetime (CD4 nadir, or AIDS-defining illness) is correlated with the risk of developing anal cancer, independent of current immune status.[23,24]

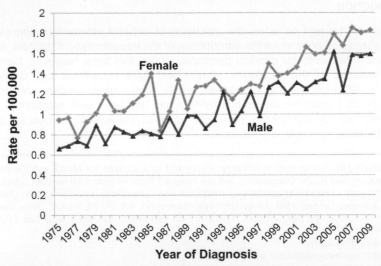

Fig. 1. Age-adjusted incidence of invasive anal cancer by gender and year of diagnosis in the United States. (*Data from* SEER fast cancer statistics, National Cancer Institute. Available at: http://seer.cancer.gov/faststats/selections.php? Accessed December 15, 2012.)

PREVENTION OF ANAL CANCERS

Primary prevention of anal cancer may be possible through widespread HPV vaccination. Recent evidence from randomized controlled vaccine trials has demonstrated a decrease in anal HPV prevalence and a decrease in the development of AIN among MSM.[25] Long-term follow-up of these vaccinated populations will be critical to establishing the impact on the incidence and mortality of anal cancer.

Secondary prevention of anal cancer through screening is a controversial topic. There are no large population-based studies defining the risk of progression of high-grade AIN to anal cancer. However, there are data demonstrating the oncogenic potential of high-grade AIN.[26–28] Some groups argue that until well-designed studies demonstrate the link between screening and the decrease in incidence and mortality of anal cancer, screening for anal cancer should not be performed.[1] These groups believe that the harms and side effects of treatment outweigh the potential population benefit. Proponents of screening argue that the link between HPV and anogenital cancers is well established and that screening is justified. These groups believe that despite the current absence of evidence from natural history studies, we cannot ignore the increased risk of anal cancer in high-risk populations when we have the tools to screen and treat precancerous anal lesions.[29]

Using prevention of HPV-related cervical cancers as a model, anal cytology testing has been used for the detection of anal high-grade squamous intraepithelial neoplasia (HSIL) lesions. For anal cytology, the anal epithelium is sampled using a polyester-fiber swab, and the cells are smeared onto a glass slide or transferred to a liquid-based medium for cytopathologic examination. Like cervical cytology, anal cytology has variable sensitivity in detecting high-grade disease. Anal cytology may be more sensitive among HIV-positive individuals.[30] A recent population-based study showed sensitivity of anal cytology in detecting precancers of 87% among HIV-positive MSM and 55% among HIV-negative MSM.[12] Although cytology performs reasonably well as a screening test, the correlation with histology can be quite low.[31,32] The detection of anal precancer in studies was strikingly lower by cytology than for colposcopically guided biopsy; this finding probably represents underdiagnosis of high-grade lesions by cytology, owing to its lower sensitivity.[33] The low sensitivity of cytology may be partly due to the large and involuted surface area of the anal canal, which is difficult to sample thoroughly with blind swabbing.

Anal cytology is usually performed in conjunction with the digital anorectal examination (DARE) as a screening test to assess for areas of induration, tenderness, or masses in the anal canal, which are often associated with dysplasias and/or cancer and which may be missed by cytology.[6]

PATHOLOGY OF ANAL INTRAEPITHELIAL NEOPLASIA

Cytologic classification of anal cytology mirrors that of cervical cytology, using Bethesda System terminology: negative for squamous intraepithelial lesion, atypical squamous cells of undetermined significance (ASC-US), low-grade squamous intraepithelial lesion (LSIL), atypical squamous cells—cannot rule out high-grade (ASC-H), high-grade squamous intraepithelial lesion (HSIL), and invasive squamous cell carcinoma (SCC). Abnormal anal cytology results should prompt further evaluation with high-resolution anoscopy (HRA). The threshold at which referral for HRA is made differs by clinical site, but the known discrepancy between cytology and histology suggests that any abnormality should be further evaluated.

HRA is a procedure similar to cervical colposcopy; a colposcope is used to visualize the anal transformation zone (AnTZ), and lesion(s) suspicious for high-grade AIN can be biopsied. Rather than a speculum, a metal or disposable plastic anoscope is used. The anoscope is inserted after cytologic sampling has been performed, and after a DARE has been performed using a combination of lubricant jelly and lidocaine gel or cream (2%–5%) to achieve lubrication and analgesia before its introduction. After insertion of the anoscope, a gauze-wrapped swab soaked in 3% to 5% dilute acetic acid is placed in the anus, and the anoscope is removed while the acetic acid is left in place for approximately 1 minute. This gauze-wrapped swab is then removed and the anoscope is reinserted. Any obscuring lidocaine gel or stool is removed and the anoscope is slowly withdrawn until the AnTZ can be visualized. Acetic acid is continually applied using cotton swabs to visualize the entire AnTZ circumferentially. The folds of the anal canal and other potential anatomic obstacles (hemorrhoids, anal papillae, and so forth) must be manipulated to satisfactorily visualize the entire AnTZ.

The colposcopic features of AIN visualized during HRA are similar to those seen in cervical colposcopy, and include acetowhitening, punctation, mosaicism, and atypical vessels (**Figs. 2–6**).[34] Lugol's iodine is used in conjunction with acetic acid to better define areas of possible high-grade AIN (these are nonstaining areas) and to better define borders of lesions (see **Fig. 4**). Any lesion that appears high-grade should be biopsied for histologic confirmation, using a small (≤3 mm) biopsy forceps (baby Tischler or ENT forceps). Multiple studies have noted a significant discrepancy between cytologic and histologic diagnoses, which reiterates the need for biopsy of lesions to confirm high-grade AIN (HGAIN).[31,32] When performed correctly, biopsy is usually well tolerated and has a low complication rate.

The histopathologic classification of low-grade AIN (LGAIN) and HGAIN corresponds to low-grade and high-grade cervical intraepithelial neoplasia (CIN). As with the cervix, LGAIN is considered to represent a productive HPV infection, not a true precursor to cancer. Anal warts, which are commonly seen during HRA (see **Fig. 5**), should be palpated and examined carefully for colposcopic features of HGAIN, and biopsied if there are any features concerning for HGAIN or cancer.[26]

TREATMENT OF ANAL INTRAEPITHELIAL NEOPLASIA

Visual and histologic confirmation of HGAIN for treatment planning is the goal of HRA. A general treatment approach is to treat all areas of HGAIN, to reduce the risk of

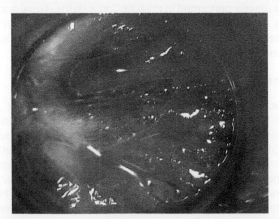

Fig. 2. High-resolution anoscopy: normal anal transformation zone. The line depicts the zone of metaplasia where the proximal columnar epithelium of the colon is transitioning to the distal squamous epithelium of the anus.

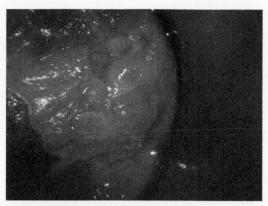

Fig. 3. High-resolution anoscopy: findings of acetowhite lesion and punctation, suggestive of high-grade anal intraepithelial neoplasia (HGAIN).

progression to anal cancer. Patients with symptomatic or cosmetically disfiguring anal or perianal condyloma should also be considered for treatment. Treatment can be patient-applied or provider-applied, medical or surgical. Advantages and disadvantages of these approaches are shown in **Table 1**.

Patients with small lesions or localized disease may be treated topically (imiquimod [indication not approved by Food and Drug Administration], 5-fluorouracil, trichloroacetic acid, and so forth) or with office-based surgical procedures such as infrared coagulation (IRC), hyfrecation, laser, or electrocautery. One of the more common therapies used by clinicians is 85% trichloroacetic acid (TCA). Data suggest that this approach is most effective for small lesions, both perianal and intra-anal, and is associated with clearance rates ranging from 35% to 65%, with better efficacy in HIV-negative than in HIV-positive individuals.[35] Perianal disease is commonly treated with liquid nitrogen, which is inexpensive, and although usually requiring 2 to 3 treatments for clearance, well tolerated overall.[36] Imiquimod cream 5%, an immunomodulator, has shown good efficacy in treating external anogenital warts in randomized controlled trials in both HIV-positive and HIV-negative populations.[37,38] There are more limited data for the use of 5% imiquimod cream to treat intra-anal condyloma

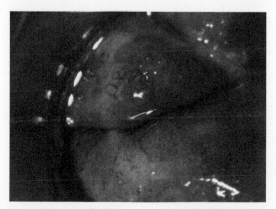

Fig. 4. High-resolution anoscopy: findings of coarse mosaicism and Lugol nonstaining lesion, which suggest a high-grade lesion. In this case, biopsy showed HGAIN.

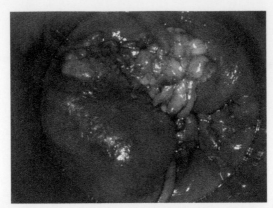

Fig. 5. High-resolution anoscopy: findings of intra-anal warts and a hemorrhoid in the posterior left lateral aspect of the visual field.

and perianal and intra-anal HGAIN, with reported clearance rates of 75%.[39,40] Studies from Europe indicate that patient-applied intra-anal imiquimod may be effective to treat intra-anal HGAIN.[41,42] 5-Fluorouracil 5% cream has also been studied in HIV-positive populations and has shown some efficacy against external and internal warts, but is less commonly used because of its side effects of erosion and ulceration, and so forth.[43,44] A more recently approved treatment for external anogenital warts is sinecatechins 15% ointment, a topical extract from green tea that has shown efficacy as a patient-applied treatment.[45]

Office-based surgical therapies include IRC, laser ablation, hyfrecation, and argon beam coagulation. IRC is a well-tolerated treatment that has been shown to be very effective for in-office treatment of HGAIN,[46] and can be performed under local anesthesia with a combination of topical and injected lidocaine. One limitation to IRC is that the equipment is not meant to be used for large lesions and can overheat for procedures that are too long. Laser and electrocautery are also office-based procedures that have been shown to be effective, producing minimal morbidity.[28,47] Potential complications of ablative therapy include painful bowel movements, bleeding, infection, abscess formation, anal sinuses, and incontinence.

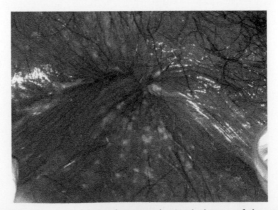

Fig. 6. High-resolution anoscopy: hyperpigmented raised plaque of the perianus, which was biopsied and found to be perianal high-grade intraepithelial lesion.

Table 1
Treatments for high-grade anal intraepithelial neoplasia (HGAIN)[a]

Treatment	Perianal Condyloma	Intra-anal Condyloma	Perianal AIN 2–3	Intra-anal AIN 2–3	Advantages	Disadvantages
Liquid nitrogen	Yes	No	Yes	No	Inexpensive	Pain, scarring, multiple visits
85% TCA	Yes	Yes	Yes	Yes	Inexpensive	Pain, scarring, multiple visits. May be less effective in HIV-positive patients
0.5% Podofilox gel	Yes	No	No	No	Patient-applied	Pain/irritation/erosions
5% Imiquimod cream	Yes	Possibly	Possibly	Possibly	Patient-applied	Pain/irritation. May be less effective in men and HIV-positive patients
5% 5-fluorouracil cream	Possibly	Possibly	Possibly	Possibly	Patient-applied	Pain/irritation/erosions
15% Sinecatechin ointment	Yes	No	No	No	Patient-applied	Pain/irritation/erosions
Infrared coagulation	Yes	Yes	Yes	Yes	May be used to treat extensive disease, relatively inexpensive. Can be performed in the office	Painful, bleeding infection
Electrocautery	Yes	Yes	Yes	Yes	Inexpensive. Can be performed in the office	Painful, bleeding infection
Laser	Yes	Yes	Yes	Yes	May be used to treat extensive disease. Can be performed in the office	Painful, bleeding infection
Scalpel excision	Yes	Yes	Yes	Yes	May be used to treat extensive disease	Painful, bleeding infection

Abbreviation: TCA, trichloroacetic acid.
[a] Not approved for all of these indications by the Food and Drug Administration.
Data from Palefsky JM. Anal cancer prevention in HIV-positive men and women. Curr Opin Oncol 2009;21(5):433–8.

Patients with widespread disease or large, extensive lesions will usually need to be treated with excision or electrocautery under anesthesia in the operating room.[6] Another approach is to do staged ablative treatments in the office for widespread HGAIN if features concerning for invasive cancer are absent. Any patient with a mass on DARE and/or suspicion for cancer on HRA but with biopsies showing HGAIN should be taken to the operating room for surgical examination and biopsies. Patients with invasive anal cancer should be referred to a medical oncologist and radiation oncologist for treatment planning.

RECURRENT RESPIRATORY PAPILLOMATOSIS

Recurrent respiratory papillomatosis (RRP) is a disease characterized by nonmalignant yet aggressive neoplasms in the upper aerodigestive tract caused by the HPV. RRP is grouped into juvenile-onset RRP (JORRP) and adult-onset RRP (AORRP), based on diagnosis before or after 12 years of age. JORRP is more common and is often more severe than AORRP.

Epidemiology of RRP

RRP has a bimodal age distribution.[48] It is seen most commonly in children younger than 5 years or in persons in the fourth decade of life. A survey in 1993 estimated there 5977 new cases of RRP occur each year in the United States, with 2354 new pediatric cases and 3623 new adult cases. The estimated incidence in children aged 14 years or younger is 4.3 cases per 100,000 persons. In adolescents older than 15 years, the incidence is approximately 1.8 cases per 100,000.[49] In JORRP the male-to-female ratio is approximately equal, but in AORRP the male-to-female ratio is estimated to be 4:1.[50] Children with JORRP are more likely to be the first-born of young mothers.[51] The majority of adult and juvenile cases involve the larynx. Papillomas, however, may develop anywhere in the respiratory tract from the nose to the lungs. Between 13% and 50% of children with RRP are reported to have distal spread of disease.[49–55]

Because RRP is uncommon and requires laryngoscopy for diagnosis, children often have symptoms for a year or more before the diagnosis is made. Children with JORRP have an average of 4.4 surgical procedures per year and 20 procedures in their lifetime.[49] Ten percent to 15% of children with RRP ultimately require tracheostomy. Malignant degeneration of papillomatous lesions to SCC occurs in less than 1% of patients with RRP, usually associated with HPV-11 disease.[56] Because of this risk of malignant transformation, it is necessary to take biopsies periodically during subsequent procedures to monitor for any malignant changes.

Pathophysiology of RRP

HPV-6 and HPV-11 cause the vast majority of cases of RRP, and the disease associated with HPV-11 infection is usually more severe. As many as 70% of children with HPV-11–associated disease require tracheostomy compared with less than 20% of children infected with HPV-6. Risk factors for JORRP include being first in birth order, vaginal delivery, having a mother younger than 20 years, and being from families of low socioeconomic status.[57] Sexual abuse should be considered in children older than 5 years who acquire RRP.

Transmission of juvenile RRP occurs from the mother to the child either in utero or at the time of birth.[48] Although data are limited, a meta-analysis has shown that up to 10% of normal-appearing oral mucosa contained high-risk HPV.[58] Of the many children exposed to HPV during the perinatal period, few develop RRP, the reasons for which are unknown. One study demonstrated that children with RRP have reduced

CD4/CD8 ratios and poor lymphocyte response to mitogen stimulation, implying that these children have deficient cell-mediated immunity.[59] Thus, a deficient host immune system likely plays a role. Patients with RRP do mount an immune response that is initially manifested by production of serum antibodies to the viruses.[60] Patients with RRP have comparable levels of CD4$^+$ T-helper cells, CD8$^+$ T-cytotoxic cells, B cells, natural killer cells, and normal responses to other pathogens relative to unaffected controls.[61] This finding suggests that the HPV-specific immune dysfunction is likely epithelial-site specific. Some molecular biological evidence suggests that the root problem is activation of suppressor immunocyte derived tolerance to HPV.[50]

It has been hypothesized that HPV is transmitted vertically from the mother to the neonate during passage through the birth canal. However, this method has not been conclusively shown to be the only mechanism of HPV infection. Findings supporting this theory include children born to mothers with active condylomata who have an increased risk of infection,[62] with this risk increased when affected primigravid mothers have increased duration of labor after rupture of the membranes.[63] Although vaginal delivery is a risk factor, cesarean delivery is not completely protective.[64] In addition, neonates may become infected before birth, as evidenced by findings that approximately 12% of neonates may develop HPV infections through transplacental transmission.[65] The transmission/disease acquisition picture is further complicated by the finding in one study that HPV was recoverable from the nasopharyngeal secretions of 30% of infants exposed to HPV in the birth canal, but all were clear within a couple of months, and the number of infants expected to manifest evidence of RRP is only a small fraction of this.[66] HPV DNA has been found in placental tissues and in umbilical cord blood, possibly related to transplacental infections.[67,68] HPV has also been found in near-term amniotic fluid, and some babies do have laryngeal lesions at birth.[69]

It is unknown whether patients with AORRP have reactivation of HPV infection acquired during birth or acquire it from exposure during adulthood. A case-control study of patients with AORRP found them more likely than adult controls to have more lifetime sexual partners and a higher frequency of oral sex.[63] However, it is well established that HPV may form subclinical or latent infections in otherwise healthy-appearing mucosa, making definitive transmission routes unclear. Gastroesophageal reflux disease, which can chronically damage the lining of the oropharynx allowing virus access to basement membranes, has also been found to be a high-risk factor for RRP.[70]

Diagnosis and Treatment of RRP

Patients with JORRP commonly present with a weak cry, and episodes of choking, hoarseness, or failure to thrive. Patients with AORRP present with hoarseness, choking spells, voice change, dyspnea, or a foreign-body sensation in the throat. Voice changes, inspiratory wheezing, stridor, or combinations of these symptoms may be found. Physical findings often are nonspecific. Chest radiography is usually unremarkable. RRP can easily be mistaken for asthma, acute laryngitis, or upper respiratory infection.

RRP is diagnosed via laryngoscopy or bronchoscopy, by observation of the characteristic growths that look very similar to genital mucous membrane condyloma acuminata. Typing of the virus by polymerase chain reaction (PCR) on fresh tissue may be helpful in determining prognosis. Pulmonary function studies may establish the presence and level of upper airway obstruction. Flow-volume loops may show the characteristic flattening of the inspiratory limb or both the inspiratory and expiratory limbs.

The goals of therapy are to relieve airway obstruction, improve voice quality, and facilitate remission. Although CO_2 laser was traditionally used, this causes more thermal injury to underlying tissue than the currently preferred angiolytic KTP and pulse-dyed lasers.[48] Today, treatment typically involves repeated debulking of the warty growths by laser or microdebridement coupled with intralesional cidofovir therapy in patients with moderate or severe disease.[52] Interferon treatment appears to slow the rate of growth without curing the disease. Some antiviral agents may slow the rate of regrowth of lesions, and several agents appear to increase the intervals between resections. These agents include intralesional cidofovir,[71] oral indole-3-carbinol,[72] interferon,[73] and photodynamic therapy.[74] None of these agents are curative, but some patients eventually enter remission. Tracheostomy may be necessary for severe disease. Compared with microdebridement and laser procedures, surgical resection may be associated with a higher risk of tracheal stenosis. Roughly 15,000 surgical procedures are performed each year on RRP patients.[75]

Because prolonged exposure to HPV following rupture of the membranes can be avoided by a cesarean section, it is possible that surgical delivery may decrease transmission, especially in mothers with a previous child with RRP. Although a planned cesarean section is now a routine surgical procedure, it still carries inherent risks and may result in increased morbidity or mortality for the mother.[76] Further studies are needed to determine the actual harms and benefits of planned cesarean section for RRP prevention. In their 2010 guidelines, the Centers for Disease Control and Prevention (CDC) recommended that because cesarean section is of unknown efficacy in preventing RRP in infants and children, cesarean delivery should not be performed solely to prevent transmission of HPV infection to the newborn.[77]

The quadrivalent HPV vaccine protects against infection and lower genital tract and anal disease associated with HPV types 6, 11, 16, and 18, and therefore has promise for decreasing the incidence of RRP. Although individuals may clearly benefit from vaccination, the effect this will have on neonatal transmission of HPV or on the overall incidence of RRP is uncertain. It has been suggested that vaccines might be of benefit to neonates via passive immunity through maternal antibodies.[78] At present, HPV vaccines are not approved for the prevention of RRP.

HEAD AND NECK CANCERS

The classic major risk factors for head and neck SCC (HNSCC) are smoking, smokeless tobacco use, betel nut chewing, and alcohol consumption.[79,80] However, many patients with oropharyngeal SCC (OPSCC), especially those found in the tonsils and base of the tongue, do not tend to have these risk factors but are associated with HPV.[81]

Epidemiology of HNSCC

In 2008 approximately 47,500 people were diagnosed with head and neck cancers in the United States, representing about 3% of new cancers that year. A little over 11,200 people died of this disease.[82] Approximately half a million people worldwide are diagnosed with HNSCC, and 298,408 people die of this disease each year.[83] These worldwide data demonstrate an incidence of head and neck cancers similar to that of cervical cancers.

The SCCs of the oropharyngeal area that are not associated with the classic risk factors have been found to be associated with high-risk HPV types, especially HPV-16 (**Box 1**).[81] The prevalence of HPV infection in OPSCC varies widely but is increasing. Although cohort studies from the 1990s suggested that about half of

---

Box 1
Characteristics of patients found to have HPV-positive oropharyngeal cancer

Younger by 5 to 10 years[86]

More likely to be nonsmokers/drinkers[86]

Men and women seem to be at equal risk[86]

More likely to have a high lifetime number of oral-sex or vaginal-sex partners, more frequent engagement in casual sex, early age at first intercourse, and infrequent use of condoms[87]

Present with more advanced stage[86]

Cystic lymph node metastases common[88]

Worse histology: poorly differentiated, basaloid histology[89]

---

oral pharyngeal cancers were attributable to HPV, more recent studies suggest that HPV accounts for 70% to 80% of these malignancies.[81,84] An analysis of the National Cancer Institute's Surveillance, Epidemiology, and End Results (SEER) data from 1973 to 2001 showed an annual increase in the incidence of cancers more commonly associated with HPV infection (tongue, palatine tonsil, and base of tongue) of 2.1%, 3.9%, and 1.7%, respectively, in 20- to 44-year-old white patients, whereas the incidence of HNSCC at other sites declined.[85]

There are multiple important differences between HNSCCs resulting from classic risk factors and HPV-associated OPSCCs (**Fig. 7**).[81,84,90,91] There is good evidence that a significant fraction of the population with no history of papillomatous disease carries latent HPV DNA in the upper airway.[92] Most studies have found that exposure to tobacco or alcohol did not seem to act synergistically with HPV positivity to increase the risk of oropharyngeal cancer (OPC).[87,93] This finding argues that there are two distinct pathways for the development of OPC; one driven predominantly by the effects of tobacco and/or alcohol and another by HPV-induced carcinogenesis. However, a larger, well-conducted, weighted critical review of the literature found that the larger more rigorous studies showed a positive association between smoking and HPV-positive OPSCCs.[94]

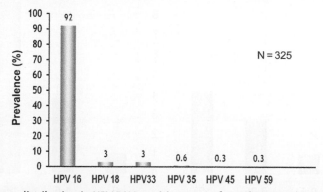

Fig. 7. HPV type distribution in HPV DNA-positive cases of oropharyngeal squamous cell carcinoma. (*Data from* Kreimer AR, Clifford GM, Boyle P, et al. Human papillomavirus types in head and neck squamous cell carcinomas worldwide: a systematic review. Cancer Epidemiol Biomarkers Prev 2005;14(2):467–75.)

Risk Factors Associated with HPV-Positive HNSCC

Case-control studies have shown an association between HPV-positive OPSCC and certain sexual behaviors such as a high lifetime number of oral-sex or vaginal-sex partners, an early age at first intercourse, and infrequent use of condoms (**Fig. 8**).[87] These factors mirror those for the risk of cervical cancer. Women with a history of high-grade lower genital tract dysplasia or cancer have an increased risk of HPV-positive OPC.[95]

A 2010 cross-sectional study of men and women aged 14 to 69 years showed a prevalence of oral HPV in exfoliated cells to be 6.9%, with a prevalence of HPV-16 of 1%.[90] The prevalence followed a bimodal distribution with peaks at age 30 to 34 years and 60 to 64 years. Prevalence was also found to be 3-fold more common in men than in women, which is consistent with the observed sex distribution for HPV-associated oral pharyngeal cancers. Oral infection with high-risk HPV has been highly associated with an increased risk of developing OPC when adjusted for alcohol and tobacco use (odds ratio [OR] 230; 95% confidence interval [CI] 44–1200).[96]

HPV-16 seropositivity is associated with an increased risk of developing HPV-positive OPCs and oral cancer.[97] A nested case-control study using serum samples from 900,000 people in Norway, Finland, and Sweden identified 292 individuals diagnosed with HNSCC and compared them with 1568 matched control individuals. After adjustment for smoking, the adjusted OR for development of an HNSCC at any site with HPV-16 seropositivity was only 2.1 (95% CI 1.4–3.2), but was 14.4 (95% CI 3.6–58.1) for OPCs.[98] A 2007 case-control study of persons diagnosed with OPC found that HPV-16 seropositivity was strongly associated in people with (OR 19.4; 95% CI 13.3–113.9) and without (OR 33.6; 95% CI 3.3–84.8) a history of smoking or drinking.[87]

Because simply detecting HPV in tumor cells or serum markers for HPV does not demonstrate that HPV actually caused the tumor, markers for transcriptionally active HPV such as E6 and E7 expression and p16 overexpression are better markers. Studies using quantitative PCR and/or in situ hybridization techniques found HPV in only a small proportion of oral cavity SCCs but in 40% to 60% of OPCs.[99–105] A 2006 meta-analysis of 17 studies found that high-risk HPV is associated most strongly with tonsillar cancers (OR 15.1, 95% CI 6.8–33.7), is intermediate for OPC (OR 4.3, 95%

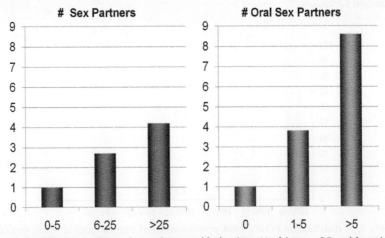

Fig. 8. Risk for HPV positivity and certain sexual behaviors. Hx, history; OR, odds ratio. (*Data from* D'Souza G, Kreimer AR, Viscidi R, et al. Case-control study of human papillomavirus and oropharyngeal cancer. N Engl J Med 2007;356:1944–56.)

CI 2.1–8.9), and is weakest for oral cancers (OR 2.0, 95% CI 1.0–4.2).[106] A 2003 International Agency for Research on Cancer study found HPV in 3.9% (95% CI 2.5–5.3) of oral cavity tumors and 18.3% of OPSCCs.[97]

There are still a lot of questions to be answered about the natural history of oral pharyngeal HPV infections. It is currently unknown as to what degree oropharyngeal HPV infections are sexually acquired, or if they cause productive infections in these areas. The degree of oral transmission of HPV is also uncertain, and the duration of infections is unknown.

Prognosis of HPV-Positive OPC

The prognosis for patients with HPV-associated OPC is significantly better than for those with HPV-negative cancer of a similar stage.[107–110] Retrospective studies have shown a 50% to 80% reduction in risk of cancer-related death for HPV-positive OPC.[99,111–113] HPV-positive OPC seems to have a better response to treatment with induction chemotherapy,[100,114,115] radiotherapy,[116] and combination chemoradiotherapy.[100,115] HPV-associated oropharyngeal cancers are more likely to present with relatively early-stage (T1/T2) primary tumors, but relatively advanced disease in the neck (N2/N3)[107,117]; they also tend to develop distant metastases later.[117]

Why do HPV-Related Cancers Arise in These Areas?

The epithelia of body openings have stratified squamous epithelium at their external borders, which often connect to columnar epithelia internally such as inside the cervical os, in the trachea, and in the rectum. There is often an area of rapidly dividing cells called the metaplastic or transformation zone that establishes a squamocolumnar junction somewhere near each body opening. It is known that areas of metaplastic epithelium are particularly susceptible to papilloma virus infection, owing to its fragile nature that allows basement-membrane access to the virus required for infection. When these areas undergo infection with high-risk HPV types, a chronic infection with potential HPV interpolation into the human genome may occur. In these areas of metaplasia, the complete life cycle of the squamous cell is not completely realized. In these areas of transforming epithelium with incomplete maturation of squamous cells, the orderly production of HPV viral expression is interrupted, possibly causing continuous overproduction of viral oncogenes and increasing human genome interpolation, resulting in the increased rates of cancer noted in these areas.[118]

The perianal area has such a squamocolumnar junction and thus might well be expected to express higher levels of HPV dysplasia, as is observed. In the upper airway digestive tract, squamous epithelium is most commonly seen in the oral cavity, which has a lower rate of HPV-related cancers, much like the vagina. However, transformation zones are seen in the nasopharynx, where HPV-related cancers are more common. Tonsillar tissue also transitions from squamous into lymphoid type tissues, producing a similar effect to that in the metaplastic areas noted earlier. It is theorized that these areas of transitional epithelium in the head and neck or more susceptible to the HPV-transforming effects than are other areas of the upper aerodigestive tract, as has been observed clinically.

Can We Screen or Test for HPV-related HNSCC?

There are several required elements if we are to have an effective cervical-style screening program for OPCs. To be most effective, there must be a premalignant face to the disease that lasts long enough to allow timely intervention to prevent cancer, although finding cancers earlier is of value. It is currently unknown whether there is a dysplastic phase to HPV-related OPCs. There must also be effective treatment during the dysplastic phase to prevent the cancer, which is also currently lacking. Tonsillectomy or superficial destruction of identifying lesions may provide the answer, but further study is needed.

We must also have an effective screening test for pharyngeal HPV-related cancers. Cytology specimens will probably not do well in this area of the body, because there is a large area that must be sampled and many of the areas (especially the tonsils) are deeply invaginated, making reliable sampling difficult. HPV testing may provide a better answer, especially with the high sensitivity of modern HPV tests. However, the odds ratios for oral HPV-16 infection and OPCs are less than that for cervical cancers, and the current HPV tests are not currently indicated (nor have they been studied) for use in the oropharyngeal area.

A subset of patients with OPSCC develops recurrence of cancer after treatment. These patients could possibly benefit from a test that detects markers associated with HPV infection for the detection of disease persistence or of early disease recurrence. A small 2008 study evaluated salivary rinsing as a possible screening test for recurrence of HPV-positive tumors after treatment, and found that detection of HPV-E6 and -E7 by reverse transcription–PCR had sensitivity of 100% and a specificity of 50% for detection of OPC recurrence.[119]

Finally, some form of HPV testing might be used to help identify the site of primary tumor in HNSCC without a known primary site of origin. A small percentage of neck masses are of unknown primary origin. Markers of HPV-associated tumors could be used to pinpoint possible origins and give prognostic information. Fine-needle aspiration biopsies of neck metastases with in situ HPV hybridization[120,121] and immunohistochemistry for p16 overexpression[120] have been shown to be predictive of an oropharyngeal primary tumor.

FUTURE DIRECTIONS

There are many questions that have yet to be answered concerning HPV-related head and neck cancers. Although we have the means to detect and treat high-grade AIN, we do not know at this time whether such treatment, or its detection using anal Pap tests, reduces the risk of anal cancer. How widely screening should be performed is also uncertain. Should we only perform anal Pap tests on HIV-infected individuals, MSM, women with high-grade lower genital tract dysplasias, and other high-risk groups? Or should it potentially include all individuals who are at much lower overall risk?

Better response rates to chemotherapy and radiation therapy, and higher survival rates, have been found in patients with HPV-related OPCs. It is been suggested that treatment protocols might be altered in patients with HPV-positive OPCs to include less aggressive induction and maintenance chemotherapy.[81] Head and neck cancers have also raised the question again about vaccination of males with prophylactic HPV vaccines. Unlike anal cancers, which are still more common in women, OPCs are more prevalent in men. If prophylactic HPV vaccines are shown to prevent these cancers, then relying on herd immunity, as opposed to direct vaccinations of males, may not be an acceptable answer.

There is a good mechanistic basis on which to assume that prophylactic quadrivalent HPV vaccination should prevent respiratory papillomatosis and that both the quadrivalent and bivalent HPV vaccines could prevent HPV-related head and neck cancers, because up to 95% of HPV-positive OPCs are associated with HPV-16 infections. However, currently there is no experimental evidence that they do so. This area will be difficult to study because at present we do not know if there is a premalignant stage to these head and neck cancers, rendering vaccine study end points difficult because cancer is not an acceptable end point. This dilemma may require clinicians to rely on observational data on prevention of head and neck cancer, which will take longer to develop.

REFERENCES

1. Machalek DA, Poynten M, Jin F, et al. Anal human papillomavirus infection and associated neoplastic lesions in men who have sex with men: a systematic review and meta-analysis. Lancet Oncol 2012;13(5):487–500.
2. Kreimer AR, Clifford GM, Boyle P, et al. Human papillomavirus types in head and neck squamous cell carcinomas worldwide: a systematic review. Cancer Epidemiol Biomarkers Prev 2005;14(2):467–75.
3. Hoots BE, Palefsky JM, Pimenta JM, et al. Human papillomavirus type distribution in anal cancer and anal intraepithelial lesions. Int J Cancer 2009;124:2375–83.
4. Available at: http://seer.cancer.gov/statfacts/html/anus.html#incidence-mortality. Accessed December 11, 2012.
5. SEER Fast Stats. Available at: http://seer.cancer.gov/faststats/selections.php?run=runit&output=1&data=1&statistic=1&year=201201&race=1&sex=1&age=1&series=cancer&cancer=34. Accessed December 11, 2012.
6. Palefsky JM. Anal cancer prevention in HIV-positive men and women. Curr Opin Oncol 2009;21(5):433–8.
7. De Vuyst H, Cliff ord GM, Nascimento MC, et al. Prevalence and type distribution of human papillomavirus in carcinoma and intraepithelial neoplasia of the vulva, vagina and anus: a meta-analysis. Int J Cancer 2009;124:1626–36.
8. Edgren G, Sparen P. Risk of anogenital cancer after diagnosis of cervical intraepithelial neoplasia: a prospective population-based study. Lancet Oncol 2007; 8:311–6.
9. Grulich AE, van Leeuwen MT, Falster MO, et al. Incidence of cancers in people with HIV/AIDS compared with immunosuppressed transplant recipients: a meta-analysis. Lancet 2007;370:59–67.
10. Daling JR, Madeleine MM, Johnson LG, et al. Human papillomavirus, smoking, and sexual practices in the etiology of anal cancer. Cancer 2004;101:270–80.
11. Crum-Cianflone NF, Hullsiek KH, Marconi VC, et al. Anal cancers among HIV-infected persons: HAART is not slowing rising incidence. AIDS 2010;24:535–43.
12. Chin-Hong PV, Berry JM, Cheng SC, et al. A population-based study of human papillomavirus-associated anal neoplasia in HIV-positive and HIV-negative men using self-collected specimens: the TPOP study. Ann Intern Med 2008;149:300–6.
13. Hernandez BY, McDuffie K, Zhu X, et al. Anal human papillomavirus infection in women and its relationship with cervical infection. Cancer Epidemiol Biomarkers Prev 2005;14(11 pt 1):2550–6.
14. Palefsky JM, Holly EA, Ralston ML, et al. Prevalence and risk factors for anal human papillomavirus infection In human immunodeficiency virus (HIV)-positive and high-risk HIV-negative women. J Infect Dis 2001;183:383–91.
15. Conley L, Bush T, Darragh TM, et al. Factors associated with prevalent abnormal anal cytology in a large cohort of HIV-infected adults in the United States. J Infect Dis 2010;202:1567–76.
16. Chin-Hong PV, Vittinghoff E, Cranston RD, et al. Age-specific prevalence of anal human papillomavirus infection in HIV-negative sexually active men who have sex with men: the EXPLORE study. J Infect Dis 2004;190:2070–6.

17. Critchlow CW, Holmes KK, Wood R, et al. Association of human immunodeficiency virus and anal human papillomavirus infection among homosexual men. Arch Intern Med 1992;152:1673–6.

18. Palefsky JM, Holly EA, Ralson ML, et al. Prevalence and risk factors for human papillomavirus infection of the anal canal in human immunodeficiency virus (HIV)-positive and HIV-negative homosexual men. J Infect Dis 1998;177:361–7.

19. De Pokomandy A, Rouleau D, Ghattas G, et al. Prevalence, clearance, and incidence of anal human papillomavirus infection in HIV-infected men: the HIPVIRG cohort study. J Infect Dis 2009;199:965–73.

20. Piketty C, Darragh TM, Da Costa M, et al. High prevalence of anal human papillomavirus infection and anal cancer precursors among HIV-infected persons in the absence of anal intercourse. Ann Intern Med 2003;138:453–9.

21. Saiag P, Bauhofer A, Bouscarat F, et al. Imiquimod 5% cream for external genital or perianal warts in human immunodeficiency virus-positive patients treated with highly active antiretroviral therapy: an open-label, noncomparative study. Br J Dermatol 2009;161(4):904–9.

22. Piketty C, Selinger-Leneman H, Grabar S, et al. Marked increase in the incidence of invasive anal cancer among HIV-infected patients despite treatment with combination antiretroviral therapy. AIDS 2008;22:1203–11.

23. Clifford G, Bertisch B, Franceschi S, et al, members of the Swiss HIV Cohort Study. Risk factors for anal cancer in persons infected with HIV: a nested case-control study in the Swiss HIV Cohort Study. Plenary presentation at 28th International Papillomavirus Conference. Puerto Rico, December 6, 2012.

24. Shiels M, Goedert JJ, Engels EA, et al. Anal cancer incidence in HIV+ women and men estimated using population-based US HIV/AIDS and cancer registry data. Plenary presentation at 28th International Papillomavirus Conference. Puerto Rico, December 6, 2012.

25. Palefsky JM, Giuliano AR, Golstone S, et al. HPV vaccine against anal HPV infection and anal intraepithelial neoplasia. N Engl J Med 2011;365:1576–85.

26. Watson AJ, Smith BB, Whitehead MR, et al. Malignant progression of anal intraepithelial neoplasia. ANZ J Surg 2006;76:715–7.

27. Pineda CE, Berry JM, Jay N, et al. High-resolution anoscopy targeted surgical destruction of anal high-grade squamous intraepithelial lesions: a ten-year experience. Dis Colon Rectum 2008;51:829–35 [discussion: 835–7].

28. Kreuter A, Potthoff A, Brockmeyer NH, et al. Anal carcinoma in HIV-positive men: results of a prospective study from Germany. Br J Dermatol 2010;162:1269–77.

29. Palefsky J, Berry JM, Jay N. Anal cancer screening. Re: Machalek et al "Anal human papillomavirus infection and associated neoplastic lesions in men who have sex with men: a systematic review and meta-analysis". Lancet Oncol 2012;13:e279–80 [author reply: e280].

30. Berry JM, Palefsky JM, Jay N, et al. Performance characteristics of anal cytology and human papillomavirus testing in patients with high-resolution anoscopy-guided biopsy of high-grade anal intraepithelial neoplasia. Dis Colon Rectum 2009;52:239–47.

31. Zhao C, Domfeh AB, Austin RM. Histopathologic outcomes and clinical correlations for high-risk patients screened with anal cytology. Acta Cytol 2012;56:62–7.

32. Jay N, Berry JM, Park I, et al. ASC-US anal cytology is highly predictive of high-grade anal intraepithelial neoplasia (HGAIN) in at-risk populations. Abstract presentation at 28th International Papillomavirus Conference. Puerto Rico, December 3, 2012.

33. Darragh TM, Winkler B. Anal cancer and cervical cancer screening: key differences. Cancer Cytopathol 2011;119:5–19.
34. Mayeaux EJ, Cox JT, editors. Modern colposcopy textbook and atlas. Philadelphia: Wolters Kluwer Health/Lippincott Williams & Wilkins; 2012.
35. Singh JC, Kuohung V, Palefsky JM. Efficacy of trichloroacetic acid in the treatment of anal intraepithelial neoplasia in HIV-positive and HIV-negative men who have sex with men. J Acquir Immune Defic Syndr 2009;52(4):474–9.
36. Scheinfeld N, Lehman DS. An evidence-based review of medical and surgical treatments of genital warts. Dermatol Online J 2006;12:5.
37. Komericki P, Akkilic-Materna M, Strimitzer T, et al. Efficacy and safety of Imiquimod versus Podophyllotoxin in the treatment of anogenital warts. Sex Transm Dis 2011;38:216–8.
38. Wagstaff AJ, Perry CM. Topical imiquimod: a review of its use in the management of anogenital warts, actinic keratoses, basal cell carcinoma and other skin lesions. Drugs 2007;67:2187–210.
39. Kreuter A, Potthoff A, Brockmeyer NH, et al. Imiquimod leads to a decrease of human papillomavirus DNA and to a sustained clearance of anal intraepithelial neoplasia in HIV-infected men. J Invest Dermatol 2008;128:2078–83.
40. Pa Fox, Nathan M, Francis N, et al. A double-blind, randomized controlled trial of the use of imiquimod cream for the treatment of anal canal high-grade anal intraepithelial neoplasia in HIV-positive MSM on HAART, with long-term follow-up data including the use of open-label imiquimod. AIDS 2010;24:2331–5.
41. Goldstone SE, Hundert JS, Huyett JW. Infrared coagulator ablation of high-grade anal squamous intraepithelial lesions in HIV-negative males who have sex with males. Dis Colon Rectum 2007;50:565–75.
42. Stier EA, Goldstone SE, Berry JM, et al. Infrared coagulator treatment of high-grade anal dysplasia in HIV-infected individuals: an AIDS malignancy consortium pilot study. J Acquir Immune Defic Syndr 2008;47:56–61.
43. Richel O, Wieland U, De Vries HJ, et al. Topical 5-fluorouracil treatment of anal intraepithelial neoplasia in human immunodeficiency virus-positive men. Br J Dermatol 2010;163:1301–7.
44. Snyder SM, Siekas L, Aboulafia DM. Initial experience with topical fluorouracil for treatment of HIV-associated anal intraepithelial neoplasia. J Int Assoc Physicians AIDS Care (Chic) 2011;10:83–8.
45. Tatti S, Stockfleth E, Beutner KR, et al. Polyphenon E: a new treatment for external anogenital warts. Br J Dermatol 2009;162:176–84.
46. Goldstone SE, Kawakek AZ, Huyett JW. Infrared coagulator: a useful tool for treating anal squamous intraepithelial lesions. Dis Colon Rectum 2005;48:1042–54.
47. Nathan M, Hickey N, Mayuranathan L, et al. Treatment of anal human papillomavirus-associated disease: a long term outcome study. Int J STD AIDS 2008;19:445–9.
48. Venkatesan NN, Pine HS, Underbrink MP. Recurrent respiratory papillomatosis. Otolaryngol Clin North Am 2012;45(3):671–94.
49. Armstrong I R, Derkay CS, Reeves WC. Initial results from the national registry for juvenile-onset recurrent respiratory papillomatosis. RRP Task Force. Arch Otolaryngol Head Neck Surg 1999;125(7):743–8.
50. Bonagura VR, Hatam LJ, Rosenthal DW, et al. Recurrent respiratory papillomatosis: a complex defect in immune responsiveness to human papillomavirus-6 and -11. APMIS 2010;118(6–7):455–70.
51. Wiatrak BJ, Wiatrak DW, Broker TR, et al. Recurrent respiratory papillomatosis: a longitudinal study comparing severity associated with human papilloma viral

types 6 and 11 and other risk factors in a large pediatric population. Laryngoscope 2004;114:1–23.

52. Schraff S, Derkay CS, Burke B, et al. American Society of Pediatric Otolaryngology members' experience with recurrent respiratory papillomatosis and the use of adjuvant therapy. Arch Otolaryngol Head Neck Surg 2004;130(9):1039–42.

53. Derkay CS. Task force on recurrent respiratory papillomas: a preliminary report. Arch Otolaryngol Head Neck Surg 1995;121:1386–91.

54. Cole RR, Myer CM, Cotton RT. Tracheotomy in children with recurrent respiratory papillomatosis. Head Neck 1989;11:226–30.

55. Lindeberg H, Elbrond O. Laryngeal papillomas: clinical aspects in a series of 231 patients. Clin Otolaryngol 1989;14:333–42.

56. Cook JR, Hill DA, Humphrey PA. Squamous cell carcinoma arising in recurrent respiratory papillomatosis with pulmonary involvement: emerging common pattern of clinical features and human papillomavirus serotype association. Mod Pathol 2000;13:914–8.

57. Shah KV, Stern WF, Shah FK, et al. Risk factors for juvenile onset recurrent respiratory papillomatosis. Pediatr Infect Dis J 1998;17(5):372–6.

58. Miller CS, Johnstone BM. Human papillomavirus as a risk factor for oral squamous cell carcinoma: a meta-analysis, 1982-1997. Oral Surg Oral Med Oral Pathol Oral Radiol Endod 2001;91(6):622–35.

59. Stern Y, Felipovich A, Cotton RT, et al. Immunocompetency in children with recurrent respiratory papillomatosis: prospective study. Ann Otol Rhinol Laryngol 2007;116(3):169–71.

60. Bonnez W, Kashima HK, Leventhal B, et al. Antibody response to human papillomavirus (HPV) type 11 in children with juvenile-onset recurrent respiratory papillomatosis (RRP). Virology 1992;188:384–7.

61. Bonagura VR, Siegal FP, Abramson AL, et al. Enriched HLA-DQ3 phenotype and decreased class I major histocompatibility complex antigen expression in recurrent respiratory papillomatosis. Clin Diagn Lab Immunol 1994;1:357–60.

62. Silverberg MJ, Thorsen P, Lindeberg H, et al. Condyloma in pregnancy is strongly predictive of juvenile-onset recurrent respiratory papillomatosis. Obstet Gynecol 2003;101(4):645–52.

63. Kashima HK, Shah F, Lyles A, et al. A comparison of risk factors in juvenile-onset and adult-onset recurrent respiratory papillomatosis. Laryngoscope 1992;102(1):9–13.

64. Kosko JR, Derkay CS. Role of cesarean section in prevention of recurrent respiratory papillomatosis—is there one? Int J Pediatr Otorhinolaryngol 1996;35(1):31–8.

65. Rombaldi RL, Serafini EP, Mandelli J, et al. Transplacental transmission of human papillomavirus. Virol J 2008;5:106.

66. Tenti P, Zappatore R, Migliora P, et al. Perinatal transmission of human papillomavirus from gravidas with latest infections. Obstet Gynecol 1999;93:475–9.

67. Gomez LM, Ma Y, Ho C, et al. Placental infection with human papillomavirus is associated with spontaneous preterm delivery. Humanit Rep 2008;23:709–815.

68. Sarkola ME, Grénman SE, Rintala MA, et al. Human papillomavirus in the placenta and umbilical cord blood. Acta Obstet Gynecol Scand 2008;87:1181–8.

69. Sedlacek TV, Lindheim S, Eder C, et al. Mechanism for human papillomavirus transmission at birth. Am J Obstet Gynecol 1989;161:55–9.

70. Pignatari SS, Liriano RY, Avelino MA, et al. Gastroesophageal reflux in patients with recurrent laryngeal papillomatosis. Braz J Otorhinolaryngol 2007;73:210–4.

71. Shehab N, Sweet BV, Hogikyan ND. Cidofovir for the treatment of recurrent respiratory papillomatosis: a review of the literature. Pharmacotherapy 2005;25(7): 977–89.
72. Rosen CA, Bryson PC. Indole-3-carbinol for recurrent respiratory papillomatosis: long term results. J Voice 2003;18:248–53.
73. Leventhal BG, Kashima HK, Mounts P, et al. Long-term response of recurrent respiratory papillomatosis to treatment with lymphoblastoid interferon alfa-N1. Papilloma Study Group. N Engl J Med 1991;325(9):613–7.
74. Shikowitz MJ, Abramson AL, Freeman K, et al. Efficacy of DHE photodynamic therapy for respiratory papillomatosis: immediate and long-term results. Laryngoscope 1998;108(7):962–7.
75. Derkay CS, Wiatrak B. Recurrent respiratory papillomatosis: a review. Laryngoscope 2008;118:1236–47.
76. Larson DA, Derkay CS. Epidemiology of recurrent respiratory papillomatosis. APMIS 2010;118(6–7):450–4.
77. CDC. Sexually transmitted diseases treatment guidelines, 2010. MMWR Recomm Rep 2010;59(RR-12):1–110.
78. Schaffer A, Brotherton J, Booy R. Do human papillomavirus vaccines have any role in newborns and the prevention of recurrent respiratory papillomatosis in children? J Paediatr Child Health 2007;43(9):579–80.
79. Muttagi SS, Chaturvedi P, Gaikwad R, et al. Head and neck squamous cell carcinoma in chronic areca nut chewing Indian women: case series and review of literature. Indian J Med Paediatr Oncol 2012;33(1):32–5.
80. Ragin CC, Modugno F, Gollin SM. The epidemiology and risk factors of head and neck cancer: a focus on human papillomavirus. J Dent Res 2007;86(2): 104–14.
81. Sturgis EM, Ang KK. The epidemic of HPV-associated oropharyngeal cancer is here: is it time to change our treatment paradigms? J Natl Compr Canc Netw 2011;9:665.
82. Jemal A, Siegel R, Ward E, et al. Cancer statistics, 2008. CA Cancer J Clin 2008; 58(2):71–96.
83. Parkin DM, Bray F, Ferlay J, et al. Global cancer statistics, 2002. CA Cancer J Clin 2005;55(2):74–108.
84. Chaturvedi AK, Engels EA, Pfeiffer RM, et al. Human papillomavirus and rising oropharyngeal cancer incidence in the United States. J Clin Oncol 2011;29: 4294.
85. Shiboski CH, Schmidt BL, Jordan RC. Tongue and tonsil carcinoma: increasing trends in the U.S. population ages 20-44 years. Cancer 2005;103:1843–9.
86. Fakhry C, Gillison ML. Clinical implications of human papillomavirus in head and neck cancers. J Clin Oncol 2006;24:2606–11.
87. D'Souza G, Kreimer AR, Viscidi R, et al. Case-control study of human papillomavirus and oropharyngeal cancer. N Engl J Med 2007;356:1944–56.
88. Goldenberg D, Begum S, Westra WH, et al. Cystic lymph node metastasis in patients with head and neck cancer: an HPV-associated phenomenon. Head Neck 2008;30:898–903.
89. Adelstein DJ, Ridge JA, Gillison ML, et al. Head and neck squamous cell cancer and the human papillomavirus: summary of a National Cancer Institute State of the Science Meeting. November 9-10, 2008, Washington, DC. Head Neck 2009; 31:1393–422.
90. Gillison ML, Broutian T, Pickard RK, et al. Prevalence of oral HPV infection in the United States, 2009-2010. JAMA 2012;307:693.

91. Näsman A, Attner P, Hammarstedt L, et al. Incidence of human papillomavirus (HPV) positive tonsillar carcinoma in Stockholm, Sweden: an epidemic of viral-induced carcinoma? Int J Cancer 2009;125:362.

92. Nunez DA, Astley SM, Lewis FA, et al. Human papilloma viruses: a study of their prevalence in the normal larynx. J Laryngol Otol 1994;108:319–20.

93. Applebaum KM, Furniss CS, Zeka A, et al. Lack of association of alcohol and tobacco with HPV16-associated head and neck cancer. J Natl Cancer Inst 2007;99:1801–10.

94. Sinha P, Logan HL, Mendenhall WM. Human papillomavirus, smoking, and head and neck cancer. Am J Otol 2012;33(1):130–6.

95. Hemminki K, Dong C, Frisch M. Tonsillar and other upper aerodigestive tract cancers among cervical cancer patients and their husbands. Eur J Cancer Prev 2000;9:433–7.

96. Hansson BG, Rosenquist K, Antonsson A, et al. Strong association between infection with human papillomavirus and oral and oropharyngeal squamous cell carcinoma: a population based case-control study in southern Sweden. Acta Otolaryngol 2005;125:1337–44.

97. Herrero R, Castellsague X, Pawlita M, et al. Human papillomavirus and oral cancer: the International Agency for Research on Cancer multicenter study. J Natl Cancer Inst 2003;95:1772–83.

98. Mork J, Lie AK, Glattre E, et al. Human papillomavirus infection as a risk factor for squamous-cell carcinoma of the head and neck. N Engl J Med 2001;344: 1125–31.

99. Gillison ML, Koch WM, Capone RB, et al. Evidence for a causal association between human papillomavirus and a subset of head and neck cancers. J Natl Cancer Inst 2000;92:709–20.

100. Fakhry C, Westra WH, Li S, et al. Improved survival of patients with human papillomavirus-positive head and neck squamous cell carcinoma in a prospective clinical trial. J Natl Cancer Inst 2008;100:261–9.

101. Schwartz SM, Daling JR, Doody DR, et al. Oral cancer risk in relation to sexual history and evidence of human papillomavirus infection. J Natl Cancer Inst 1998;90:1626–36.

102. Klussmann JP, Gultekin E, Weissenborn SJ, et al. Expression of p16 protein identifies a distinct entity of tonsillar carcinomas associated with human papillomavirus. Am J Pathol 2003;162:747–53.

103. Ritchie JM, Smith EM, Summersgill KF, et al. Human papillomavirus infection as a prognostic factor in carcinomas of the oral cavity and oropharynx. Int J Cancer 2003;104:336–44.

104. Syrjänen S. Human papillomavirus (HPV) in head and neck cancer. J Clin Virol 2005;32(Suppl 1):59–66.

105. Kim SH, Koo BS, Kang S, et al. HPV integration begins in the tonsillar crypt and leads to the alteration of p16, EGFR and c-myc during tumor formation. Int J Cancer 2007;120:1418–25.

106. Hobbs CG, Sterne JA, Bailey M, et al. Human papillomavirus and head and neck cancer: a systematic review and meta-analysis. Clin Otolaryngol 2006; 31:259–66.

107. Ang KK, Harris J, Wheeler R, et al. Human papillomavirus and survival of patients with oropharyngeal cancer. N Engl J Med 2010;363:24.

108. Rischin D, Young RJ, Fisher R, et al. Prognostic significance of p16INK4A and human papillomavirus in patients with oropharyngeal cancer treated on TROG 02.02 phase III trial. J Clin Oncol 2010;28:4142.

109. Lorch JH, Goloubeva O, Haddad RI, et al. Induction chemotherapy with cisplatin and fluorouracil alone or in combination with docetaxel in locally advanced squamous-cell cancer of the head and neck: long-term results of the TAX 324 randomised phase 3 trial. Lancet Oncol 2011;12:153.

110. Posner MR, Lorch JH, Goloubeva O, et al. Survival and human papillomavirus in oropharynx cancer in TAX 324: a subset analysis from an international phase III trial. Ann Oncol 2011;22:1071.

111. Weinberger PM, Yu Z, Haffty BG, et al. Molecular classification identifies a subset of human papillomavirus-associated oropharyngeal cancers with favorable prognosis. J Clin Oncol 2006;24:736–47.

112. Mellin H, Friesland S, Lewensohn R, et al. Human papillomavirus (HPV) DNA in tonsillar cancer: clinical correlates, risk of relapse, and survival. Int J Cancer 2000;89:300–4.

113. Ritta M, De Andrea M, Mondini M, et al. Cell cycle and viral and immunologic profiles of head and neck squamous cell carcinoma as predictable variables of tumor progression. Head Neck 2009;31:318–27.

114. Kumar B, Cordell KG, Lee JS, et al. EGFR, p16, HPV Titer, Bcl-xL and p53, sex, and smoking as indicators of response to therapy and survival in oropharyngeal cancer. J Clin Oncol 2008;26:3128–37.

115. Worden FP, Kumar B, Lee JS, et al. Chemoselection as a strategy for organ preservation in advanced oropharynx cancer: response and survival positively associated with HPV16 copy number. J Clin Oncol 2008;26:3138–46.

116. Lassen P, Eriksen JG, Hamilton-Dutoit S, et al. Effect of HPV-associated p16INK4A expression on response to radiotherapy and survival in squamous cell carcinoma of the head and neck. J Clin Oncol 2009;27:1992–8.

117. Huang SH, Perez-Ordonez B, Liu FF, et al. Atypical clinical behavior of p16-confirmed HPV-related oropharyngeal squamous cell carcinoma treated with radical radiotherapy. Int J Radiat Oncol Biol Phys 2012;82:276.

118. Evans M, Powell NG. The changing aetiology of head and neck cancer: the role of human papillomavirus. Clin Oncol (R Coll Radiol) 2010;22(7):538–46.

119. Chang F, Syrjänen S, Kellokoski J, et al. Human papillomavirus (HPV) infections and their associations with oral disease. J Oral Pathol Med 1991;20:305–17.

120. Begum S, Gillison ML, Nicol TL, et al. Detection of human papillomavirus-16 in fine-needle aspirates to determine tumor origin in patients with metastatic squamous cell carcinoma of the head and neck. Clin Cancer Res 2007;13:1186–91.

121. Zhang MQ, El-Mofty SK, Davila RM. Detection of human papillomavirus-related squamous cell carcinoma cytologically and by in situ hybridization in fine-needle aspiration biopsies of cervical metastasis: a tool for identifying the site of an occult head and neck primary. Cancer 2008;114:118–23.

Cervical Cancer Screening in Immunocompromised Women

Minh Ly Nguyen, MD, MPH[a], Lisa Flowers, MD[b],*

KEYWORDS

- Cervical cancer screening • HIV or AIDS • Solid organ transplant
- Combined antiretroviral therapy

KEY POINTS

- Immunocompromised women are at an increased risk of squamous intraepithelial lesion (SIL) and cervical cancer.
- There is an increased risk of oncogenic and nononcogenic human papillomavirus (HPV) infection, infection with multiple HPV subtypes, and persistence of HPV infection in human immunodeficiency virus–infected women.
- The effect of combined antiretroviral therapy on HPV infection and rates of cervical cancer is inconclusive.
- Vigilance in screening for SIL and cancer in immunocompromised women is warranted.

INTRODUCTION

Immunocompromised women encompass a variety of populations, the largest being human immunodeficiency virus (HIV)–infected women. Approximately 17 million women worldwide are HIV-infected, with US estimates at 280,000.[1,2] Women who belong to the other immunocompromised populations are solid organ transplant recipients and patients with conditions requiring chronic immunosuppressive therapies such as systemic lupus erythematosus (SLE), inflammatory bowel disease (IBS), and other conditions requiring chronic immunosuppressive therapies. Cervical cancer screening in these populations has been debated and insufficiently investigated except in the HIV-infected population. Limited numbers of studies and conflicting data have made it challenging to develop evidence-based guidelines for cervical cancer screening. This article discusses the data and the current guidelines for cervical cancer screening in the immunocompromised population.

[a] Division of Infectious Disease, Department of Internal Medicine, Emory University School of Medicine, 341 Ponce de Leon Northeast, Atlanta, GA 30308, USA; [b] Division of Gynecologic Oncology, Department of Gynecology and Obstetrics, Emory University School of Medicine, 49 Jesse Hill Jr. Drive, Emory University Faculty Office Building 3rd Floor, Atlanta, GA 30303, USA
* Corresponding author.
E-mail address: lflowe2@emoryhealthcare.org

Obstet Gynecol Clin N Am 40 (2013) 339–357
http://dx.doi.org/10.1016/j.ogc.2013.02.005
0889-8545/13/$ – see front matter © 2013 Published by Elsevier Inc.

CERVICAL CANCER SCREENING IN WOMEN INFECTED WITH HIV
HIV and Human Papillomavirus Interaction

Human papillomavirus (HPV), a nonenveloped DNA virus, has been identified as the cause of anogenital cancers. In the 1990s, a subset of HPV was identified as a necessary, but not sufficient, cause of cervical cancer. This subset was called oncogenic HPV or high-risk HPV (hrHPV) and included HPV subtypes 16, 18, 31, 33, 35, 39, 45, 51, 52, 56, 58, 59, 66, and 68.[3] In the immunocompetent host, it is estimated that hrHPV infection causes high-grade precancerous lesions (CIN3) to develop slowly over many years (7–8 years), and causes CIN3 to become invasive cervical cancer (ICC) over an additional 5 to 7 years.[3] However, in HIV-infected women the time to progression to ICC is much shorter. In a cancer–acquired immunodeficiency syndrome (AIDS) registry linkage study from 11 sites in the United States (1995–1998), Frisch and colleagues[4] reported that the mean age difference from in-situ cervical cancer to ICC was 3.2 years for women with an AIDS diagnosis compared with 15.7 years for women in the general population. It has been shown that HIV-infected women have a higher prevalence of non-16 and non-18 hrHPV, a higher risk of multiple HPV infections, a higher persistence of HPV infections, as well as an increased risk of progression to precancerous or cancerous cervical lesions compared with HIV-uninfected women.[5,6] In a meta-analysis of 20 studies published between January 1989 and June 2005, with a total of 5578 HIV-infected women with available baseline cervical Papanicolaou (Pap) test and HPV genotyping throughout the world, the investigators reported a baseline rate of normal cytology in 58%, atypical squamous cell of undetermined significance (ASCUS) or low grade squamous intraepithelial lesion (LSIL) in 37% and high grade squamous intraepithelial lesion (HSIL) in 5% of HIV-infected women (WHIV). In addition, they showed that the rate of HPV prevalence increased with the degree of cytologic abnormality: 36.3% for those with normal cytology, 69.4% for ASCUS/LSIL, and 84.1% for HSIL. Multiple HPV infection prevalence was 11.9% for normal cytology, 34.7% for ASCU/LSIL, and 41.1% for HSIL. Among those with normal cytology at baseline, the prevalence of HPV was 57.4% in South/Central America, 56.6% in Africa, 32.4% in Europe, 31.4% in North America, and 31.1% in Asia. Among those with HSIL, the prevalence of any HPV was similar to that in the general population (84.1% for WHIV compared with 84%). However, the rate of multiple HPV infections was higher for WHIV than in the general population (41.4% vs 6.7%). In addition, there is a lower prevalence of HPV16 among HIV-infected women with HSIL (odds ratio [OR] = 0.6, 95% confidence interval [CI] 0.4–0.7) and a higher prevalence of HPV18, 33, 51, 52, and 58 than in the general population.

Molecular studies have shown that, in the HPV-infected cell, the viral early proteins E6 and E7 interact with intracellular growth–regulating host cell proteins (p53 and retinoblastoma protein), which leads to a disturbance of the regulation of DNA replication, repair, and cellular growth.[7,8] Moreover, in vitro data have shown that the transactivator of transcription (tat) protein may enhance the expression of E6 and E7 proteins,[9] although this has not been shown in in vivo models.

Palefsky[10] proposed a pathogenesis model in WHIV in which, early in the HPV infection, the specific immune response to HPV plays a major role in the control of HPV infection as well as the development of squamous intraepithelial lesions (SILs) or cervical intraepithelial neoplasia (CIN) but, later on, cellular genetic change and chromosomal instability would play a predominant role in the transformation of advanced precancerous lesions to ICC. In this model, as long as the effects of immunosuppression from HIV remained minimal, the HPV infection would be limited with little epithelial abnormality. As immunosuppression progresses with a more advanced stage of HIV infection, there is increased HPV replication with more epithelial damage and development of CIN grades 1 to 3. However, progression from CIN3 to ICC would be determined more by host genetic change and chromosomal instability than by the systemic HPV response of the local tissues immunity. Based on that model, as long as antiretrovirals are started early and the immune system reconstituted before the so-called genetic point of no return[10] is reached, ICC can be prevented and tissue abnormalities reversed.

Data from multiple studies of adult WHIV have shown a clear relationship between immunosuppression as measured by lower CD4+ cell count (<500/mm^3) and increased prevalence of cervical HPV infection and increased HPV DNA levels, with many studies showing even higher risk among those with CD4+ cell counts less than 200/mm^3.[11-13] Along with higher HPV DNA levels, there is also a relationship between lower CD4+ cell count and increased number of HPV types in cervical specimens of HIV-infected women.[13] Moreover, immunosuppression among WHIV is associated with higher prevalence of CIN and faster progression to high-grade CIN.[14] With the immunosuppressive state, the higher rate of HPV infection and the presence of multiple HPV subtypes, an environment of vulnerability develops, leading to the development of CIN3 and ICC.

Effect of Combined Antiretroviral Therapy on Cervical Cancer Incidence in Developed Countries

Although combined antiretroviral therapy (cART) has led to reductions in the incidence of 2 of the AIDS-defining cancers (Kaposi sarcoma and non-Hodgkin lymphoma) among HIV-infected individuals, it has not reduced the incidence of ICC, which has remained almost unchanged (**Table 1**).[15-17] A population-based, AIDS-cancer record-linkage study in 472,378 individuals with AIDS from 1960 to 2006 showed a stable cumulative 5-year incidence of ICC (0.63 for 1980–1989, the pre-cART era; 0.73 for 1990–1995; and 0.64 for 1996–2006, the cART era).[18] A systematic review of published literature on population-based studies showed no significant changes in ICC incidence in the preantiretroviral and postantiretroviral eras.[19] The prospective cohort of WHIV adds more information on the effect of cART on the incidence of ICC. In a report from a French HIV cohort of patients with HIV during the period of 1998 to 2006 with a median follow-up of 4.9 years (interquartile range (IQR) 1.7–9 years), the relative risk (RR) of ICC decreases with increased CD4+ cell count and increased time on cART. In a multivariate analysis of factors associated with cervical cancers based on Poisson regression models, there was an inverse relationship of risk of cancer and CD4+ cell count (RR = 0.7; 95% CI = 0.6–0.8), as well as duration of cART of more than 6 months (RR = 0.5; 95% CI = 0.3–0.9) and an increase of cancer risk for each decade after the age of 30 years until the age of 60 years.[20] Two US cohorts that followed HIV-infected patients prospectively reported conflicting results. The first was derived from the Women's Interagency HIV study (WIHS) comparing 1760 WHIV with 472 HIV-uninfected women enrolled from 1994 and followed for a median of 10.3 and 11.3 years respectively.[21] The investigators reported no significant difference in ICC incidence rate between HIV-infected and HIV-uninfected women (21.4/100,000 patient-years vs 0/100,000 patient-years, $P = .59$). The calculated standardized incidence rate ratio (SIR) compared with the Surveillance, Epidemiology and End Results (SEER) data was not significantly different at 1.32 (95% CI = 0.27–3.85). The investigators concluded that, among WHIV enrolled in a care program that included regular cervical cancer prevention measures, the incidence of ICC was not

Table 1
ICC rates in the eras before and after the advent of highly active antiretroviral therapy (HAART) from population-based studies

Authors	Study	Population	Pre-HAART	HAART	
Biggar et al,[84] 2007	Linkage HIV/ AIDS-cancer registry United States	325,516 AIDS	IR = 64/100,000 py	IR = 86/100,000 py RR = 1.4 (0.8–2.5)	No statistically significant impact of CD4+ cell count on rate
Patel et al,[16] 2008	Outpatient HIV cohort ASD/HOPS	54,780 HIV	1992–1995: SRR = 12 (7–19)	2000–2003: SRR = 10 (6–16)	—
Engels et al,[17] 2008	Linkage HIV/ AIDS-cancer registry United States	114,700 HIV	1986–1996: SIR = 3.1 (1.1–6.7)	1997–2004: SIR = 2.9 (1.8–4.4)	—
Dal Maso et al,[85] 2009	Linkage AIDS- cancer registries Italy	21,951 AIDS	1991–1996: SIR = 51 (23–97)	1996–2002: SIR = 41.5 (28–59)	—
Chaturvedi et al,[86] 2009	Linkage HIV/ AIDS-cancer registry United States	499,230 AIDS	1990–1995: IR = 89/100,000 py	1996–2004: IR = 90.4/ 100,000 py RR = 1.03 (0.7–1.5)	—

Abbreviations: ASD, adult and adolescent spectrum of HIV disease; HOPS, HIV outpatient study; IR, incidence rate; py, person-years; RR, relative risk; SIR, standardized incidence rate ratio; SRR, standardized rate ratio.

significantly higher than in HIV-uninfected women or in the general population. However, another study from the North American AIDS Cohort Collaboration on Research and Design (NA-ACCORD),[22] a prospective multicenter cohort of HIV-infected and uninfected persons enrolled from 1996 to 2010 followed for a median of 4.5 years (WHIV) and 5 years (HIV-uninfected), showed that the rate of ICC was significantly higher in 13,690 WHIV compared with 12,021 HIV-uninfected women (incidence rate of 26 and 6 per 100,000 person-years). The risk of ICC increases with the degree of immunosuppression: 2.3 times increase in incidence compared with HIV-uninfected women for those with baseline CD4+ cell count greater than 350 cells/mm³, 3.0 times for those with CD4+ cell count between 200 and 349 cells/mm³, and 7.7 times for those with CD4+ cell count less than 200 cells/mm³ (*P* trend = .001). Similar risk trends were reported using CD4+ cell count 18 months before cancer diagnosis or CD4+ cell count cancer diagnosis. The overall SIR was 4.1 (1.3–9.3) in WHIV compared with the cohort in the SEER data.[22] The difference observed in the two studies may stem from the design of the two cohorts. In the WIHS cohort, women received regular cervical cancer screening every 6 months, whereas, in the NA-ACCORD, some women may have only been receiving HIV care, or may not have been engaged in regular care. Six of the 17 incident cases in the NA-ACCORD cohort had no evidence of cervical cancer screening within the 5 years before diagnosis.

Therefore, in the cART era, the incidence of ICC among WHIV remained stable, possibly for 2 reasons. Because WHIV survive longer with cART, they reach an age when ICC is more prevalent, and have time for HPV-associated diseases to progress to advanced cancer and thus increase the burden of ICC in WHIV. This effect may be offset by the beneficial effect of combined antiretroviral therapy (cART) and regular cervical cancer screening for WHIV in care. Antiretroviral therapy would have an indirect effect on HPV infection by reconstituting the cell mediated immune system as well as a direct effect as some protease inhibitors were shown to inhibit HPV proliferation and cellular replication.[23,24] In addition, WHIV in care also benefitted from counseling in avoidance of HPV-infection prone behaviors,[25] as well as regular cervical cancer screening that would allow early detection and treatment of precancerous lesions. Finally, the stable ICC rate could also be explained by the increasing number of WHIV due to improved survival which would mask an increase of absolute number of cervical cancers.

Effect of cART on HPV Persistence and Evolution of Precancer Lesions

Two systematic reviews of published studies until 2009 on the impact of cART on HPV infection and HPV-associated cervical dysplasia showed inconsistent and conflicting results.[19,26,27] The investigators pointed out the heterogeneity among the studies in terms of study design, methods of screening, molecular testing methods for HPV, the different lengths of follow-up, as well as the varying definition of regression and progression of cervical lesions, which precludes an overall conclusion about the impact of cART on HPV cervical diseases. Although studies have shown an inverse association between depressed CD4+ cell count and prevalence of HPV infection (any type or oncogenic type) and squamous intraepithelial lesion (SIL),[28–32] the evolution of HPV infection or SIL in the era of cART is not fully elucidated. In **Table 2**, a comparison of recently published studies addressing this question is listed. For the effect of cART on the persistence of HPV in WHIV, some studies[33,34] showed a protective effect against new HPV infections and an improved clearance of HPV. Another study showed an effect of cART on HPV clearance among WHIV who had SIL but not in those with normal cytology.[35] In terms of evolution of SIL lesions, data are more supportive of an effect of cART on the progression of SIL lesions.[33,36] Minkoff and colleagues[37] showed that, among 286 women enrolled in the WIHS cohort who initiated cART, adherence to cART resulted in a significant reduction of SIL (OR = 2.25; 95% CI = 1.03–4.93) compared with before cART.

Further longitudinal studies with more uniform methods and outcome definitions are needed to assess the effect of cART on HPV infection as well as SIL progression, persistence, or regression.

Pap Test and HPV Cotesting in HIV-infected Women

The Pap test is an effective, low-cost screening test for detecting abnormal cytology or neoplasia in exfoliated epithelial cells. Since 1995, HIV treatment guidelines issued by the United States Public Health Services (USPHS) and the Infectious Diseases Society of America (IDSA) have recommended that all WHIV receive cervical cancer screening (via Pap tests) twice during the year after the HIV diagnosis or at enrollment in care and annually thereafter if the tests are negative. The initial biennial screening Pap test for WHIV was recommended given the low sensitivity of Pap tests and concern that a high-grade lesion may be missed with a single Pap test. The results of the Pap test performed on WHIV indicate that 20% to 40% have cytologic cervical abnormalities.[38,39] The role of hrHPV DNA testing in WHIV is uncertain because of the high prevalence of HPV and the transient HPV infections in many instances. Although the guidelines for testing for HIV-uninfected women have been updated and recommendations made for less frequent screening as well as using HPV cotesting with Pap tests

Table 2
Effect of cART on HPV and SIL

Authors	Study Question	Population	HPV Testing Method	Follow-up Duration	cART Use (%)	HPV Incidence	HPV Clearance	SIL Incidence	SIL Clearance	SIL Progression
Minkoff et al,[37] 2010	Effect of cART on HPV and SIL clearance	WIHS: 286 women on cART	Cervicovaginal lavage HPV PCR	At least 2.5 y after cART initiation	100	ANY HPV: (cART vs pre-cART) OR = 0.69 (P = .02) HR HPV: (cART vs pre-cART) (OR = 0.49, P = .006)	ANY HPV: (cART vs pre-cART) (OR = 1.28, P = .06) HR HPV: (cART vs pre-cART) (OR not available)	ANY HPV: (cART vs pre-cART) (OR = 068, P = .45) HR HPV: (cART vs pre-cART) (OR = 0.72, P = .48).	ANY HPV: (cART vs pre-cART) (OR = 2.25, P = .04) HR HPV: (cART vs pre-cART) (OR = 2.352, P = .03)	—
Heard et al,[31] 2012	HR HPV clearance in WHIV in Europe	MACH cohort: 518 WHIV HrHPV = 49.5%	HC2 (liquid Pap or cervical brush)	29 mo	70	—	77% any HPV cleared within 2 y 55.8% with persistence of HR HPV	—	—	—

Study	Topic	n	Sample / HPV test	mo	Result 1	Result 2
Paramsothy et al,[35] 2009	Effect of cART on HPV clearance and SIL clearance	HERS: 537 WHIV	Cervicovaginal lavage HPV PCR	46	cART associated with clearance of HPV in SIL lesions but not with normal or ASCUS	cART associated with SIL regression (HR = 1.3; 1–1.7) CD4+ cell count per 100-cell increase associated with regression (HR = 1.1, 1–1.2)
Zeier et al,[36] 2012	Progression/persistence of LSIL in WHIV	Tygerberg Hospital, South Africa: 1720 with LSIL as first abnormal Pap 3 groups: HIV+, HIV- and never tested	Cervicovaginal lavage HPV PCR	HIV+ 17.5 (5.4–35.6) mo	59	MVA: duration of ART, excision of LSIL, age: • HR = 1.71 (1.29–2.27) if ART before first LSIL • HR = 0.77 (0.61–0.97) if started after first LSIL

MVA: duration of ART, excision of LSIL, age:
• HR = 0.66 (0.54–0.81) if ART before first LSIL
• No difference if ART after LDIL

Abbreviations: HC2, digene hybrid capture 2; HERS, HIV epidemiologic research study; MACH, management of abnormal cytology in HIV-infected women; MVA, multivariate analys s; PCR, polymerase chain reaction assay; WIHS, women's interagency HIV study.

to lengthen the screening interval, there has been little change in cervical cancer screening for WHIV in the past 2 decades (**Table 3**). The use of HPV DNA tests in conjunction with Pap tests for primary screening endorsed in the general population may be less specific in immunocompromised women and thus might not be as efficient for screening because of the high prevalence and persistence of HPV infection among WHIV.[38]

Recent published studies may assist in identifying subsets of WHIV who may need less frequent cervical cancer screening. Massad and colleagues[40] recently reported on the negative predictive value (NPV) of a negative baseline Pap test among 942 HIV-infected women who were in care and 520 HIV-uninfected participants in the WIHS cohort who had no prior history of abnormal Pap tests, cervical cancer, or cervical treatment. The participants had conventional Pap tests every 6 months per study protocol. The outcome was development of precancer lesions, defined as a composite of cervical cytology (HSIL, atypical glandular cells favoring neoplasia or adenocarcinoma in situ) as well as histology from cervical biopsies histology (CIN2 or CIN3 or adenocarcinoma in situ). Among the WHIV the baseline Pap test had a sensitivity of 68% and sensitivity of 78% and a positive predictive value of 6% to develop a precancer lesion within 15 months, and sensitivity of 44% and specificity of 78% with a positive predictive value of 11% to develop a precancer lesion within 39 months. For the WHIV who had 3 consecutive negative Pap tests, none developed precancer in the subsequent 15 months and 10 (2%) developed precancer within 39 months. The investigators further reported that, at 15 months, the negative predictive value (NPV) improved from 99.2% to 100%, and, at 39 months, from 95.8% to 98.1% with 3 consecutive negative Pap tests. In addition, Firnhaber[41] conducted a study among 1193 WHIV in South Africa screened using 3 methods: conventional Pap test, HPV DNA (by hybrid capture or HC2), and visual inspection with acetic acid (VIA). The investigators showed that the NPV for CIN2+ with cytology alone was 89.7% and, using combined cytology and HC2, was 95.5% (93.1%–98%), and for CIN3+ it was 99.2% (98.6%–99.9%) for cytology alone and 100% (99.9%–100%) for combined cytology and HC2. Based on these data, a subgroup of WHIV who are in care without prior history of abnormal Pap tests may be candidates for longer screening interval if they have 3 consecutive negative Pap tests.

Two studies have evaluated the cumulative incidence of cytologic and histologic cervical abnormalities among women with initial normal Pap tests and negative

Table 3
Guideline recommendations for cervical cancer screening in HIV-uninfected and HIV-infected women

	HIV-negative Women[87,88]	HIV-positive Women[83]
Age to start (years)	21	—
Testing frequency: 21–29 years old (Pap alone) 30–64 years old (Pap alone) 30–64 years old (Pap and HPV cotesting)	 Every 3 y Every 3 y Every 5 y if both normal	Every 6 mo for the first year after HIV diagnosis or first entry into care and yearly thereafter if negative
Age to stop (years)	65 after adequate screening	Not addressed
After hysterectomy for benign reason with removal of cervix	Discontinue if no dysplasia or cancer	Not addressed
Screening after HPV vaccination	Not addressed	Not addressed

high-risk HPV. The first women enrolled in the WIHS study from before the highly active antiretroviral therapy (HAART) era between 1994 and 1995 (855 HIV-infected and 343 HIV-uninfected) and were followed for a median of 7 years.[42] Among the women who had a negative HPV DNA test in their cervicovaginal lavage, the investigators reported a 2-year cumulative incidence of SIL that was similar between the HIV-infected (9% for CD4+ cell count <500 cells/mm^3 and 4% for CD4+ cell count >500 cells/mm^3) compared with 3% for HIV-uninfected women. However, for the same group, the 3-year cumulative incidence of any SIL was higher in the HIV-infected women (29% for CD4+ cell count <200 cells/mm^3, 14% for CD4+ cell count between 200 and 499 cells/mm^3 and 6% for CD4+ cell count >500 cells/mm^3) compared with 5% among the HIV-uninfected women. There was no HSIL or cervical cancer reported during the 3-year follow-up. For the women whose cervicovaginal lavage was negative for oncogenic HPV, the 2-year cumulative incidence of any SIL was 21% for CD4+ cell count less than 200 cells/mm^3, 15% for CD4+ cell count 200 to 499 cells/mm^3, and 5% for CD4+ cell count greater than 500 cells/mm^3, which is similar to the low rate in HIV-uninfected women. This rate persists at 3 years for WHIV without oncogenic HPV infection (9% vs 6%). Another follow-up study enrolled women in the WIHS cohort in 2001 to 2002[43] and followed them for at least 5 years (420 HIV-infected women and 297 HIV-uninfected women). There was no statistically significant difference in the 5-year cumulative incidence for HSIL for HIV-infected women (0.3%) and HIV-uninfected women (0.4%), CIN2+ for HIV-infected women (5%) and HIV-uninfected women (5%), or CIN3+ for HIV-uninfected women (0.5%) and HIV-uninfected women (0.7%). There was no significant difference in the 5-year cumulative rate according to immune status for HSIL or CIN2+. However, CD4+ cell count levels inversely affected the 5-year cumulative incidence of any SIL: 25% for CD4+ cell count less than or equal to 350 cells/mm^3, 11% for CD4+ cell count greater than or equal to 350 cells/mm^3, and 6% for HIV-uninfected women. The two studies highlighted that WHIV with a normal Pap test and without oncogenic HPV on cervicovaginal lavage at presentation had the same rate of precancer (HSIL) and cancer as HIV-uninfected women over a 3-year to 5-year follow-up.

Therefore, WHIV in care, no prior abnormal Pap, and with regular cervical screening, 3 consecutive negative Pap tests may allow longer intervals between cervical cancer screenings. In addition, a baseline normal Pap test with a negative HPV DNA test might allow longer screening intervals if these results are confirmed by larger cohorts in regular HIV clinics.

Cervical Cancer Screening in Adolescents

The data on cervical screening in the HIV adolescent are limited. Little is known about the natural history of HPV infection in adolescents with perinatally acquired HIV infection or behaviorally acquired HIV infection. In the Reaching for Excellence in Adolescent Health Care (REACH) study,[14] a national study of HIV infection involving 16 US sites, 133 HIV-positive and 55 HIV-negative adolescent girls were screened for HPV DNA using polymerase chain reaction (PCR) and Pap test during baseline visits to detect HPV infection and SIL disease. At baseline visits, HPV DNA was detected in 78% of HIV-infected patients compared with 54% of HIV-uninfected adolescent girls. High-risk HPV infection was more prevalent among HIV-infected compared with HIV-uninfected adolescents (RR = 1.8; 95% CI = 1.2–2.7) than low-risk HPV (RR = 1.2; 95% CI = 0.4–3.9). Among those with HPV infection, 30% of HIV-infected, compared with 70% of HIV-uninfected, adolescents had normal Pap tests. In a multivariate analysis, CD4+ cell count and viral load were not predictors for HPV infection or SIL disease. In a subsequent study, participants of the REACH cohort of adolescent girls between 13 and 18 years of age with without evidence of HSIL cervical cytology at study entry were enrolled and followed for HSIL disease. In this study, 172 HIV-infected and 84 HIV-uninfected adolescents were enrolled from February 1996 to December 1999 and followed until November 2000 with Pap tests every 6 months.[44] The incidence of HSIL was higher for HIV-infected (21.5%) than HIV-uninfected (4.8%) subjects. In addition, the occurrence of HSIL was significantly associated with persistent LSIL and a positive HPV test. Setse and colleagues[45] reported the prevalence of abnormal Pap tests among sexually active girls and young women (13–24 years of age) followed in the Longitudinal Epidemiologic Study to Gain Insight into HIV/AIDS in Children and Youth (LEGACY) cohort between November 2005 and June 2007. There were 231 eligible participants, 46% perinatally infected and 54% behaviorally infected, of whom 49% had at least 1 Pap test. Of those participants with at least 1 Pap test, 42.5% had normal cervical cytology, 37% had low-grade lesions or atypical cells, and 2% had HSIL or CIN 3 lesions. The prevalence of SIL was 57.5% for both populations. The concerning issue was that cervical cancer screening in this study population was low, especially in the perinatally infected HIV cohort. Another study from the WIHS cohort[46] reported on 132 young women (45 HIV-infected and 87 HIV-uninfected women) aged 16 to 20 years, who were followed for at least 3 years with 18% being on cART at enrollment. None had high-grade cervical disease (HSIL or CIN2+) at baseline. The investigators showed that the incidence rate for HSIL/CIN2+ was not statistically different among HIV-infected and HIV-uninfected women (incidence rate for HSIL/CIN2+ of 4.8/100 person-years in HIV-infected and 1.6/100 person-years in HIV-uninfected subjects, $P = .13$). Despite the higher rate of high-grade cervical disease in the HIV-positive adolescents, cervical cancer was not observed during the follow-up period in either group. It would be interesting to evaluate the persistence or clearance of HPV infection or of SIL in the adolescent HIV-infected group because, in immunocompetent adolescents, HPV infection is usually transient and most SIL lesions regress.[47] Further studies are needed to assess the appropriate intervals to screen the HIV-infected adolescent population, because of their higher prevalence of SIL as well as the effect of cART on cervical lesions in this population. Until then, annual cervical screening as in the HIV-infected adult should be performed.

Cervical Cancer Screening in HIV-infected Women After Hysterectomy

There is a paucity of data on the natural history of HPV infection in the vagina and vaginal cancer in HIV-positive women after hysterectomy. There is a high incidence of cervical cancer and vaginal cancer in the HIV-infected population compared with their HIV-uninfected counterparts and current recommendations suggest annual cervical screening to prevent cancer.[48] However, vaginal cancer is rare[49] and, in the event of a hysterectomy for benign reasons, in the general healthy population the current recommendation is to cease cervical cancer screening except in high-risk populations[50] (eg, immunocompromised women). Whether vaginal cancer decreases sufficiently to warrant decreased cytologic screening of the vagina after hysterectomy in HIV-infected women is not certain. In the WIHS, a cohort of 86 HIV-infected women and 17 HIV-uninfected women who underwent a hysterectomy were tested for oncogenic and nononcogenic HPV DNA before and after the hysterectomy. Long-term follow-up of this cohort of women revealed that HIV-infected women, compared with their HIV-uninfected counterparts, had significantly higher rates of HPV infection before the hysterectomy (59% vs 12%; $P<.001$) as well as afterward (56% vs 6%; $P<.001$), with the prevalence of HPV infection higher in those with lower CD4+ cell counts. However, hysterectomy was significantly associated with a reduction of

HPV infection in both groups using women as their own controls (OR = 0.71; 95% CI = 0.59–0.85) and this effect was observed for the prevalence of oncogenic HPV infection (OR = 0.50; 95% CI = 0.37–0.68), not with nononcogenic types. The investigators inferred that oncogenic HPV may have a preference toward the cervix compared with the vaginal epithelium, and hence lower rates of vaginal cancer.[51] Massed and colleagues,[52] using a cohort of HIV-infected and HIV-uninfected women from the WIHS study, evaluated women with abnormal vaginal cytology after hysterectomy and histologically confirmed vaginal intraepithelial neoplasia (VAIN) disease. Abnormal vaginal cytology was found in 29% of 3700 visits from HIV-infected women (95% CI = 25%–33%) compared with 4% of 763 visits from HIV-uninfected women (95% CI = 2%–8%; $P<.001$). In addition, HSIL Pap abnormalities were found in HIV-infected women (10 out of 3700) and there were none in the HIV-uninfected women (0 out of 763; $P<.001$). Also, the 5-year clearance rate of abnormal cervical cytology was significantly lower in the HIV-infected women than in the HIV-uninfected women, and lower CD4+ cell counts resulted in less chance of clearance. In this study, 2 HIV-infected women were diagnosed with stage II vaginal cancers. In light of the higher rates of HPV infection and rates of vaginal cancer in HIV-infected women compared with their HIV-uninfected counterparts, these women need close follow-up despite hysterectomy.[49] At present, annual cervical cytology is recommended until further studies show similar disease risk with increased intervals of screening.

CERVICAL CANCER SCREENING IN OTHER IMMUNOCOMPROMISED WOMEN
Organ Transplant Recipients

Organ transplant patients are at an increased risk for HPV-related malignancies because of the requirement of lifelong immunosuppressive therapy. There is a clear link between the dose and duration of immunosuppressive therapy and the development of cancers after transplantation.[53–55] Most posttransplant immunosuppressive therapy entails an adjunctive agent (azathioprine), a corticosteroid, and a calcineurin inhibitor (cyclosporine). These agents have increased survival and reduced acute rejection by 10% to 15%.[30] However, azathioprine and cyclosporine have carcinogenic properties such as the production of growth factors and inhibiting DNA repair leading to cancer.[56]

Most of the research supporting an increased risk of HPV-related malignancies has been in renal transplant recipients (RTRs).[57,58] RTRs have a higher risk of acquiring HPV infections.[32] Whether newly acquired or reactivated latent infection, the incidence of mucosal HPV infections can range between 22% and 63%.[32,59–64] RTRs present with a higher rate of multifocal HPV infections than the general population and hrHPV DNA is detected in a high percentage of these infections. Veroux and colleagues[64] detected HPV DNA in the cervicovaginal brushings of 62.8% of RTRs, and 59% of these women were positive for the hrHPV genotype. Brown and colleagues[60] examined the HPV subtypes present in premalignant and malignant tissue from the cervix, vulva, and vagina of RTRs, immunocompetent patients, and normal samples of immunocompetent controls. There was a significantly higher rate of HPV-positive specimens in the RTRs compared with the immunocompetent patients.[60] It has recently been shown that these multifocal anogenital lesions showed different HPV subtypes and types not generally seen in the immunocompetent patient population.[65] However, there are studies that report low or similar prevalence rates of HPV cervical infection in RTRs and the general population.[66,67] Further studies with larger numbers and longer follow-up with new molecular assays for detection of the different HPV subtypes are needed to show the prevalence of HPV infection in RTR.

In most population-based studies, the incidence of cancers in RTRs is 3-fold to 5-fold higher than in the general population and cervical cancer has been shown to be higher in RTRs than in their immunocompetent counterparts.[53,68] In female kidney transplant recipients in Korea, the risk of cervical cancer was 10 times higher than in the general Korean population. The incidence of cervical cancer in the Korean study was significantly higher than in studies conducted in Western countries; however, the prevalence of HPV infection in the general population of Korea is higher at 43.7% to 44.8%.[69] In a national study of UK solid organ transplant recipients, cervical cancer rates in RTRs were significantly higher than in the general population, with an SIR of 2.3 (95% CI = 1.4, 3.5).[70] This excess in cancers among solid organ transplant recipients is thought to be caused by the effects of immunosuppressive drugs, oncogenic viruses, and immunologic surveillance.

ICC after renal transplantation can present significant challenges in treatment because RTRs with advanced cervical cancer need radiotherapy, which can compromise the transplant. In addition, in patients undergoing surgical management of their cervical cancer, sampling the pelvic nodes can be difficult depending on the placement of the transplanted kidney. Therefore cervical cancer screening recommendations are needed in this population, similar to the HIV-infected population, to capture premalignant lesions, which are easier to treat and result in successful management of cervical neoplasia. Several organizations have developed best practices or recommended guidelines for cervical cancer screening in the organ transplant population.[71,72] The American College of Obstetrics and Gynecology provides a comment that this population may require more frequent screening. The Expert Group on Renal Transplantation and the American Society of Transplantation recommend annual Pap tests and pelvic examinations in all women with renal transplants.[71] Although evidence for optimal frequency of screening has not been established, most recommend annual Pap tests similar to the HIV-infected population. This seems reasonable, because studies comparing cancer rates among HIV-infected and organ transplant recipients show significantly increased rates of cervical cancer compared with the general population for both groups.[61,73] The risk factors of immunosuppression and increased risk of virus-related cancers are reflected in the common pattern of cancer risk among both populations.[61,73,74] A meta-analysis of cancer incidence in 444,172 subjects with HIV/AIDS and 31,977 immunocompromised transplant recipients showed SIRs of 5.82 (95% CI = 2.98–11.3) and 2.13 (95% CI = 1.37–3.30) respectively compared with age-matched controls[73] for cervical cancer.

It has been suggested that this population can be screened as for the general population. Contrary to most studies, a large US population-based study of solid organ transplants (kidney, liver, heart and lung) showed no difference in the rates of cervical and vaginal cancers among transplant recipients and their immunocompetent counterparts.[75] However, there was an increased rate of cancers associated with oncogenic viruses other than in the cervix and vagina.[75] A nationwide cohort study in Sweden revealed similar results, with no significant difference in the rates of cervical cancer among patients with solid organ transplants.[76] There were significant increases in other HPV-related cancers such as vulva, vagina, and anal cancer.[76] The investigators hypothesized that it was most likely secondary to effective screening (Pap test) and treatment of precancerous lesions. In a study by Meeuwis and colleagues,[65] in which there was a 5-fold increased risk of cervical cancer in RTRs compared with controls, there was poor cervical cancer screening in the renal transplant population before transplantation. This finding emphasizes the need for regular cervical cancer screening in all women. However, there is insufficient evidence that cervical screening as an intervention reduces cancer risk and is cost-effective in this population. In light of the newly revised screening guidelines for the general population, additional studies are needed in immunocompromised women to determine appropriate screening intervals, the usefulness of hrHPV testing and HPV genotyping, and the cost-effectiveness of such programs. At present, it seems prudent to start screening at age 21 years and perform yearly cervical cytology after transplantation in conjunction with pelvic examination to evaluate other areas (vagina, vulva) at risk for increased anogenital cancers.

Systemic Lupus Erythematous

There has been conflicting evidence of the effect of SLE or immunosuppressive treatment on the risk of cervical cancer in women with SLE. Several small cohort studies of patients with SLE with long-term follow-up have not shown an increase risk of cervical cancer compared with the general population. However in a large cohort study by Hemminki and colleagues, patients with discoid lupus erythematous demonstrated an increase risk of cervical cancer, SIR 3.34.[77,78] In some of these studies, dose and duration of immunosuppressive therapy were not recorded and compliance with screening recommendations was not evident. Studies have shown that SLE is associated with a higher risk of HPV infection and CIN disease compared with the general population.[79,80,81] The use of immunosuppressive therapy in patients with SLE resulted in an increased risk of CIN disease compared with patients with SLE not on therapy and the general population.[79,80–82] Tam and colleagues[80] showed increased abnormal cervical cytology in patients with SLE (OR = 3.1; 95% CI = 1.6–6.2) independent of duration or dose of immunosuppressive therapy after adjusting for hrHPV infection. Whether this increased prevalence of CIN and abnormal cervical cytology translate into a higher risk of cervical cancer is yet to be determined. Therefore, cervical cancer screening in this population should be encouraged; however, increased surveillance similar to that recommended for the HIV-infected population may be warranted in those on immunosuppressive therapy.

SUMMARY

Over the years, cervical cancer screening has been reviewed, debated, and has undergone several revisions in the general population. Challenges still exist in the best approach for screening immunocompromised women in an evidence-based and cost-effective manner. The data suggest that the immunocompromised populations are at higher risks for HPV-related cancers, especially the HIV-infected population.[73] However, studies in the solid organ transplant population and other populations on chronic immunosuppressive therapy have also shown higher rates of oncogenic viral-induced cancers such as those caused by HPV.[53,57,58,65] Newly revised recommendations for the general population[50] do not address screening in the immunocompromised populations and there is still a concern for the lack of data to justify increased screening intervals in these high-risk populations. Current recommendations for women infected with HIV suggest annual Pap tests after 2 screening Pap tests are conducted at the initial encounter.[48,83] Massad and colleagues[40] showed that performing 2 Pap tests 6 months apart before proceeding to annual screening may not be necessary. To date, the data on the effect of cART on the prevalence and persistence of HPV and the evolution of SIL in HIV-infected women are inconclusive. Further longitudinal studies with more uniform methods of HPV DNA measurements, more consistent cervical sampling, and comparable defined outcomes are needed to assess the impact of cART in cervical precancerous lesions. In addition, further studies are needed to identify the subset of HIV-infected women who are on cART and have regular gynecologic follow-up who may be candidates for longer cervical cancer screening intervals. In this subset, cotesting with HPV DNA may help identify those who do not need yearly Pap tests. Among adolescents who are sexually active, as well as individuals who are immunocompromised for reasons other than HIV, annual cervical cancer screening is warranted. Also, thorough periodic examination of the anogenital tract (cervix, vagina, vulva, and anus) for HPV-related lesions that may require follow-up or treatment is critical in the care of these immunocompromised women.

REFERENCES

1. UNAIDS Reports on the global AIDS epidemic 2012. Available at: http://www. unaids.org/en/media/unaids/contentassets/documents/epidemiology/2012/gr2012/20121120_UNAIDS_Global_Report_2012_with_annexes_en.pdf. Accessed January 15, 2013.
2. HIV among women. Center for Diseases and Prevention-National Center for HIV/AIDS, Viral Hepatitis, STD, and TB Prevention, Division of HIV/AIDS Prevention. Available at: http://www.cdc.gov/Features/WomenGirlsHIVAIDS/. Accessed January 15, 2013.
3. Anderson Jean EL, Sanghvi H, Kibwana S, et al. Cervical cancer screening and prevention for HIV-infected women in the developing world. Cancer prevention - from mechanisms to translational benefits. Available at: http://www.jhpiego.org/files/CECAP_Mechanisms_Translation_Benefits_Ch9.pdf. Accessed January 15, 2013.
4. Frisch M, Biggar RJ, Goedert JJ. Human papillomavirus-associated cancers in patients with human immunodeficiency virus infection and acquired immunodeficiency syndrome. J Natl Cancer Inst 2000;92(18):1500–10.
5. Denny L. Cytological screening for cervical cancer prevention. Best Pract Res Clin Obstet Gynaecol 2012;26(2):189–96.
6. Clifford G, Franceschi S, Diaz M, et al. Chapter 3: HPV type-distribution in women with and without cervical neoplastic diseases. Vaccine 2006;24(Suppl 3). S3/26–34.
7. Havre PA, Yuan J, Hedrick L, et al. p53 inactivation by HPV16 E6 results in increased mutagenesis in human cells. Cancer Res 1995;55(19):4420–4.
8. Jones DL, Thompson DA, Munger K. Destabilization of the RB tumor suppressor protein and stabilization of p53 contribute to HPV type 16 E7-induced apoptosis. Virology 1997;239(1):97–107.
9. Vernon SD, Hart CE, Reeves WC, et al. The HIV-1 tat protein enhances E2-dependent human papillomavirus 16 transcription. Virus Res 1993;27(2):133–45.
10. Palefsky J. Biology of HPV in HIV infection. Adv Dent Res 2006;19(1):99–105.
11. Krajden M, Karunakaran K, So S, et al. Prevalence of human papillomavirus 16 and 18 neutralizing antibodies in prenatal women in British Columbia. Clin Vaccine Immunol 2009;16(12):1840–3.
12. Palefsky JM. Anal squamous intraepithelial lesions: relation to HIV and human papillomavirus infection. J Acquir Immune Defic Syndr 1999;21(Suppl 1):S42–8.
13. Sun XW, Kuhn L, Ellerbrock TV, et al. Human papillomavirus infection in women infected with the human immunodeficiency virus. N Engl J Med 1997;337(19): 1343–9.
14. Moscicki AB, Ellenberg JH, Vermund SH, et al. Prevalence of and risks for cervical human papillomavirus infection and squamous intraepithelial lesions in

adolescent girls: impact of infection with human immunodeficiency virus. Arch Pediatr Adolesc Med 2000;154(2):127–34.

15. Clifford GM, Gallus S, Herrero R, et al. Worldwide distribution of human papillomavirus types in cytologically normal women in the International Agency for Research on Cancer HPV prevalence surveys: a pooled analysis. Lancet 2005; 366(9490):991–8.

16. Patel P, Hanson DL, Sullivan PS, et al. Incidence of types of cancer among HIV-infected persons compared with the general population in the United States, 1992-2003. Ann Intern Med 2008;148(10):728–36.

17. Engels EA, Biggar RJ, Hall HI, et al. Cancer risk in people infected with human immunodeficiency virus in the United States. Int J Cancer 2008;123(1):187–94.

18. Simard EP, Pfeiffer RM, Engels EA. Cumulative incidence of cancer among individuals with acquired immunodeficiency syndrome in the United States. Cancer 2011;117(5):1089–96.

19. Vajdic CM, van Leeuwen MT, McDonald SP, et al. Increased incidence of squamous cell carcinoma of eye after kidney transplantation. J Natl Cancer Inst 2007;99(17):1340–2.

20. Guiguet M, Boue F, Cadranel J, et al. Effect of immunodeficiency, HIV viral load, and antiretroviral therapy on the risk of individual malignancies (FHDH-ANRS CO4): a prospective cohort study. Lancet Oncol 2009;10(12):1152–9.

21. Massad LS, Seaberg EC, Watts DH, et al. Long-term incidence of cervical cancer in women with human immunodeficiency virus. Cancer 2009;115(3):524–30.

22. Abraham AG, Strickler HD, Jing Y, et al. Invasive cervical cancer risk among HIV-infected women: a North American multi-cohort collaboration prospective study. J Acquir Immune Defic Syndr 2013;62(4):405–13.

23. Hampson L, Kitchener HC, Hampson IN. Specific HIV protease inhibitors inhibit the ability of HPV16 E6 to degrade p53 and selectively kill E6-dependent cervical carcinoma cells in vitro. Antivir Ther 2006;11(6):813–25.

24. Palefsky J. HIV protease inhibitors to prevent progression of cervical intraepithelial neoplasia to cervical cancer: therapeutic opportunities and challenges. AIDS 2012;26(8).1035–6.

25. Gravitt PE, Paul P, Katki HA, et al. Effectiveness of VIA, Pap, and HPV DNA testing in a cervical cancer screening program in a peri-urban community in Andhra Pradesh, India. PLoS One 2010;5(10):e13711.

26. Adler DH. The impact of HAART on HPV-related cervical disease. Curr HIV Res 2010;8(7):493–7.

27. Levine AM, Seaberg EC, Hessol NA, et al. HIV as a risk factor for lung cancer in women: data from the Women's Interagency HIV Study. J Clin Oncol 2010;28(9): 1514–9.

28. Moloney FJ, Comber H, O'Lorcain P, et al. A population-based study of skin cancer incidence and prevalence in renal transplant recipients. Br J Dermatol 2006; 154(3):498–504.

29. Palefsky J. Human papillomavirus infection in HIV-infected persons. Top HIV Med 2007;15(4).130–3.

30. Moloney FJ, Kelly PO, Kay EW, et al. Maintenance versus reduction of immunosuppression in renal transplant recipients with aggressive squamous cell carcinoma. Dermatol Surg 2004;30(4 Pt 2):674–8.

31. Heard I, Cubie H, Mesher D, et al. Characteristics of HPV infection over time in European women who are HIV-1 positive. BJOG 2012;120(1):41–9.

32. Fairley CK, Sheil AG, McNeil JJ, et al. The risk of ano-genital malignancies in dialysis and transplant patients. Clinical Nephrology 1994;41(2):101–5.

33. Budde K, Sommerer C, Becker T, et al. Sotrastaurin, a novel small molecule inhibiting protein kinase C: first clinical results in renal-transplant recipients. Am J Transplant 2010;10(3):571–81.

34. Lillo FB, Ferrari D, Veglia F, et al. Human papillomavirus infection and associated cervical disease in human immunodeficiency virus-infected women: effect of highly active antiretroviral therapy. J Infect Dis 2001;184(5):547–51.

35. Paramsothy P, Jamieson DJ, Heilig CM, et al. The effect of highly active antiretroviral therapy on human papillomavirus clearance and cervical cytology. Obstet Gynecol 2009;113(1):26–31.

36. Zeier MD, Botha MH, van der Merwe FH, et al. Progression and persistence of low-grade cervical squamous intraepithelial lesions in women living with human immunodeficiency virus. J Low Genit Tract Dis 2012;16(3):243–50.

37. Minkoff H, Zhong Y, Burk RD, et al. Influence of adherent and effective antiretroviral therapy use on human papillomavirus infection and squamous intraepithelial lesions in human immunodeficiency virus-positive women. J Infect Dis 2010; 201(5):681–90.

38. Heard I. Prevention of cervical cancer in women with HIV. Curr Opin HIV AIDS 2009;4(1):68–73.

39. Clifford GM, Goncalves MA, Franceschi S, HPV and HIV Study Group. Human papillomavirus types among women infected with HIV: a meta-analysis. AIDS 2006;20(18):2337–44.

40. Massad LS, D'Souza G, Tian F, et al. Negative predictive value of pap testing: implications for screening intervals for women with human immunodeficiency virus. Obstet Gynecol 2012;120(4):791–7.

41. Firnhaber C, Mayisela N, Mao L, et al. Validation of cervical cancer screening methods in HIV positive women from Johannesburg South Africa. PLoS One 2013;8(1):e53494.

42. Harris TG, Burk RD, Palefsky JM, et al. Incidence of cervical squamous intraepithelial lesions associated with HIV serostatus, CD4 cell counts, and human papillomavirus test results. JAMA 2005;293(12):1471–6.

43. Ortiz AP, Colon-Lopez V, Girona-Lozada G, et al. Report of the 2012 capacity building for HIV-HPV clinical trials recruitment among minority underserved populations of Hispanic origin in Puerto Rico. P R Health Sci J 2012;31(3): 185–7.

44. Moscicki AB, Ellenberg JH, Crowley-Nowick P, et al. Risk of high-grade squamous intraepithelial lesion in HIV-infected adolescents. J Infect Dis 2004; 190(8):1413–21.

45. Setse R, Siberry GK, Moss WJ, et al. Cervical pap screening cytological abnormalities among HIV-infected adolescents in the LEGACY cohort. J Pediatr Adolesc Gynecol 2012;25(1):27–34.

46. Dantal J, Berthoux F, Moal MC, et al. Efficacy and safety of de novo or early everolimus with low cyclosporine in deceased-donor kidney transplant recipients at specified risk of delayed graft function: 12-month results of a randomized, multicenter trial. Transpl Int 2010;23(11):1084–93.

47. Laing ME, Moloney FJ, Kay EW, et al. Malignant melanoma in transplant patients: review of five cases. Clin Exp Dermatol 2006;31(5):662–4.

48. ACOG Committee on Practice Bulletins–Gynecology. ACOG Practice Bulletin No. 117: gynecologic care for women with human immunodeficiency virus. Obstet Gynecol 2010;116(6):1492–509.

49. Jemal A, Siegel R, Ward E, et al. Cancer statistics, 2008. CA Cancer J Clin 2008; 58(2):71–96.

50. Saslow D, Solomon D, Lawson HW, et al. American Cancer Society, American Society for Colposcopy and Cervical Pathology, and American Society for Clinical Pathology screening guidelines for the prevention and early detection of cervical cancer. J Low Genit Tract Dis 2012;16(3):175–204.

51. Minkoff H, Feldman JG, Strickler HD, et al. Relationship between smoking and human papillomavirus infections in HIV-infected and -uninfected women. J Infect Dis 2004;189(10):1821–8.

52. Massad LS, Xie X, Greenblatt RM, et al. Effect of human immunodeficiency virus infection on the prevalence and incidence of vaginal intraepithelial neoplasia. Obstet Gynecol 2012;119(3):582–9.

53. Birkeland SA, Storm HH, Lamm LU, et al. Cancer risk after renal transplantation in the Nordic countries, 1964-1986. Int J Cancer 1995;60(2):183–9.

54. Jensen P, Moller B, Hansen S. Skin cancer in kidney and heart transplant recipients and different long-term immunosuppressive therapy regimens. J Am Acad Dermatol 2000;42(2 Pt 1):307.

55. Buell JF, Brock GN. Risk of cancer in liver transplant recipients: a look into the mirror. Liver Transpl 2008;14(11):1561–3.

56. Jensen P, Hansen S, Moller B, et al. Are renal transplant recipients on CsA-based immunosuppressive regimens more likely to develop skin cancer than those on azathioprine and prednisolone? Transplant Proc 1999;31(1–2):1120.

57. Penn I. Cancers of the anogenital region in renal transplant recipients. Analysis of 65 cases. Cancer 1986;58(3):611–6.

58. Porreco R, Penn I, Droegemueller W, et al. Gynecologic malignancies in immunosuppressed organ homograft recipients. Obstet Gynecol 1975;45(4):359–64.

59. Alloub MI, Barr BB, McLaren KM, et al. Human papillomavirus infection and cervical intraepithelial neoplasia in women with renal allografts. BMJ 1989; 298(6667):153–6.

60. Brown MR, Noffsinger A, First MR, et al. HPV subtype analysis in lower genital tract neoplasms of female renal transplant recipients. Gynecol Oncol 2000; 79(2):220–4.

61. Busnach G, Piselli P, Arbustini E, et al. Immunosuppression and cancer: a comparison of risks in recipients of organ transplants and in HIV-positive individuals. Transplant Proc 2006;38(10):3533–5.

62. Gentile G, Formelli G, Orsoni G, et al. Immunosuppression and human genital papillomavirus infection. Eur J Gynaecol Oncol 1991;12(1):79–81.

63. Halpert R, Fruchter RG, Sedlis A, et al. Human papillomavirus and lower genital neoplasia in renal transplant patients. Obstet Gynecol 1986;68(2):251–8.

64. Veroux M, Corona D, Scalia G, et al. Surveillance of human papilloma virus infection and cervical cancer in kidney transplant recipients: preliminary data. Transplant Proc 2009;41(4):1191–4.

65. Meeuwis KA, Melchers WJ, Bouten H, et al. Anogenital malignancies in women after renal transplantation over 40 years in a single center. Transplantation 2012;93(9):914–22.

66. Pietrzak B, Mazanowska N, Ekiel AM, et al. Prevalence of high-risk human papillomavirus cervical infection in female kidney graft recipients: an observational study. Virol J 2012;9:117.

67. Morrison EA, Dole P, Sun XW, et al. Low prevalence of human papillomavirus infection of the cervix in renal transplant recipients. Nephrol Dial Transplant 1996;11(8):1603–6.

68. Vajdic CM, McDonald SP, McCredie MR, et al. Cancer incidence before and after kidney transplantation. JAMA 2006;296(23):2823–31.

69. Hwang JK, Moon IS, Kim JI. Malignancies after kidney transplantation: a 40-year single-center experience in Korea. Transpl Int 2011;24(7):716–21.
70. Collett D, Mumford L, Banner NR, et al. Comparison of the incidence of malignancy in recipients of different types of organ: a UK Registry audit. Am J Transplant 2010;10(8):1889–96.
71. Kasiske BL, Zeier MG, Chapman JR, et al. KDIGO clinical practice guideline for the care of kidney transplant recipients: a summary. Kidney Int 2010;77(4): 299–311.
72. EBPG Expert Group on Renal Transplantation. European best practice guidelines for renal transplantation. Section IV: Long-term management of the transplant recipient. IV.6.3. Cancer risk after renal transplantation. Solid organ cancers: prevention and treatment. Nephrol Dial Transplant 2002;17(Suppl 4):32, 4–6.
73. Inserra P, Abrahamsen M, Papenfuss M, et al. Ethnic variation of the P53 codon 72 polymorphism, HPV persistence, and cervical cancer risk. Int J STD AIDS 2003;14(12):800–4.
74. Dugue PA, Rebolj M, Garred P, et al. Immunosuppression and risk of cervical cancer. Expert Rev Anticancer Ther 2013;13(1):29–42.
75. Engels EA, Pfeiffer RM, Fraumeni JF Jr, et al. Spectrum of cancer risk among US solid organ transplant recipients. JAMA 2011;306(17):1891–901.
76. Adami J, Gabel H, Lindelof B, et al. Cancer risk following organ transplantation: a nationwide cohort study in Sweden. Br J Cancer 2003;89(7):1221–7.
77. Iuri Usêda Santana, Alline do Nascimento Gomes, Leomar D'Cirqueira Lyrio, et al. Systemic lupus erythematous, human papilomavirus infection, cervical pre-malignant and malignant lesions: a systemic review. Clinical Rheumatology 2011;30:665–72.
78. Hemminki K, Liu X, Ji J, et al. Effect of autoimmune diseases on risk and survival in female cancers. Gynecol Oncol 2012;127(1):180–5.
79. Bernatsky SR, Cooper GS, Mill C, et al. Cancer screening in patients with systemic lupus erythematosus. J Rheumatol 2006;33(1):45–9.
80. Tam LS, Chan AY, Chan PK, et al. Increased prevalence of squamous intraepithelial lesions in systemic lupus erythematosus: association with human papillomavirus infection. Arthritis Rheum 2004;50(11):3619–25.
81. Klumb EM, Pinto AC, Jesus GR, et al. Are women with lupus at higher risk of HPV infection? Lupus 2010;19(13):1485–91.
82. Bateman H, Yazici Y, Leff L, et al. Increased cervical dysplasia in intravenous cyclophosphamide-treated patients with SLE: a preliminary study. Lupus 2000; 9(7):542–4.
83. Mofenson LM, Brady MT, Danner SP, et al. Guidelines for the prevention and treatment of opportunistic infections among HIV-exposed and HIV-infected children: recommendations from CDC, the National Institutes of Health, the HIV Medicine Association of the Infectious Diseases Society of America, the Pediatric Infectious Diseases Society, and the American Academy of Pediatrics. MMWR Recomm Rep 2009;58(RR-11):1–166.
84. Biggar RJ, Chaturvedi AK, Goedert JJ, et al, Study HACM. AIDS-related cancer and severity of immunosuppression in persons with AIDS. J Natl Cancer Inst 2007;99(12):962–72.
85. Dal Maso L, Polesel J, Serraino D, et al. Pattern of cancer risk in persons with AIDS in Italy in the HAART era. Br J Cancer 2009;100(5):840–7.
86. Chaturvedi AK, Madeleine MM, Biggar RJ, et al. Risk of human papilomavirus-associated cancers among persons with AIDS. J Natl Cancer Inst 2009; 101(16):1120–30.

87. Saslow D, Solomon D, Lawson HW, et al. American Cancer Society, American Society for Colposcopy and Cervical Pathology, and American Society for Clinical Pathology screening guidelines for the prevention and early detection of cervical cancer. Am J Clin Pathol 2012;137(4):516–42.
88. Moyer VA, Force USPST. Screening for cervical cancer: U.S. Preventive Services Task Force recommendation statement. Ann Intern Med 2012;156(12):880–91, W312.

Vulvar and Vaginal HPV Disease

Erin L. Nelson, MD[a], Colleen K. Stockdale, MD, MS[b],*

KEYWORDS

- Human papillomavirus • Condyloma • Genital wart • Vulvar intraepithelial neoplasia
- Vaginal intraepithelial neoplasia

KEY POINTS

- HPV infection of the lower genital tract is common and its effects variable. Most infections are transient and the related pathology is self-resolving.
- Condyloma accuminatum is caused predominantly by HPV 6 and 11 and can be managed with medical therapy (imiquimod, sinechetins, trichloroacetic acid, podofilox) or surgical therapy (laser, excision).
- VIN is a treatable precursor to vulvar cancer with two main forms: one related to HPV, the other to chronic vulvar inflammatory conditions.
- VaIN is a treatable precursor to vaginal cancer, and is highly related to HPV.
- Use of a quadrivalent HPV vaccine has the potential to decrease HPV-related lower genital disease burden substantially.

INTRODUCTION

In excess of 120 types of the human papilloma virus (HPV) exist, of which 40 affect the anogenital tract. Most HPV virus infections are asymptomatic, subclinical, and transient in nature. It is estimated that more than 50% of sexually active persons become infected with HPV at least once in their lifetime.[1] Peak prevalence of HPV occurs in the age groups 17 to 33 years, with peak incidence in persons aged 20 to 24 years.[2] On initiating sexual activity with a male partner the 1-year cumulative incidence of first HPV infection was 28.5% and increased to almost 50% by 3 years in a study of virginal female college students.[3]

HPV is associated with a multitude of lower genital tract diseases in women in addition to cervical cancer, including genital warts (90% associated with nononcogenic subtypes HPV types 6 and 11) and vulvar intraepithelial neoplasia (VIN), vaginal intraepithelial neoplasia (VaIN), and some vulvar, vaginal, and anal cancers that are

[a] Department of Obstetrics & Gynecology, University of Texas, 7703 Floyd Curl Drive, San Antonio, TX 78229, USA; [b] Department of Obstetrics & Gynecology, University of Iowa, 200 Hawkins Drive, Iowa City, IA 52242, USA
* Corresponding author.
E-mail address: colleen-stockdale@uiowa.edu

Obstet Gynecol Clin N Am 40 (2013) 359–376
http://dx.doi.org/10.1016/j.ogc.2013.03.003
0889-8545/13/$ – see front matter Published by Elsevier Inc.

obgyn.theclinics.com

associated with oncogenic subtypes (primarily HPV 16, 18, and 45). The degree to which HPV manifests pathology depends on viral type, host immune response, and local environmental factors. Most HPV infections are transient with 60% to 70% clearing within 1 year[4] and 91% clearing within 2 years.[5] We review the evaluation and management of the following vulvar and vaginal HPV diseases: (1) condyloma, (2) VIN, and (3) VaIN. Also included is a brief discussion of the association with vulvar and vaginal cancer.

CONDYLOMATA ACCUMINATUM/GENITAL WART

Condyloma accuminatum is the most common sexually transmitted disease in the United States, with approximately 500,000 to 1 million new cases diagnosed each year. The incidence of condyloma has been reported as 3.4% (0.87 cases per 100 person-years at risk) based on analysis of the placebo arm of three randomized controlled phase III trials for the quadrivalent HPV vaccine.[6] HPV DNA was detected in 90.8% of these women (predominant subtypes 6 and 11, 86%).[6] Population-based studies of sexually active persons place the prevalence of condylomata in the United States at 1%.[7,8] HPV is a very contagious virus with reported transmission rates of 65%.[9] Risk factors for condyloma include infection with HPV types 6 and 11, higher numbers of sexual partners, unprotected intercourse, history of sexually transmitted infections, smoking, the use of oral contraceptives, and immunodeficiency.

Clinical Presentation

Condyloma accuminatum present clinically as flat, papular, or pedunculated growths occurring in the genital area. Common areas affected include the introitus, perianum, and vulva. Condylomas are often asymptomatic, but depending on location and size can exhibit symptoms of pruritis, burning, and pain (**Fig. 1**).

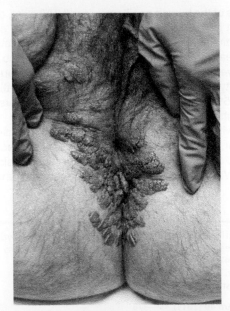

Fig. 1. Vulvar/perianal condyloma. (*Courtesy of* Alan Waxman, MD, Albuquerque, New Mexico.)

Diagnostic Evaluation

Diagnosis can be made by direct visual inspection. This may be aided with magnification and bright lighting, especially in the case of smaller lesions.[10] If the diagnosis is uncertain or lesions do not respond to appropriate therapy biopsy is warranted. When a patient is diagnosed with genital warts, she should undergo testing for other sexually transmitted infections (gonorrhea, Chlamydia, HIV, syphilis, hepatitis B and C) and cervical cancer screening based on available published guidelines.[11]

Natural Course

If left untreated condyloma generally resolve (30%–40%); remain unchanged; or increase in size or number. Therapy centers on removing or destroying the lesion, rather than eliminating the causative HPV viral infection. Available therapies involve tissue destruction (podofilox, cryotherapy, bichloroacetic or trichloroacetic acid); surgical excision; or immune modulation (imiquimod, sinecatechins). Therapy options vary in terms of cost, duration of therapy, dosing, discomfort, pain, and success rates. At this time, no evidence exists to recommend one therapy over others. The choice of treatment is based on patient or provider preference, size and location of warts, cost of treatment, convenience, and experienced adverse effects. There is a high incidence of recurrence (13%–65%) with condyloma, and multiple treatments or use of multiple therapeutic modalities is often required. Additionally, the impact is considerable because condyloma causes significant psychosocial distress and anxiety to patients and treatment of this condition can be painful and costly. The estimated total lifetime cost in 2003 associated with new cases of condyloma per year in the United States was $171 million dollars.[12]

Treatment Options

Although most patients desire treatment for symptom resolution, it is important to note the role of expectant management. There is a 30% incidence of spontaneous regression,[13] thus making expectant management an acceptable alternative for some patients.

Pharmacologic

a. Bichloroacetic and trichloroacetic acid (80% solution): Chemical coagulation of proteins; nontoxic, although burning occurs in the treated areas. Applied by provider, washed off after 6 hours. May treat at 1- to 2-week intervals until resolution of condyloma. Side effects include pain, burning, and local irritation. Can be used in pregnancy, children, in the vagina, inside the anal canal, perianally, and on the urethral meatus. May be used in pregnancy.
b. Podophyllin (0.5% solution): Antimitotic agent; induces local tissue necrosis. Applied by patient; may also be applied as a 10% to 25% resin by provider, washed off after 4 hours. Applied twice a day for 3 days; then patient goes 4 days without therapy. May repeat the cycle up to four times. Inexpensive, safe, easy to use. Side effects include pain and local irritation. Should not be used in pregnancy; children; or in the vagina, inside the anal canal, or on thinned, ulcerated skin. It is not recommended in pregnancy because of neurotoxicity.
c. Imiquimod 5% cream (Aldara): Immune enhancer, stimulating local production of cytokines. Applied by patient once daily (bedtime) 3 days a week. Washed off in morning after 8 hours. Maximum length of treatment is 16 weeks. Side effects include redness, irritation, vesicles, and hypopigmentation. Not approved for

treatment of urethral, vaginal, cervical, rectal, or intra-anal disease. Safety in pregnancy is unknown.

d. Botanic (sincechatechin 15% ointment [Veregen]): Green tea extract. Mechanism of action not clear, thought to be antioxidant, immune enhancer. Applied by patient three times a day for up to a maximum duration of 16 weeks. Side effects include burning, pain, ulceration, and vesicular rash. Should not be used by HIV-infected, immunocompromised patients, or those with active genital herpes because safety and efficacy of therapy in these settings has not been determined. Approved for treatment of external genital warts including perianal warts in immunocompetent patients 18 years and older. Safety in pregnancy is unknown.[14]

Surgical treatment options (all surgical modalities are considered safe during pregnancy)

a. Cryotherapy: Destroys warts by thermal-induced cytolysis using liquid nitrogen. Applied directly to the wart (either by cotton-tipped applicator or sprayed on). Freezing can also be accomplished using cryotweezers or a metal probe containing liquid nitrogen. Generally does not require anesthetic. Generally does not cause scarring. Success rates 60% to 100% with recurrence varying between 38% and 73%.[15] The use of cryosurgery should be avoided in the vagina.

b. Excision: Scalpel removal of affected tissue. Helpful for raised or pedunculated lesions. Requires anesthetic or anesthesia. A 19% to 29% recurrence rate.[15]

c. Electrosurgery: High-frequency electrical current (thermal coagulation or electrocautery) to burn or destroy lesion. Requires local anesthetic. May cause scarring. A 14% to 22% recurrence rate.[15]

d. CO_2 laser: Heats or vaporizes tissues. Requires special equipment and training and is more expensive. Must control depth and extent of vaporization to destroy the wart only, and not the underlying tissue. Often used for recurrent, widespread disease. Associated with pain, bleeding, burning, and potential scarring postprocedure. Requires anesthetic or anesthesia. Cure rates of 60% to 100% with recurrence rates up to 80% (**Table 1**).[16]

Treatment Resistance and Complications

Pain, irritation, and superficial skin ulcerations are the most common complications associated with therapies for condyloma. Surgical therapies may induce scarring, pain, disfigurement, and sexual dysfunction. Poor response to treatment is generally addressed by choosing another therapeutic modality. A biopsy should be considered for condyloma that do not respond to treatment or any concerning lesions.

Evaluation of Outcome and Long-term Recommendations

Prevention of most condyloma is possible by vaccination. A quadrivalent (HPV 6, 11, 16, and 18) vaccine (Gardasil) is given as a series of three shots over 6 months. Vaccine trial studies demonstrate 99% effectiveness in preventing genital warts from viral strains included in the vaccine in a naive (HPV) population. Because 90% of condyloma is caused by HPV 6 or 11 a significant impact could be made with this intervention. The most common adverse reactions include mild injection site reactions (erythema, pain, swelling, pruritis); headache; and dizziness. The quadrivalent vaccine is pregnancy class B. Other recommendations to decrease the risk of contracting condyloma include abstinence or limiting the number of sexual partners. Correct and consistent condom use may decrease transmission of HPV. However, this is not fully protective because HPV is often multifocal and can infect areas not covered by the condom.

Table 1
Treatment of genital warts

Therapy	Treatment	Application	Use in Pregnancy	Recurrence Rates[a]
Patient-applied	Imiquimod 5% cream	Apply at bedtime three times a week for up to 16 wk. The area treated should be washed with soap and water 6–10 h after use.	Safety not established	9%–19%
	Podofilox 0.5% solution and gel	Apply twice daily for 3 d followed by 4 d without therapy; the cycle may be repeated up to four times. The total wart area treated should not exceed 10 cm², and the total volume should be limited to 0.5 mL per d.	Safety not established	4%–91%
	Sinecatechins (15% ointment)	Applied by patient three times per day, maximum length 16 wk.	Safety not established	6%–9%[b]
Provider-applied	Cryotherapy	Liquid nitrogen or cryoprobe. May repeat applications every 1–2 wk.	Yes	21%
	Podophyl in resin 10%–25% in compound of tincture of benzoin	Carefully applied to the wart and then washed off by the patient between 1 and 4 h after application. May repeat weekly if needed. To avoid toxicity, (1) application should be limited to <0.5 mL podophyllin or an area of <10 cm² warts treated per session and (2) no open lesions or wounds present in treatment area.	Safety not established	23%–65%
	Trichloroacetic or bichloroacetic acid 80%–90%	First, coat the surrounding normal epithelium with a protective substance (eg, 5% licocaine gel) and then use a small cotton-tipped applicator to apply medication to the wart. Allow to dry before patient sits or stands. If excess acid used, treated area should be powdered with talc, sodium bicarbonate, or liquid soap preparations. May repeat weekly, if needed.	Yes	63%
	CO₂ laser		Yes	0%–80%
	Surgical removal	Tangential scissor excision, tangential shave excision, curettage or electrosurgery.	Yes	19%–29%

[a] *Adapted from* Kennedy CM, Boardman LA. New approaches to external genital warts and vulvar intraepithelial neoplasia. Clin Obstet Gynecol 2008;51(3):518–26.
[b] Tatti S, Swinehart JM, Thielert C, et al. Sinecatechins, a defined green tea extract, in the treatment of external anogenital warts: a randomized controlled trial. Obstet Gynecol 2008;111:6):1371–9.

Special Situations with Pregnant Patients with Condyloma

Genital warts can proliferate during pregnancy. Although treatment can be considered, resolution is often incomplete (because of pregnancy-induced immunosuppression) until the postpartum period. Rarely, HPV types 6 and 11 can cause respiratory papillomatosis in infants and children. However, the route of transmission is not understood and whether cesarean section prevents respiratory papillomatosis in infants and children is unclear. Thus, the Centers for Disease Control and Prevention recommends cesarean delivery for women with genital warts only if the outlet is obstructed or if vaginal delivery would result in excessive bleeding.[13]

VULVAR INTRAEPITHELIAL NEOPLASIA

VIN is a high-grade squamous lesion of the vulva, considered a precursor to invasive vulvar cancer. This condition is associated with a high risk of recurrence and the potential to progress to vulvar cancer. In a large case review series van Seters and colleagues[17] found 9% of untreated patients with VIN III developed invasive cancer in 12 to 96 months. In contrast, Jones and Rowan[18] found seven (87.5%) of eight women with untreated VIN III developed cancer within 8 years. Additionally, Jones and coworkers[19] found 3.8% of treated patients later went on to develop invasive cancer. The incidence of VIN seems to be increasing, particularly in younger women. Although VIN is considered to be a premalignant condition, spontaneous regression (11%)[19] can occur and has been documented. Risk factors for VIN include infection with oncogenic HPV subtypes, cigarette smoking, an immunocompromised host, other genital neoplasia, and chronic inflammation.

The diagnosis of VIN has historically been made by histologic evaluation of a vulvar biopsy specimen, using the classifications of low grade (VIN1) and high grade (VIN2/3). The lower anogenital squamous terminology (LAST) standardization project for HPV-associated lesions recently revised a unified terminology for HPV-associated squamous lesions of the lower anogenital tract.[20] This was done in part to improve communication between clinicians and pathologists and to improve the accuracy of histologic diagnoses. Essential recommendations for vulvar and vaginal HPV-associated disease include a unified histopathologic nomenclature for all preinvasive HPV-associated squamous lesions, and a two-tiered nomenclature (LSIL, low-grade [IN 1]; HSIL, high-grade [IN 2, 3]). Condyloma is a low-grade lesion, whereas VIN is a high-grade lesion.

In 2004, the International Society for the Study of Vulvovaginal Disease modified the classification system to reflect the two clinically distinct types of VIN, one related to HPV (usual) and one that is not (differentiated). Thus, the 2012 College of American Pathologists guidelines as noted previously refer to VIN (usual type) as classified by the International Society for the Study of Vulvovaginal Disease:

a. Usual-type VIN (warty, basaloid, and mixed VIN), which are associated with HPV. Often multifocal. Invasive potential: 9% of untreated patients with usual type VIN

Epidemiology of VIN

Incidence[21]: 1.2 per 100,000 annually from 1999 to 2004

Peak age[21]: 45 to 49 years

Race[21]: White greater than black (relative risk, 0.7). Non-Hispanic greater than Hispanic (relative risk, 0.5)

Overall HPV prevalence[22]: 80.4% with HPV 16 most common subtype (71.2%), then HPV 33.

progress to invasive cancer within 1 to 8 years and 3.3% progress after treatment.[17] Risk factors include oncogenic HPV subtypes, cigarette smoking, immunocompromised host, and younger age.

b. Differentiated VIN: Not associated with HPV. More commonly seen with vulvar dermatologic conditions (lichen sclerosus), older age, and histology of keratinizing type.

Note that VIN1 (flat lesions with basal atypia and koilocytic changes) are also considered condyloma in the current International Society for the Study of Vulvovaginal Disease classification system and are excluded from this discussion.

Clinical Presentation

On examination, a visible lesion is noted. The lesions are variable in appearance. They can be brown, white, gray, or red in color. Topography can be flat, raised, or eroded. Common symptoms include vulvar itching, burning, pain, and dyspareunia. The patient may be asymptomatic and present with no symptoms at all, with the lesion being noted on routine examination (**Fig. 2**).

Diagnostic Evaluation

Direct visual and colposcopic examination and histologic examination of vulvar biopsy is called for. A complete evaluation includes assessment of cervix, vagina, and perianal areas because of the frequency of multicentric and concomitant disease. VIN may be found in association with vulvar carcinoma; therefore, this must be ruled out (biopsy) before the diagnosis and treatment of VIN. Treatment is indicated for all cases of VIN.[23]

Treatment Options

Pharmacologic
Topical medical therapies for VIN generally fall into two different categories. One group acts by enhancing the immune system (imiquimod, cidofovir, α-interferon) to fight against HPV. The other group acts by destruction of affected cells (5-fluorouracil

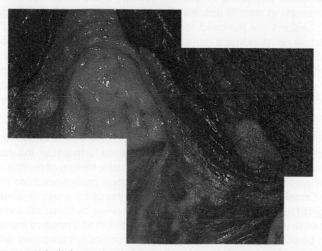

Fig. 2. Vulvar intraepithelial neoplasia. (*Courtesy of* Alan Waxman, MD, Albuquerque, New Mexico.)

[5-FU], bleomycin). Because of extreme side effects and lack of proved benefit to patients, 5-FU and bleomycin are no longer recommended or used in the therapeutic management of VIN. Furthermore, pharmacologic treatments for VIN have not been approved by the Food and Drug Administration (FDA) for this use.

In a randomized controlled trial published by Mathiesen and colleagues,[24] topical 5% imiquimod versus placebo applied once a week for 2 weeks, then twice weekly for 2 weeks and, if tolerated, three times a week for the last 12 weeks was studied. This regimen was associated with a complete response in 81%. A small randomized controlled trial by van Seters and colleagues[25] used application of 5% imiquimod or placebo twice weekly for 16 weeks with complete response in 35% and partial response in 46%; responders remained disease free at 12-month follow-up.[26] However, recurrence was noted in 1 (9%) of 11 complete responders. Residual lesions required surgical ablation or excision.

Nonpharmacologic treatment

This entails topical or systemic application of 5-aminolevulinic acid followed by application of nonthermal light from a laser. The light interacting with protoporphyrin IX results in generation of radicals capable of producing a local cytotoxic effect. This procedure can be performed in the outpatient setting. Results of one retrospective study were consistent with a complete response in 52% of patients receiving photodynamic therapy; however, 48% later had recurrence.[27]

Surgical

Ablative CO_2 laser ablation is used in cases when cancer is not suspected. It can be used for single or multiple lesions. It uses focused (by micromanipulator with depth gauge) application of laser energy according to published guidelines to destroy the VIN lesion. For non–hair-bearing areas, it is recommended that therapy extend through the dermis (1–2 mm). For hair-bearing areas, therapy should extend to a depth of 3 mm. A small margin of normal-appearing skin adjacent to the lesion should also be treated. A power setting of 750 to 1250 W/cm^2 is required to avoid deep coagulation injury. Acetic acid is typically used to assist in the delineation of lesion margins.

Cavitational ultrasonic surgical aspiration (CUSA) has been previously used for intraoperative tumor debulking of ovarian cancer. It allows for removal of affected areas while preserving normal tissue and provides a specimen (cytology) to be sent to pathology. Lesions are removed to the depth of the reticular layer of the dermis. Common ablative posttreatment complications include pain, delayed wound healing, scarring, discharge, ulceration, vaginal stenosis, and sexual dysfunction. In a randomized controlled trial comparing CUSA with laser ablation, postoperative pain and scarring were decreased with CUSA.[28] There was no statistically significant difference in recurrence rates at 1 year of follow-up with reported recurrence rates of 22% to 35%.

Excisional Wide local excision (WLE) is the preferred therapy in cases where invasive cancer is suspected. Microscopic disease may extend further than the visible acetowhite changes used to judge surgical excision and thus a margin of normal tissue should be excised in addition to the lesion. Clinical practice guidelines from the Society of Gynecologic Oncologists recommend local excision of all gross disease with a 0.5- to 1-cm margin of normal tissue.[29] A retrospective review by Modesitt and colleagues[30] reported that 66% women treated with surgical excision had positive margins. Of those patients with positive margins, 46% suffered recurrence, compared with 17% with negative margins. Margin negativity conferred a three-time lower risk of recurrence and a longer disease-free interval. An occult squamous cancer was found at the time of initial treatment in 22% of patients. These would have been missed had ablation been performed, which emphasizes caution in patient selection for ablative therapy.

Vulvectomy, the surgical excision of all vulvar skin, is rarely necessary. It is associated with high morbidity and may require use of skin flaps to cover the defect. Vulvectomy has been useful in cases with confluent or multifocal lesions.

Postsurgical treatment considerations Surgical therapies can be potentially disfiguring and have negative psychosexual impact on patients,[31] thus consideration of counseling and referral may be warranted. Fifty percent of women treated surgically require at least one further treatment by the 14th year.[19]

Comparisons among different therapeutic modalities have been limited. One retrospective study of 93 patients with VIN[27] reviewed CO_2 laser, photodynamic therapy, WLE, and vulvectomy therapy modalities for VIN. Recurrence rates were 40.4% for laser, 48.1% photodynamic therapy, 42% for WLE, and 0% for vulvectomy. A subsequent smaller (N = 29) study on comparative therapy modalities found a higher recurrence with excision (50%) compared with imiquimod and laser (0%).[32] The most recent study published in 2012 (N = 303 patients) notes a higher rate of recurrence with CO_2 laser compared with excision and topical imiquimod (**Table 2**).[33]

Prognosis

There is a high incidence of recurrence[18] (30%–50% for all methods, higher if positive margins) and treatment failure for VIN. This high rate of recurrence is likely caused by the fact the underlying cause (persistent HPV infection) has not been cleared. The potential for progression of disease to frank vulvar cancer is important to note in the counseling of patients with VIN.

Identified risk factors for VIN recurrence were smoking, larger lesion size, and positive margins in a recent retrospective study of 303 patients comparing clinical outcomes and recurrence for VIN. Patients in this trial were treated with laser, excision, and imiquimod.[33] Factors potentially associated with risk of invasive vulvar carcinoma in women with VIN are HPV infection, smoking, chronic inflammation, vulvar dystrophies, and other genital tract neoplasia.[34]

Table 2
Treatment of VIN[a]

Study	Treatment	Application	Numbers of Patients in Study	Response Rates
Mathiesen et al,[24] 2007	Imiquimod 5% cream	Once a week for 2 wk, then twice weekly for 2 wk and, if tolerated, three times a wk for the last 12 wk	32	81%
van Seters et al,[25] 2008	Imiquimod 5% cream	Twice weekly for 16 wk	52	Partial 46% Complete 35%
Hillemanns et al,[27] 2006	Aminolevulinic acid photodynamic therapy	Topical or systemic application of aminolevulinic acid followed by application of nonthermal light from a laser	27	52%

[a] These therapies are not FDA approved for use for VIN or in pregnancy.
Data from Refs.[24,25,27]

Treatment Resistance and Complications

Pain, irritation, and superficial ulcerations are the most common complications associated with medical therapies for VIN. Surgical therapies may induce scarring, pain, disfigurement, and sexual dysfunction. Treatment resistance generally is addressed by choosing another therapeutic modality. Given the risk of progression to cancer, excisional treatment or biopsy confirmation is warranted in cases of recurrent VIN.

Although no consensus as to the optimal therapeutic approach can be made, in cases where malignancy is suspected excision is recommended. In cases where occult invasion is not a concern, VIN can be treated with excision, laser, or topical imiquimod.

Evaluation of Outcomes and Long-term Recommendations

Because of the high risk of recurrence (30%–50% with all methods), treatment failures, and risk of progression to vulvar carcinoma, posttreatment follow-up is essential. Re-examination at 6 months and 12 months posttherapy, and then annually is recommended by American College of Obstetricians and Gynecologists.[23] In a review of 3322 patients with VIN III, 3.2% of patients were diagnosed with occult vulvar carcinoma during their treatment and follow-up for VIN.[17]

Prevention

Immunization with HPV vaccination (quadrivalent or bivalent) could potentially prevent 70%[7,35] of VIN. The bivalent vaccine does not have FDA indication for prevention of vulvar or vaginal disease. However, in theory, since most HPV related VINs are due to HPV type 16 it should afford protection. Smoking cessation and treatment of vulvar dermatologic disorders are other interventions recommended to decrease the likelihood of VIN.

VAGINAL INTRAEPITHELIAL NEOPLASIA

VaIN is a premalignant condition of the vaginal epithelium. It is defined as the presence of squamous cell atypia involving the vaginal epithelium. As noted for VIN, terminology for all HPV-associated squamous lesions was recently revised cosponsored by the College of American Pathologists and the American Society for Colposcopy and Cervical Pathology. Thus, VaIN is now reported using a two-tiered nomenclature: LSIL for low-grade disease (formerly VaIN 1) and HSIL for high-grade disease (formerly VaIN 2/3).[20]

VaIN is much less common than cervical intraepithelial neoplasia (CIN) or VIN with an incidence of 0.1 per 100,000 annually.[21] To put this into perspective, the frequency of VaIN is approximately 100-fold less than that of CIN.[36] The average patient diagnosed with VaIN is from 43 to 60 years of age with a peak of 70 to 79 years. The frequency of VaIN diagnoses is increasing because of improved screening (cytology) and thorough colposcopic evaluation. VaIN is frequently associated with previous or

---

Epidemiology of VaIN

Incidence[21]: 0.1 per 100,000 annually

Peak age[21]: 70 to 79 years

Race[21]: not mentioned in most studies (blacks more than whites)

Overall HPV prevalence[22]: 92.6% in VaIN 2/3 and 98.5% VaIN3; most common subtype HPV 16 (65.8%).

concurrent neoplasia elsewhere in the lower genital tract, most commonly the cervix or vulva. Most VaIN is actually diagnosed by colposcopy done to assess CIN.[37] The main risk factor for VaIN is HPV, with reported HPV prevalence of 92.6% in VaIN 2/3 and 98.5% VaIN3.[22] The most common subtype found is HPV 16 (65.8%).[22] Other risk factors include prior pelvic irradiation (generally seen after treatment of cervical cancer)[36]; a history of in utero exposure to diethylstilestrol[38,39]; a history of vaginal condylomata; and having had a prior hysterectomy for CIN.[36,40]

Clinical Presentation

VaIN is usually asymptomatic, although some patients may have postcoital spotting or report vaginal discharge. The most common presentation is abnormal cytology (pap smear) in a patient who has previously undergone hysterectomy with a history of cervical dysplasia or cervical cancer. Additionally, VaIN may manifest in a patient with abnormal cytology who has no identifiable cervical disease at the time of colposcopy (with VaIN being the ultimate explanation as the source of abnormal cytology). The most frequent location for VaIN is in the upper one-third of the vagina. In a patient with a history of CIN who has undergone hysterectomy, a high level of suspicion for VaIN should be kept in mind. The incidence of VaIN after hysterectomy for CIN ranges from 0.9%[41] to 7.4%.[42]

Diagnostic Evaluation

Direct visual and colposcopic examination of the vagina and histologic examination of vaginal biopsy should be made. A complete examination including assessment of cervix, vagina, vulvar, and perianal areas must be performed because of the frequency of multifocal and concomitant disease. Specific attention to posthysterectomy lateral fornices and the use of a skin hook may assist in assessing for disease at the time of colposcopy. Colposcopic features of VaIN include white lesions (flat or raised) (**Fig. 3**); granular appearance; vascular punctuation; spiky surface changes; and non-staining areas with application of Lugol iodine.[43] Invasive disease (vaginal cancer) must be excluded before therapy for VaIN, especially if medical and ablative therapy is used. The main risk associated with VaIN is the risk of progression to vaginal cancer of 2% to 5%.[36,44]

Therapy

Low-grade VaIN (condyloma) may resolve with expectant management and may be managed with close clinical follow-up. High-grade VaIN is preinvasive; therefore,

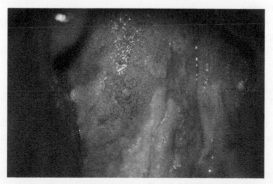

Fig. 3. Vaginal intraepithelial neoplasia 3. (*Courtesy of* Alan Waxman, MD, Albuquerque, New Mexico.)

treatment is recommended. Pharmacologic treatment options are not specifically FDA-approved for vaginal use including VaIN. As noted previously, the use of cryosurgery should also be avoided in the vagina. Additionally, surgical excision is essential if invasion is suspected or cannot be excluded.

Pharmacologic Treatment Options

Available studies of 5-FU quote effectiveness of 75% to 92%.[45,46] Published regimens were varied: 1 to 2 mL of 5% cream applied once weekly[47] or 5 g of 5% 5-FU cream applied nightly for 5 nights.[45] The application of 5-FU is discontinued when the lesion surface sloughs. Common side effects include pain, burning, and superficial ulcerations.

Imiquimod is described only in very small case studies. Using a regimen of vaginal application of 5% cream one to three times per week for up to 8 weeks, a recurrence rate of 22% to 29% was reported.[48,49] Common side effects include pain and local burning sensation.

Trichloroacetic acid in a small study of 28 patients showed 53% efficacy for VaIN 2/3[50] and 100% in VaIN1. Common side effects include pain and burning.

Nonpharmacologic Treatment Options

Radiation

Radiation therapy has success rates similar to other modalities in the treatment of VaIN. It is associated with higher morbidity as compared with other therapies; therefore, most reserve it as a secondary form of therapy for poor surgical candidates or treatment failures. The ill effects of irradiation on ovarian function and the occasional fibrosis of the vaginal vault make this treatment currently unacceptable except in very rare cases resistant to conservative therapy.[51]

High-, medium-, and low-dose brachytherapy have been described for intracavitary radiation. Most existing data come from the United Kingdom, where it has been used as standard therapy. Because of heterogeneous dosing regimens, study designs, and small numbers of patients it is difficult to draw conclusions regarding efficacy and toxicity of radiotherapy for VaIN. One study noted medium-dose intracavitary brachytherapy was 77% effective,[52] whereas another noted low-dose brachytherapy was 93% effective in treating VaIN3.[53]

Complications of radiotherapy include atrophy, stenosis, and shortening of the vagina. Because of close physical proximity, the bowel and bladder may also be affected.

Combination therapies

Small studies (N = 27 patients) have reported presurgical administration of topical therapies (5-FU) to reduce lesion size and improve ease of excision. This "chemosurgery" has a reported efficacy of 70%.[36] Pain and pruritis were the most common side effects.

Surgical Treatment Options

Excision

Surgical excision of varying amounts of vaginal mucosa is an option. Depending on amount of tissue removed, vaginal shortening, pain, and stenosis have been described.

a. Wide local excision (WLE): Removal of entire visible lesion and a small margin (usually 5 mm) of normal tissue. WLE offers histologic confirmation of diagnosis and delineation of margin status. Success rates between 66% and 83%.

b. Loop electrical excision procedure (LEEP): Use of a hot wire loop to excise lesion. It is not recommended because it may cut too deep and carries a potential to cause injury to bladder or rectum and other underlying structures.

c. Partial or total upper vaginectomy: Because larger amounts of tissue are excised it is associated with a higher morbidity compared with WLE. Partial or total vaginectomy is effective, but it may leave the patient with little or no sexual function because of scarring or stenosis.[51] Vaginectomy is most commonly used for cases of extensive or multifocal disease and in cases where VaIN is located in posthysterectomy suture recesses and is therefore inaccessible.

Ablation

CO_2 laser ablation entails focused laser destruction of identified lesions. The depth (1.5 mm) and width of destruction are carefully controlled. CO_2 laser ablation is restricted to lesions that are visible and accessible and where malignancy has been ruled out by colposcopic-directed biopsy. Success rates are generally quoted as 75%. Recurrence rate is 38%.[44] Treated areas generally heal well, and therapy is well tolerated. Approximately one-third of patients require more than one treatment. Laser ablation is a good option for multifocal disease in a younger woman or those who do not desire excision.

One retrospective study of CUSA reported a recurrence rate of 19.8%.[54] A second, smaller retrospective study reported a cure rate of 66%.[55] Benefits of CUSA include a similar efficacy compared with other modalities without the associated scarring, pain, stenosis, and sexual side effects.

Other described ablative therapies include fulguration and cryotherapy, but these are not commonly used in the management of VaIN because of their less precise nature and potential to cause injury. No randomized controlled trials comparing therapy modalities for VaIN have been performed. However, a recent review[56] of 21 available studies on VaIN therapeutic modalities found cure rates were similar for excision, ablation, and CUSA (69%–87.5%). Vaginectomy and radiation cure rates were also comparable with each other and slightly better than excision, ablation, and CUSA (80%–100%).

Treatment Resistance and Complications

Pain, irritation, and superficial ulcerations are the most common complications associated with medical therapies for VaIN. Surgical therapies may induce scarring, pain, disfigurement, and sexual dysfunction. Treatment resistance generally is addressed by choosing another therapeutic modality.

Evaluation of Outcome and Long-term Recommendations

In general, there is no consensus as to the optimal therapeutic approach or follow-up posttherapy for VaIN. This is multifactorial because of the low incidence of VaIN, limited evidence with retrospective studies using small numbers of patients, and also because choice of therapy is individualized with patients often receiving more than one therapeutic modality. Choice of therapy depends on extent of disease, level of certainty for exclusion of invasive disease, overall health status of the patient, future desire for sexual function, and whether or not the patient has received any other therapy modality for VaIN. Factors identified with higher incidence of recurrence include multifocal lesions, immunosuppression, and VaIN associated with other anogenital neoplasias.[36] Given the potential for recurrence and progression to invasive vaginal cancer, a reasonable follow-up posttreatment plan is cytology with or without colposcopic examination every 6 months until two normal results have been obtained with

Table 3
HPV positivity and prevalent subtypes found in lower genital disease

	Condyloma	VIN	VaIN	Vulvar Cancer	Vaginal Cancer
Overall HPV positivity[a,22]	90%	80.4%	92.6%	40.1%	65.5%
Predominant subtypes[22]	HPV 6 and 11	HPV 16, much less 33	HPV 16	HPV 16	HPV 16
Vaccine efficacy[7] (naive population)	99%	100%	100%		

[a] Note: The rates of HPV detection vary based on sensitivity of HPV detection method and how it was used for testing. This HPV positivity summarized in the table comes from the meta analysis of 67 studies performed by Smith and coworkers.[22]
Data from Refs.[7,22]

continued surveillance at less frequent intervals for 20 years similar to that followed for post-CIN treatment.

Prevention

Immunization with HPV vaccination (quadrivalent or bivalent) could potentially prevent approximately 70% of VaIN.[7,35] Smoking cessation and complete or proper treatment of CIN, VIN, and adenocarcinoma in situ are other interventions recommended to decrease the likelihood of VaIN (**Table 3**).

SUMMARY

HPV infection of the lower genital tract is common and its effects are highly variable. Fortunately, most infections are transient and the related pathology is often self-resolving.

In the United States, initial approval for a quadrivalent HPV vaccination (HPV types 6, 11, 16, and 18) was granted by the FDA in 2006 for prevention of anogenital warts, CIN, adenocarcinoma in situ of the cervix, VIN, VaIN, and cervical cancer. In 2008, the label was expanded to include prevention of vulvar and vaginal cancer.[57] In 2009, the FDA approved a bivalent HPV vaccine (HPV 16 and 18) for the indication of cervical cancer prevention.

Randomized controlled trial data of the quadrivalent vaccine (HPV types 6, 11, 16, and 18) places the prophylactic efficacy in a naive population of 96% for CIN1, 99% for CIN2/3 or adenocarcinoma in situ, 100% for VIN/VaIN1, and 99% for condylomata.[7] The bivalent vaccine (HPV 16 and 18) shows a prophylactic efficacy against CIN3+ and adenocarcinoma in situ from HPV 16/18 of 100%.[58] The contribution of HPV types 6, 11, 16, and 18 in the development of condyloma, VIN, and VaIN is roughly 90%, 80%, and 93%. The overall HPV prevalence in vulvar cancer is 40.1% (range, 40%–51%); for vaginal cancer this number is 65.5% (range, 40%–65.5%).[20,59,60] In vulvar and vaginal cancer HPV 16 is the most common subtype identified.

The potential impact for prevention of these entities by vaccination is substantial and the vaccines have been FDA approved for use in girls and women aged 9 to 26 years. The degree to which future lower genital disease burden can be reduced depends on a multitude of factors including acceptance and use of vaccination, length of immunity conferred, amount of cross-protection from other oncogenic HPV subtypes, and whether or not the critical mass to obtain herd effect by vaccination will be reached.

Lifestyle modifications including smoking cessation, limiting one's number of sexual partners, and consistent correct use of condoms provide opportunities to prevent and decrease the burden of HPV. Regular screening to detect HPV-related lower genital tract disease, diagnosis and treatment of preinvasive conditions (VIN, VaIN), and treatment of chronic vulvar dermatoses provide additional areas to mitigate the burden of HPV-related lower genital disease.

Treatment of condyloma, VIN, and VaIN is costly (economic and psychosocially); painful; and associated with high rates of recurrence. The goals in treating these conditions should be to improve quality of life for patients, minimize potential treatment sequelae, and prevent disease progression.

REFERENCES

1. Myers ER, McCrory DC, Nanda K, et al. Mathematical model for the natural history of human papillomavirus infection and cervical carcinogenesis. Am J Epidemiol 2000;151:1158–71.
2. Dunne EF, Unger ER, Sternberg M, et al. Prevalence of HPV infection among females in the United States. JAMA 2007;297(8):813–9.
3. Winer RL, Feng Q, Hughes JP, et al. Risk of female human papillomavirus acquision associated with first male sex partner. J Infect Dis 2008;197:279–82.
4. Rodriguez AC, Schiffman M, Herrero R, et al. Rapid clearance of human papillomavirus and implications of clinical focus on persistent infections. J Natl Cancer Inst 2008;100:513–7.
5. Gravitt PE. The known unknowns of HPV natural history. J Clin Invest 2011; 121(12):4593–9.
6. Garland SM, Steben M, Sings HL, et al. Natural history of genital warts: analysis of the placebo arm of 2 randomized phase iii trials of a quadrivalent vaccine. J Infect Dis 2009;199:805–14.
7. Futurel/II Study Group. Four year efficacy of prophylactic human papillomavirus quadrivalent vaccine against low grade cervical, vulvar, and vaginal intraepithelial neoplasia and anogenital warts: randomized controlled trial. BMJ 2010;340: c3493.
8. Koutsky L. Epidemiology of genital human papillomavirus infection. Am J Med 1997;102:3–8.
9. Lacey CJ, Lowndes C, Shah K. Burden and management of noncancerous HPV related-conditions; HPV 6/11 disease. Vaccine 2006;24(Suppl 3):S35–41.
10. Beutner KR, Richwald GA, Wiley DJ, et al. External genital warts: report of the American Medical Association Consensus Conference. AMA Expert Panel on External Genital Warts. Clin Infect Dis 1998;27(4):796–806.
11. American College of Obstetricians and Gynecologists. Cervical Cytology Screening. ACOG Practice Bulletin No 131. Obstet Gynecol 2012;120:1222–38.
12. Hu D, Goldie S. The economic burden of noncervical human papillomavirus disease in the United States. Am J Obstet Gynecol 2008;198:500.o1 7.
13. Kennedy CM, Boardman LA. New approaches to external genital warts and vulvar intraepithelial neoplasia. Clin Obstet Gynecol 2008;51(3):518–26.
14. Centers for Disease Control and Prevention. Sexually transmitted diseases treatment guidelines 2010. MMWR Recomm Rep 2010;59(RR-12):1–117.
15. Wiley DJ, Douglas J, Beutner K, et al. External genital warts: diagnosis, treatment and prevention. Clin Infect Dis 2002;35(Suppl 2):S10–24.
16. Beutner KR, Wiley DJ, Douglas JM, et al. Genital warts and their treatment. Clin Infect Dis 1999;28:S37–56.

17. van Seters M, van Beurden M, deCraen AJ. Is the assumed natural history of vulvar intraepithelial neoplasia III based on enough evidence? A systematic review of 3322 published patients. Gynecol Oncol 2005;97:645–51.
18. Jones RW, Rowan DM. Vulvar intraepithelial neoplasia III: a clinical study of the outcome in 113 cases with relation to the later development of invasive vulvar carcinoma. Obstet Gynecol 1994;84:741–5.
19. Jones RW, Rowan DM, Stewart AW. Vulvar intraepithelial neoplasia: aspects of the natural history and outcome in 405 women. Obstet Gynecol 2005;106(6): 1319–26.
20. Darragh TM, Colgan TJ, Cox JT, et al. The lower anogenital squamous terminology standardization project for HPV-associated lesions: background and consensus recommendations from the College of American Pathologists and the American Society for Colposcopy and Cervical Pathology. Arch Pathol Lab Med 2012;136:1–32.
21. Watson M, Saraiya M, Wu X. Update of HPV-associated female genital cancers in the United States, 1999-2004. J Womens Health 2009;18(11):1731–8.
22. Smith JS, Backes DM, Hoot BE, et al. Human papillomavirus type-distribution in vulvar and vaginal cancers and their associated precursors. Obstet Gynecol 2009;113(4):917–24.
23. American College of Obstetricians and Gynecologists. Management of vulvar intraepithelial neoplasia. Committee Opinion No 509. Obstet Gynecol 2011; 118:1192–4.
24. Mathiesen O, Buus SK, Cramers M. Topical imiquimod can reverse vulvar intraepithelial neoplasia: a randomized, double-blinded study. Gynecol Oncol 2007; 107(2):219–22.
25. van Seters M, van Beurden M, ten Kate FJ, et al. Treatment of vulvar intraepithelial neoplasia with topical imiquimod. N Engl J Med 2008;358(14): 1465–73.
26. Terlou A, van Seters M, Ewing PC, et al. Treatment of vulvar intraepithelial neoplasia with topical imiquimod: seven years median follow-up of a randomized clinical trial. Gynecol Oncol 2011;121:157–62.
27. Hillemanns P, Wang X, Staehle S, et al. Evaluation of different treatment modalities for vulvar intraepithelial neoplasia (VIN): CO2 laser vaporization, photodynamic therapy, excision and vulvectomy. Gynecol Oncol 2006;100:271–5.
28. von Gruenigen VE, Gibbons HE, Gibbins K, et al. Surgical treatments for vulvar and vaginal dysplasia: a randomized controlled trial. Obstet Gynecol 2007; 109(4):942–7.
29. Society of Gynecologic Oncologists Medical Practice and Ethics Committee. SGO clinical practice guidelines: management of gynecologic cancers. Chicago: Society of Gynecologic Oncologists; 1996.
30. Modesitt SC, Waters AB, Walton L, et al. Vulvar intraepithelial neoplasia III: occult cancer and the impact of margin status on recurrence. Obstet Gynecol 1998;92:962–6.
31. Thueson B, Andreasson B, Bock JE. Sexual function and somatopsychic reactions after local excision of vulvar intra-epithelial neoplasia. Acta Obstet Gynecol Scand 1992;71(2):126–8.
32. Riberio F, Figueiredo A, Paula T, et al. Vulvar intraepithelial neoplasia: evaluation of treatment modalities. J Low Genit Tract Dis 2012;16(3):313–7.
33. Wallbillich JJ, Rhodes HE, Milbourne AM, et al. Vulvar intraepithelial neoplasia (VIN 2/3): comparing clinical outcomes and evaluating risk factors for recurrence. Gynecol Oncol 2012;127(2):312–5.

34. Edwards CL, Tortolero-Luna G, Linares AC, et al. Vulvar intraepithlial neoplasia and vulvar cancer. Obstet Gynecol Clin North Am 1996;23:295–324.
35. Joura EA, Leodolter S, Hernandez-Avila M, et al. Efficacy of a quadrivalent prophylactic human papillomavirus (types 6, 11, 16, and 18) L1 virus-like-particle vaccine against high-grade vulval and vaginal lesions: a combined analysis of three randomised clinical trials. Lancet 2007;369(9574):1693–702.
36. Sillman FH, Fruchter RG, Chen YS, et al. Vaginal intraepithelial neoplasia: risk factors for persistence, recurrence and invasion and its management. Am J Obstet Gynecol 1997;176:93–9.
37. Woodruff JD. Carcinoma in situ of the vagina. Clin Obstet Gynecol 1981;24: 485–501.
38. Bornstein J, Kaufman RH, Adam E, et al. Human papillomavirus associated with vaginal intraepithelial neoplasia in women exposed to diethylstilbesterol in utero. Obstet Gynecol 1987;70:75–80.
39. Robboy SJ, Noller KL, Obrien P, et al. Increased incidence of cervical and vaginal dysplasia in 3,980 diethylstilbestrol-exposed young women. JAMA 1984;252(21): 2979–83.
40. Manetta A, Gutrecht EL, Berman ML, et al. Primary invasive carcinoma of the vagina. Obstet Gynecol 1990;76:639–42.
41. Gemmell J, Holmes DM, Duncan ID. How frequently need vaginal smears be taken after hysterectomy for cervical intraepithelial neoplasia? Br J Obstet Gynaecol 1990;97:58–61.
42. Schockeart S, Poppe W, Arbyn M, et al. Incidence of vaginal intraepithelial neoplasia after hysterectomy for cervical intraepithelial neoplasia: a retrospective study. Am J Obstet Gynecol 2008;199:113.e1–5.
43. Gagne HM. Colposcopy of the vagina and vulva. Obstet Gynecol Clin North Am 2008;35:659–69.
44. Dodge JA, Eltabbakh GH, Mount SL, et al. Clinical features and risk of recurrence among patients with vaginal intraepithelial neoplasia. Gynecol Oncol 2001;83:363–9.
45. Caglar H, Hertzog RW, Hreshchyshyn MM. Topical 5-fluorouracil treatment of vaginal intraepithelial neoplasia. Obstet Gynecol 1981;58:580–3.
46. Kirwan P. Topical 5-fluorouracil in the treatment of vaginal intraepithelial neoplasia. Br J Obstet Gynaecol 1985;92:287–91.
47. Audet-LaPoint P, Body G, Vauclar R, et al. Vaginal intraepithelial neoplasia. Gynecol Oncol 1990;36:232–9.
48. Haidopoulos D, Diakomanolis E, Rodolakis A, et al. Can local application of imiquimod cream be an alternative mode of therapy for patients with high-grade intraepithelial lesions of the vagina? Int J Gynecol Cancer 2005;15: 898–902.
49. Diakomanolis E, Haidopoulos D, Stefanidis K. Treatment of high-grade vaginal intraepithelial neoplasia with imiquimod cream. N Engl J Med 2002;347:374.
50. Lin J, Juang EY, Chang HY, et al. Therapeutic effect of topical applications of tricholoracetic acid for vaginal intraepithelial neoplasia after hysterectomy. Jpn J Clin Oncol 2005;35(11):651–4.
51. Hoskins W, Perez C. Treatment of VaIN. In: Hoskins WJ, Perez CA, Young RC, editors. The principles and practice of gynecologic oncology. 3rd edition. New York: Lippincott, Williams, and Wilkins; 2000. p. 820–1.
52. Graham K, Wright K, Cadwallader B, et al. 20-year retrospective review of medium dose rate intracavitary brachytherapy in VAIN3. Gynecol Oncol 2007; 106:105–11.

53. Blanchard P, Monnier L, Dumas I, et al. Low dose rate definitive brachytherapy for high-grade vaginal intraepithelial neoplasia. Oncologist 2011;16:182–8.
54. Matsuo K, Chi DS, Walker LD, et al. Ultrasonic surgical aspiration for vaginal intraepithelial neoplasia. Int J Gynaecol Obstet 2009;105:71–3.
55. Robinson JB, Sun CC, Bodurka-Bevers D, et al. Cavitational ultrasonic surgical aspiration for the treatment of vaginal intraepithelial neoplasia. Gynecol Oncol 2000;78:235–41.
56. Gurumurthy M, Curickshank M. Management of vaginal intraepithelial neoplasia. J Low Genit Tract Dis 2012;16(3):306–12.
57. Diaz ML. Prevention of cervical, vaginal and vulval cancers: role of the quadrivalent human papillomavirus (6, 11, 16, 18) recombinant vaccine. Int J Womens Health 2009;1:119–29.
58. HPV PATRICIA Study Group. Overall efficacy of HPV 16/18 ASO4-adjuvanted vaccine against grade 3 or greater cervical intraepithelial neoplasia; 4-year end-of-study analysis of the randomised double-blind PATRICIA trial. Lancet Oncol 2012;13(1):89–99.
59. DeVuyst H, Clifford GM, Nascimento MC, et al. Prevalence and type distribution of human papillomavirus in carcinoma and intraepithelial neoplasia of the vulva, vagina and anus: a meta-analysis. Int J Cancer 2009;124:1626–36.
60. Chaturvedi AK. Beyond cervical cancer: burden of other HPV-related cancers among men and women. J Adolesc Health 2010;46:S20–6.

Human Papillomavirus Testing in Cervical Cancer Screening

Philip E. Castle, PhD, MPH[a],*, Miriam Cremer, MD, MPH[b,c]

KEYWORDS

- Human papillomavirus (HPV) • Pap testing • Visual inspection after acetic acid (VIA)
- Cervical cancer • Cervical intraepithelial neoplasia • Vaccination • Screening
- Low-resource settings

KEY POINTS

- Persistent infection by certain types of human papillomavirus (HPV) is the cause of virtually all cervical cancer worldwide.
- The discovery that HPV is the necessary cause of cervical cancer has led to the development of prophylactic HPV vaccines and molecular tests for the detection of HPV.
- HPV testing is more sensitive but less specific than a Papanicolaou (Pap) test for identifying women with precancerous lesions. Thus, HPV testing is a useful screen to rule out disease in the general population and then, as desired, a more specific test, like Pap, can be applied to identify precancer.
- There are now a variety of options for cervical cancer screening, including lower-cost HPV tests, which can be used to expand screening coverage, especially to those not currently being screened by Pap programs.

BACKGROUND

For more than 50 years, cervical cytology, first using the conventional Papanicolaou (Pap) smear and more recently also liquid-based cytologic methods, has been the standard of care for cervical cancer screening.[1] Where cytology-based screening programs have been implemented effectively, cervical cancer rates have been reduced by 50% to 90%.[1] Although there are no clinical trials to establish a direct evidential link between cytology and the reduction of cancer incidence, there is little dispute

Disclosures: P.E. Castle serves as a member of a Data and Safety Monitoring Board to review data on HPV vaccines for Merck. P.E. Castle is as paid consultant to BD, GE Healthcare, and Cepheid. P.E. Castle has received a speaker's honorarium from Roche. P.E. Castle has received HPV test reagents and testing for research from Qiagen, Roche, MTM, and Norchip at a reduced or no cost. M. Cremer has received a speaker's honorarium from Roche.
[a] Global Cancer Initiative, 100 Radcliffe, Dr Chestertown, MD 21620, USA; [b] Department of Obstetrics and Gynecology, University of Pittsburgh, Pittsburgh, PA, USA; [c] The Mount Sinai Medical Center, Basic Health International, One Gustave, Levy Place, Box 1170, New York, NY 10029-6574, USA
* Corresponding author. 4318 South 8th Street, Arlington, VA 22204.
E-mail address: castle.philip@gmail.com

Obstet Gynecol Clin N Am 40 (2013) 377–390
http://dx.doi.org/10.1016/j.ogc.2013.03.002
0889-8545/13/$ – see front matter © 2013 Elsevier Inc. All rights reserved.

that cytology-based screening and timely follow-up and treatment of women who screen positive have been the cause for these reductions in cervical cancer incidence.

The discovery that human papillomavirus (HPV) causes cervical cancer has revolutionized our understanding of the causes of cervical cancer. Over the past 30 years, laboratory scientists, epidemiologists, clinicians, and public health advocates have worked collaboratively in an unparalleled effort to understand mechanistically how HPV causes cervical cancer. We now understand that certain types of persistent HPV infections are an essential cause of cervical cancer and precancer but that most HPV infections are benign and do not cause cancer or precancer. The natural history has been simplified from an old lock-and-key model based on the thickness of the transformed epithelium to 4 reliably measured stages[2,3]: HPV acquisition, HPV persistence, progression to precancer, and invasion.

The median time from any newly acquired HPV infection to invasive cervical cancer appears to be approximately 20 to 25 years.[3] The longest sojourn between stages of cervical carcinogenesis is the transition from precancerous lesions to invasion. It is this long duration of the precancerous state that has permitted successful implementation of screening-and-treatment interventions to prevent cancer. The natural history of HPV-induced cervical carcinogenesis follows the same time course for any newly acquired infection at any age. Incident infections must persist, progress, and invade along the same causal pathway. Prevalent infections represent more risk because they have already persisted for some unknown duration.[4]

The discovery that persistent cervical infections by specific HPV genotypes cause virtually all cervical cancer and its immediate precursor lesions (eg, cervical intra-epithelial neoplasia grade 3 [CIN3]) has revolutionized cervical cancer prevention strategies by directly targeting the causal agent.[3] These interventions include (1) prophylactic HPV vaccines for primary prevention in younger, HPV-naive women and (2) molecular testing for high-risk HPV for secondary prevention in older women who are at risk of cancer. When applied in an age-appropriate manner based on the natural history of HPV, both are efficacious, provide excellent population benefits, and are cost-effective. To maximize disease prevention, it is most effective to administer prophylactic HPV vaccines several years before the median age of sexual debut, and initiative screening approximately 15 years after the median age of sexual debut for a given population.

RATIONALE OF MOVING FROM PAP TO HPV TESTING FOR CERVICAL CANCER SCREENING

There is substantial and consistent evidence that high-risk HPV DNA detection is 20% to 45% more sensitive for precancer and early cancer of the cervix (CIN3+) than cytology-based methods.[5–11] These precancerous lesions found by HPV testing and missed by cytology are clinically significant. Earlier detection of precancerous lesions by HPV testing, compared with cytology, reduces the incidence of CIN3+ within 4 to 5 years,[12] and cervical cancer-related mortality within 8 years.[13] A subcohort of women who test high-risk HPV positive at a single point in time continue to accumulate disease for more than 15 years while abnormal cytology predicts disease for only a year or two.[14]

HPV testing provides excellent negative predictive value because of high sensitivity as well as slow progression from incident infection to cancer.[8,10,13,15,16] Women who test high-risk HPV negative at one-time point have a 2-fold to 3-fold lower subsequent risk of cervical precancer and cancer compared with a negative cytology at any follow-up time. Reassurance from a single negative high-risk HPV test lasts longer than reassurance from a single negative cytology. Therefore, a negative HPV test safely permits longer intervals between screens than a negative cytology.

This finding has an important clinical implication for high-risk HPV testing. High-risk HPV-negative populations are many years from being at significant risk of invasive cancer and therefore should not be rescreened too soon. Screening too frequently identifies primarily benign, transient high-risk HPV infections, which are better left undetected as it potentially increases the harms of screening and only slightly reduces the cancer risk. The screening interval should be selected so as to achieve equipoise between rescreening too soon and finding mostly irrelevant infections and not waiting so long that risk of cancer exceeds the acceptable threshold.

Given the success of cytology-based programs, what is the rationale for changing from cytology-based to high-risk HPV-based screening? How good is good enough? How much added value can be achieved? Is it worth it? In places where cytology is successfully established or there is acceptance of cytology as the standard of care, there is resistance to adopting an HPV-based screening program. The reasons for this resistance range from a lack of knowledge to maintaining the status quo because of cytology's proven track record, and stakeholders' perceptions of the standard of care.

Moving from a cytology-based to a high-risk HPV-based screening approach requires a fundamental paradigm shift in the philosophy and purpose of screening. It requires shifting from a medical perspective of finding women with disease to a public health perspective of ruling out disease in the healthy population and identifying a subpopulation at higher risk who then need further clinical follow-up. In screening for any disease, the target disease has to be sufficiently prevalent to justify screening efforts. In the case of cervical cancer screening, the prevalence of precancerous lesions (CIN2/3) of the cervix in the general population is less than 5%, and in well-screened populations around 1%. Thus, the entire process of population-based screening is inefficient: (1) more than 95% of women in the general population do not have clinically relevant disease (CIN2+); (2) approximately 80% of screen-positive women do not have CIN2+; and (3) only 30% of CIN3 if left untreated becomes invasive cancer over a 30-year period.[17] The current lifetime risk of cervical cancer has been estimated to be approximately 0.68% in the United States (http://seer.cancer.gov/statfacts/html/cervix.html) Assuming that the cervical cancer screening program in the United States has been 70% to 90% effective, the lifetime risk without screening is 2.3% to 6.8%, meaning that 1 in 44 to 1 in 14 women would develop cancer in the absence of screening. High-risk HPV testing should be used to screen out those who do not need further clinical attention for a period of time, and clinical resources for diagnostic follow-up should be focused on an at-risk population who need further intervention.

It is difficult for any single test to both effectively rule out and rule in disease. Tests that rule out disease label women who are unlikely to develop disease as positive. Conversely, tests that are specific for disease cannot identify women who have HPV infections that will subsequently persist and progress to disease. Such is the case for HPV versus Pap (ie, approximately twice the number of women test positive by HPV DNA testing as by cytology).[5–11,18,19] It therefore may not be desirable to refer all HPV-positive women to colposcopy. A secondary, triage test is then used to decide who needs immediate diagnostic evaluation by colposcopy or treatment intervention ("positive triage") versus monitoring for evidence of a persistent HPV infection ("negative triage"), which strongly predicts who has or will have CIN3+,[20,21] would be valuable.

Cytology testing among HPV-positive women is the most commonly suggested triage method because it is the most familiar test, although new strategies based on biomarkers are emerging.[22] This new strategy implies a shift in who receives Pap testing from everyone to 5% to 15% of the population who test positive for high-risk HPV, the casual factor of cervical cancer. To be effective, testing must be performed only for high-risk HPV types. Tests for low-risk HPV test have no clinical relevance. As direct consequence of an HPV testing–first approach, the positive predictive value of cytology testing improves because the prevalence of disease is increased approximately 5-fold to 10-fold, and cytomorphologic changes (eg, HPV-negative equivocal or atypical squamous cells of undetermined significance [ASC-US]), which are mostly unrelated to cervical carcinogenesis, are not observed.

COST-EFFECTIVENESS OF HPV TESTING

Several health econometric studies have found the use of HPV testing in primary screening to be cost-effective. One comprehensive analysis[23] found that cytology with HPV triage of ASC-US starting at either age 21 or 25 years and then switching to HPV testing with cytology triage at age 30 or 35 years every 3 to 5 years was cost-effective. It was less cost-effective to start screening with HPV testing for primary screening at an earlier age.

The assumption in this study of cytology sensitivity for CIN2/3 was 80%, which is higher than generally achievable; with an occasional notable exception,[10] specificity was assumed to be 95%. If a more typical, lower sensitivity for cytology was used in these models (around 50%[5]), HPV would be shown to be an even better value.

A recent analysis focused on Europe[24] found that, in most scenarios, HPV testing for primary cervical cancer screening every 5 years was more cost-effective than cytology every 5 years. The exception was those circumstances in which the costs of conducting cytology were low (with the assumption of good cytology performance) or HPV prevalence was high and HPV testing was expensive.

IMPLEMENTATION OF HPV TESTING: THE US EXPERIENCE

The United States was an early adopter of HPV testing in the screening and management of women undergoing cervical cancer screening. In 2001, primarily based on the strength of evidence from ALTS (the ASCUS LSIL Triage Study),[25] reflex HPV testing for the triage of equivocal (ASC-US) cytology was recommended.[26]

In 2003, the US Food and Drug Administration (FDA) approved the Hybrid Capture 2 (HC2) (Qiagen, Gaithersburg, MD) for concurrent HPV and Pap/cytology (cotesting) to screen women aged 30 years and older. Since that time, several US programs, including Kaiser Permanente of Northern California (KPNC, Oakland, CA) have adopted cotesting into routine practice, with 3-year intervals between cotests. In early 2003, KPNC initiated a shift from annual Pap smear testing to cotesting with HC2 and Pap smear testing over a 2-year phase-in period. The shift from Pap testing to cotesting was partially motivated by a lack of confidence in the safety against cancer in a 3-year interval after a negative Pap result latter even after following 3 consecutive negative Pap smears. Annual Pap tests continued to be available as a screening option. By early 2007, 95% of screening participants elected cotesting at 3-year intervals in preference to annual Pap testing. Management of women who tested HPV positive and Pap negative (HPV+/Pap–) evolved from annual follow-up with retesting, to recommending colposcopy after 2 HPV+/Pap– screens in 2006, to mandatory colposcopy after 2 HPV+/Pap– screens in 2008, as recommended by an interim guidance.

In a retrospective observational analysis of 330,000 women aged 30 years and older who were the first to undergo cotesting from 2003 to 2005 at KPNC, the following observations were made[19]: (1) the 5-year risk of CIN3+ after a negative cotest was comparable with the 3-year risk after negative Pap test (irrespective of the HPV result); (2) a positive cotest only marginally increased the identification of women who have or will have CIN3+ compared with a positive HPV test (irrespective of the cytology result); (3) a negative cotest only marginally increased the reassurance against CIN3+ and cervical cancer compared with a negative HPV test (irrespective of the cytology result); (4) HPV+/Pap– results identified more women who had or developed adenocarcinoma in situ or adenocarcinoma than HPV+/greater than or equal to ASC-US; (5) as noted earlier, the second round of screening after a preceding negative cotest resulted in significantly lower yields and positive predictive values for CIN3+, suggesting that a 3-year interval may be too frequent; and (6) the subset of women with a second consecutive negative cotest had similar risks of CIN3+ compared with the entire group of women with the initial negative cotest, suggesting that there may be a level of irreducible risk.

The strength of the analysis, aside from the large sample size, was that it was based on real-world practice, without the constraints and biases inherent to randomized clinical trials to evaluate efficacy. That is, all non-pregnant women aged 30 years and older with an intact cervix and without a history of cervical cancer were screened at KPNC, without additional exclusions. Although the prevalence of disease may vary between populations, and thereby affect the predictive values of test results, the results from KPNC are consistent with several randomized trials suggesting that the patterns of performance are generalizable.

US Guidelines

The American Cancer Society (ACS) first recommended cotesting as an acceptable alternative to routine cervical cytology alone for cervical cancer screening in 2002.[27] The ACS recommendations included extending the screening interval to not less than 3 years for those women who tested negative by cotest. Subsequently, other organizations, including the American College of Obstetricians and Gynecologists (ACOG),[28] adopted similar guidelines for cotesting.

In 2012, a joint review conducted by the ACS, American Society for Colposcopy and Cervical Pathology (ASCCP), and American Society for Clinical Pathology (ASCP) and one by the US Preventative Services Task Force (USPSTF) were concluded. The ACS-ASCCP-ASCP review judged that women ages 30 to 64 years should be screened with cytology and HPV testing (cotesting) every 5 years (preferred) or cytology alone every 3 years (acceptable).[29,30] Screening is discontinued at the age of 65 years if preceded by normal results (eg, 3 normal Pap tests or 2 negative cotests) in the preceding 10 years.

However, the ACS-ASCCP-ASCP review deemed that there was insufficient evidence to recommend for or against the use of HPV testing alone (at a 5-year interval) for primary cervical cancer screening for most clinical settings. The primary concern regarding HPV testing alone for screening was that the potential harms were poorly quantified. Although primary HPV-based screening approaches appeared promising, the guidelines committee concluded that the lack of a well-defined and evaluated management strategy for positive tests precluded their practical implementation in most clinical settings in the United States at this time. There are no data to estimate how the clinical performance of cytology (as a follow-up test) would be affected by a priori knowledge of positive HPV status. The lack of an internal standard for specimen adequacy for some HPV assays may provide false reassurance among a few women whose negative screening results are a function of specimen inadequacy rather than absence of disease.

ACOG has largely adopted the ACS-ASCCP-ASCP/USPSTF guidelines for cervical cancer screening.[31] As of 2012, most of the major professional medical organizations (ASCP, ACS, ASCCP, and ACOG) and USPSTF have adopted comparable guidelines. It is hoped that uniform guidelines will lead to consistent care through improved clinician compliance, which has been less than ideal as described below.

Compliance with Guidelines

One of the challenges in implementing HPV testing in the United States has been compliance with professional guidelines. One recent report[32] found that most (~2/3) clinicians who use HPV testing for screening would order HPV testing for women who had a negative cotest at a frequency less than every 3 years (the recommended screening interval at the time of the study). Another study[33] found that many clinicians, and especially obstetricians/gynecologists, order both high-risk and low-risk HPV testing despite the lack of benefit of the latter to patients. These clinicians also order HPV testing for women with high-grade squamous intraepithelial lesion (HSIL) cytology, most of whom test HPV positive, and all of whom need colposcopy regardless of HPV status, because of the high risk of CIN3+ among those with HPV-negative HSIL cytology.[34]

Issues of inappropriate test use in the United States are not limited to HPV testing and have been well documented for Pap testing as well.[35] Improper use of tests leads not only to significant added expense to health care delivery, including extra clinical visits, extra tests ordered, and clinical follow-up of benign HPV infections, but also to unnecessary excision treatment linked to negative reproductive outcomes.[36] In the case of HPV testing, inappropriate use could lead to inadequate follow-up of high-risk, albeit HPV-negative, women. For example, HPV-negative HSIL or ASC cannot rule out HSIL [atypical squamous cells, cannot rule out high-grade squamous intraepithelial lesion] cytology[34] or excessive testing costs without patient benefit.

Reaching the Underserved: Self-Collection and HPV Testing

Cervical cancer is now an uncommon cancer in the United States, ranking 13th among all female cancers,[37] as a result of widespread implementation of cervical cancer screening and treatment programs. Despite this success, cervical cancer remains high in poor, immigrant, and minority women. More than half of all cervical cancer occurring in the United States is found in medically underserved populations (http://www.uspreventiveservicestaskforce.org/uspstf11/cervcancer/cervcancerart.htm). Cervical cancer occurs mainly in these populations as part of a complex of diseases linked to poverty and racial/ethnic disparities.[38] Low socioeconomic status in the United States is linked to late-stage diagnosis of cervical cancer and increased mortality.[39] These underserved populations inhabit places like Mississippi Delta, Deep South, Appalachia, central valley of California, United States-Mexico Border region, and the US Associated Pacific Islands. There are likely to be underserved populations in most major metropolitan areas as well. To decrease the cervical cancer burden in the United States, it is essential to target these populations.[40]

A practical way to increase screening within these underserved populations is self-collection of samples. The increased sensitivity of HPV testing makes the use of self-collected cervicovaginal specimens feasible. Many studies have found that self-collection and HPV testing is equally as sensitive for CIN2+ and CIN3+ as expert cytology. This finding was shown in a recent pooled analysis of self-collection studies performed in more than 10,000 women living in China.[41] A recent study conducted in the United States reached a similar conclusion.[42] There are many advantages and potential advantages to using self-collected specimens, such as fewer clinical visits and pelvic examinations and empowerment of women. A self-collected sample does not have the same clinical sensitivity as a physician-collected specimen for HPV testing. However, it does offer a method of screening that has at least comparable for CIN2+ and CIN3+ with a current standard of care, Pap testing.

To increase the number of women who are screened in Western countries with high-coverage cytology programs, several large pilot studies (n >1000) of self-collection and HPV testing have targeted nonattendees.[43–47] Several studies reported 5% to 25% increased participation more than what was achieved by sending a reminder/reinvitation. In addition, several studies revealed greater diagnostic yields of CIN2+ in those nonattendees than in a comparable population undergoing routine screening. This finding suggests that non-participation in screening leads to higher risk, or that self-collection with HPV testing was more sensitive for CIN2+ than cytology, or both. Another, smaller study[48] found that underscreened women living in the Mississippi Delta were more likely to choose self-collection and HPV testing over cytology screening, when given a choice via door-to-door outreach. Furthermore, those women who chose self-collection were more likely to complete their sampling than women who chose free cytology screening.

GLOBAL VIEW

Despite the success of cytology-based programs, cervical cancer remains the third most common female cancer and third most common cause of female cancer-related mortality globally, with an annual incidence of 530,000 and mortality of 275,000, respectively.[49] This seeming contradiction is explained by the fact that the cervical cancer incidence and mortality is approximately 10-fold greater in low-income and middle-income countries (LMICs). LMICs make up most of the world's population and have technical and financial barriers to implementing cytology-based programs.[1,50] After 50 years of implementing cytology-based programs, it seems a foregone conclusion that one size does not fit all for cervical cancer screening. Alternative prevention strategies must be considered if the global burden of cervical cancer is to be addressed.

In lower-resource settings, there is often a severe lack of health care infrastructure, including adequate medical records. Basic laboratory procedures, quality-control measures, and safety precautions are not routinely practiced. The improvement of laboratory structure is not possible without significant financial and political investment (eg, President's Emergency Plan for AIDS Relief). In our opinion, relying on cytology as the primary cervical cancer screening test is impractical and is not working in many countries that have tried to implement and improve cytology programs. Repeated screening by cytology to achieve programmatic sensitivity is difficult to accomplish. Many areas lack the clinics to handle the volume of women needed to achieve good population coverage using any clinic-based screening strategy. Furthermore, the already overburdened cytopathologists would be unable to handle increased volume.

Thus, robust and simplified HPV tests are necessary to implement any cervical cancer prevention program. Several promising tests designed for the lower-resource setting are being validated. One is careHPV (Qiagen), a DNA test that detects the 13 carcinogenic HPV genotypes and HPV66 in aggregate.[51] careHPV is a manual test that is based on similar chemistry as the FDA-approved HC2 but performed on a paramagnetic bead matrix to increase the efficiency of mixing and washing, thereby reducing the assay time (3–3.5 hours) by approximately 50% of HC2. careHPV is anticipated to cost $5 per test. careHPV has shown promising results. It has high, albeit lower, sensitivity than HC2 and comparable specificity with HC2. careHPV has also shown good performance using self-collected specimens.[51] A research-only test using the same platform, "careHPV16/18/45" has also shown promising results as a secondary, triage test for HPV-positive women. The results are consistent with the recommendation for the use of HPV16 or HPV16/18 detection for the management of HPV-positive, Pap-negative women in the United States.[30] In 2012, careHPV received regulatory approval from China (Chinese FDA) and the European Union (CE Marked), which should provide the impetus and political acceptability for wider dissemination.

A second test, a protein test for HPV E6 oncoprotein (Avantage HPV E6 Test, Arbor Vita, Fremont, CA),[52] is also being evaluated in China. The test is a lateral flow test that captures and detects HPV E6 from HPV16, 18, or 45 from lysed cervical specimens using a sandwich assay based on E6-specific monoclonal antibodies. The non-batch test can be completed in 2 hours and requires simple equipment such as microcentrifuge and rotating shaker. It uses visual readouts, although scanning of the assay strips remains a possibility. Preliminary results show the expected sensitivity for prevalent CIN3 ($\sim 70\%$) and positive predictive values of $\sim 30\%$ to 35%. Because this test is still being evaluated in research studies and is not yet commercialized, the pricing has not been established.

Despite the relative simplicity of tests like careHPV and the E6 Test, significant challenges remain in implementing them. Basic laboratory acumen, such as compliance with good laboratory practices and safety precautions and reporting of testing errors, must be taught. Dedicated personnel must run the assays routinely to achieve and maintain good performance. For some assays, the specimens also must be tested in batches to be cost effective so that, in most cases, multiple clinic visits are necessary to achieve screening and treatment, potentially leading to losses in follow-up of screen positives.

Other lower-cost molecular assays are under development. With most of the world's medically underserved now living in upper lower-income and middle-income countries, centralized processing with high throughput and good quality control is a possibility. Belinson and colleagues[53] reported that polymerase chain reaction (PCR) amplification with a matrix-assisted laser desorption/ionization-time of flight (MALDI-TOF) detection could achieve excellent performance. Although such an approach would require significant investment in equipment and in developing PCR-safe laboratories where they may not currently exist, the potential upside is testing that costs less than $5.00. Coupled with self-collection, such an approach can minimize the costs of screening and allow high-volume screening.[53] Alternatively, new, fully automated, FDA-approved tests might provide robust solutions if made affordable through tiered-pricing schemes in which the net positive margin of profit per test is lower than for Western countries. Setting up centralized testing offers the benefit of having to establish and maintain fewer high-quality laboratories but requires good specimen transportation and laboratory information systems as well as timely transmittal of test results to the clinicians for follow-up of the screen positives.

The laboratory component of the cervical cancer screening program may be the least of the challenges. The prescreening activities (eg, subject education, recruitment, and participation and specimen collection, handling, and processing), postscreening activities (eg, tracking and follow-up of screen positives, clinical management of screening positives, which might include colposcopy and biopsy with a histopathologic diagnosis or treatment by ablation using cryotherapy or tissue excision), and communication of the results to the clinician/health worker represent significant challenges to the lower-resource setting. Poor follow-up and completion of any screening intervention can significantly reduce its effectiveness and cost- effectiveness. However, the challenge is the opportunity. Improving these systems for cervical cancer prevention would strengthen the delivery of many critical health services.

FINAL COMMENTS

Although HPV vaccines may be the ultimate cervical cancer prevention modality, especially if the next generation of HPV vaccines targeting 7 HPV genotypes proves to be effective over a long duration, they will not greatly benefit the 2 generations that have already been exposed to causal HPV infections. Some have or will develop cancer in the absence of secondary prevention through timely detection and treatment of precancerous lesions.[54] The first benefit of vaccination programs to be realized will be a reduction of preinvasive lesions and a multitude of unimportant cervical epithelial changes that spontaneously resolve but are often the source of great patient anxiety and inappropriate treatment. Given that the natural history time course of developing cervical cancer is on average 25 years, it will be several decades before the benefits of HPV vaccination are experienced. This observation holds true even if universal vaccine coverage could be implemented now. Thus, cervical cancer screening and treatment must be considered in any comprehensive cervical cancer prevention program to reduce the burden of cervical cancer.

Testing using validated HPV assays[55,56] provides an objective measure of cervical cancer risk that can be implemented effectively in high-resource and potentially lower-resource settings. Visual inspection after acetic acid (VIA) and Pap tests require that external quality control measures be implemented to maintain a good performance. In many cases, building these quality-control measures requires significantly more money and labor than is fully appreciated. The scalability and immediate and long-term impact of HPV testing on cervical cancer risk has been shown. Although the evidence for VIA is lacking and the success of Pap/cytology programs remains primarily in high-resource settings, HPV testing can be used as a first screen to rule out disease in the mostly healthy population, followed by a more specific test like Pap or VIA for identifying those women who need immediate clinical follow-up. The program has to be designed to meet local needs and capacities as well as take into consideration the local sensitivities related to cancer risk versus overscreening and treatment. In addition, the more the community is involved in the screening process, such as by self-collection programming, the more human and financial resources can be put toward medical management of the positives.

It should be recognized that different strategies may need to be employed to meet the needs of diverse populations, even within a single country. Fortunately, there is a menu of options for cervical cancer screening, management, and treatment (**Table 1**).[54] There is no single right answer for secondary cervical cancer prevention provided that the screening is performed well, there is good population coverage, and the follow-up management of screen positives is timely. Countries and regions interested in implementing screening programs should make an informed decision as to what is feasible and appropriate, based on economic, cultural, social, and political factors.

The introduction of HPV testing does not mean that other programs already in place should be disregarded or stopped. Rather, HPV testing can be introduced to complement current effective programs to expand coverage. Affordable HPV testing is clearly the way of the future for cervical cancer screening in both the United States and globally. It can be used to make current effective programs more efficient or reach those

Table 1
A hypothetical menu of options for secondary cervical cancer prevention: screening, management, and treatment. The strengths and weaknesses of the listed options are based on the authors' and do not reflect a general consensus about these methods, nor does the order represent a ranking or strength of evidence

Step	Options	Strengths	Issues/Limitations
Patient sampling	Clinician-collected cervical specimen	Highest Se and Sp; can be used for Pap testing	Requires most personnel, disposables (eg, speculums), clinic time and space; patient transportation
	Clinician-collected cervicovaginal specimen at clinic	No speculum; performed by trained personnel	Requires clinic time and space; patient transportation; lower Se and Sp
	Clinician-collected cervicovaginal specimen at home	No speculum; performed by trained personnel; no clinic	Lower Se and Sp
	Self-collected cervicovaginal specimen at clinic	No speculum	Patient acceptability; still requires clinic; lower Se and Sp
	Self-collection cervicovaginal specimen at home	No speculum; no clinic needed	Patient acceptability; lower Se and Sp
	Urine	No genital sampling	Unproved; specimen volume and transportation (if performed at home)
Testing	Pap/cervical cytology	Well-accepted; considered standard of care; testing costs are not exported to diagnostic companies; higher Sp	Difficult to establish and maintain; specialized facilities, personnel, and chemicals; requires clinician-collected cervical specimen; more labor intensive; laboratory and laboratory systems required
	HPV DNA	Best Se; adaptable for cervicovaginal specimens (self-collection)	Lower Sp than Pap ($\sim$2x positivity); costs; laboratory and laboratory systems required
	VIA	Lowest cost (ie, no assay costs); well suited to screen and treat strategy	Detects only the largest and most obvious lesions; reliability; unproved scalability
	Biomarkers (eg, E6, p16[INK4A] immunocytochemistry)	May provide a good trade-off of Se and Sp	Large-scale validation needed; more specific = less long-term predictive value; better suited for triage of HPV positives?

(continued on next page)

Step	Options	Strengths	Issues/Limitations
Management	Colposcopy	Well-accepted; diagnostic confirmation	Requires trained personnel and equipment: colposcopy misses small precancerous lesions
	Triage to colposcopy	Reduces colposcopy	Requires a more Sp test that still has reasonably high Se; losses to follow-up
	Treatment	Limits losses to follow-up	Overtreatment
	Triage to treatment	Reduces overtreatment	Losses to follow-up
Treatment	Loop electrosurgical excision procedure	Most efficacious (90%–95%)	Requires trained personnel; possible cases of excessive bleeding
	Cryotherapy	Can be implemented by any health worker	Lower efficacy; requires assessing cryotherapy eligibility, which may not be reliable; risk of human immunodeficiency virus infection?; medical acceptability; N_2O gas has been used in most studies and clinical practices often use CO_2, which is unproved
	Cold coagulation	Insufficient data to assess	

Table 1
(continued)

Abbreviations: Se, sensitivity; Sp, specificity.

who are not being screened for this mostly preventable cancer. Given the huge global disparities in cervical cancer burden, it seems implausible that cytology programs will meet the needs of all populations. Limiting access to effective alternative strategies to Pap testing for those who need cervical cancer prevention the most is doing the same thing over and over (relying only on Pap screening) and expecting a different result. It is certainly the definition of insanity.

REFERENCES

1. Cervix cancer screening. IARC Handbooks of cancer prevention, vol. 10. Lyons (France): IARC Press; 2005.
2. Wright TC Jr, Schiffman M. Adding a test for human papillomavirus DNA to cervical-cancer screening. N Engl J Med 2003;348(6):489–90.
3. Schiffman M, Castle PE, Jeronimo J, et al. Human papillomavirus and cervical cancer. Lancet 2007;370(9590):890–907.
4. Rodriguez AC, Schiffman M, Herrero R, et al. Longitudinal study of human papillomavirus persistence and cervical intraepithelial neoplasia grade 2/3: critical role of duration of infection. J Natl Cancer Inst 2010;102(5):315–24.
5. Cuzick J, Clavel C, Petry KU, et al. Overview of the European and North American studies on HPV testing in primary cervical cancer screening. Int J Cancer 2006;119(5):1095–101.

6. Mayrand MH, Duarte-Franco E, Rodrigues I, et al. Human papillomavirus DNA versus Papanicolaou screening tests for cervical cancer. N Engl J Med 2007; 357(16):1579–88.
7. Naucler P, Ryd W, Tornberg S, et al. Human papillomavirus and Papanicolaou tests to screen for cervical cancer. N Engl J Med 2007;357(16):1589–97.
8. Ronco G, Giorgi-Rossi P, Carozzi F, et al. Efficacy of human papillomavirus testing for the detection of invasive cervical cancers and cervical intraepithelial neoplasia: a randomised controlled trial. Lancet Oncol 2010;11(3):249–57.
9. Anttila A, Kotaniemi-Talonen L, Leinonen M, et al. Rate of cervical cancer, severe intraepithelial neoplasia, and adenocarcinoma in situ in primary HPV DNA screening with cytology triage: randomised study within organised screening programme. BMJ 2010;340:c1804. http://dx.doi.org/10.1136/bmj.c1804.
10. Rijkaart DC, Berkhof J, Rozendaal L, et al. Human papillomavirus testing for the detection of high-grade cervical intraepithelial neoplasia and cancer: final results of the POBASCAM randomised controlled trial. Lancet Oncol 2012;13(1):78–88.
11. Castle PE, Fetterman B, Poitras N, et al. Variable risk of cervical precancer and cancer after a human papillomavirus-positive test. Obstet Gynecol 2011;117(3): 650–6.
12. Arbyn M, Ronco G, Anttila A, et al. Evidence regarding human papillomavirus testing in secondary prevention of cervical cancer. Vaccine 2012;30(Suppl 5): F88–99. http://dx.doi.org/10.1016/j.vaccine.2012.06.095.
13. Sankaranarayanan R, Nene BM, Shastri SS, et al. HPV screening for cervical cancer in rural India. N Engl J Med 2009;360(14):1385–94.
14. Castle PE, Glass AG, Rush BB, et al. Clinical human papillomavirus detection forecasts cervical cancer risk in women over 18 years of follow-up. J Clin Oncol 2012;30(25):3044–50.
15. Sherman ME, Lorincz AT, Scott DR, et al. Baseline cytology, human papillomavirus testing, and risk for cervical neoplasia: a 10-year cohort analysis. J Natl Cancer Inst 2003;95(1):46–52.
16. Dillner J, Rebolj M, Birembaut P, et al. Long term predictive values of cytology and human papillomavirus testing in cervical cancer screening: joint European cohort study. BMJ 2008;337:a1754.
17. McCredie MR, Sharples KJ, Paul C, et al. Natural history of cervical neoplasia and risk of invasive cancer in women with cervical intraepithelial neoplasia 3: a retrospective cohort study. Lancet Oncol 2008;9(5):425–34.
18. Castle PE, Fetterman B, Poitras N, et al. Five-year experience of human papillomavirus DNA and Papanicolaou test cotesting. Obstet Gynecol 2009;113(3): 595–600.
19. Katki HA, Kinney WK, Fetterman B, et al. Cervical cancer risk for women undergoing concurrent testing for human papillomavirus and cervical cytology: a population-based study in routine clinical practice. Lancet Oncol 2011;12(7): 663–72.
20. Castle PE, Rodriguez AC, Burk RD, et al. Short term persistence of human papillomavirus and risk of cervical precancer and cancer: population based cohort study. BMJ 2009;339:b2569.
21. Kjaer SK, Frederiksen K, Munk C, et al. Long-term absolute risk of cervical intraepithelial neoplasia grade 3 or worse following human papillomavirus infection: role of persistence. J Natl Cancer Inst 2010;102(19):1478–88.
22. Cuschieri K, Wentzensen N. Human papillomavirus mRNA and p16 detection as biomarkers for the improved diagnosis of cervical neoplasia. Cancer Epidemiol Biomarkers Prev 2008;17(10):2536–45.

23. Goldhaber-Fiebert JD, Stout NK, Salomon JA, et al. Cost-effectiveness of cervical cancer screening with human papillomavirus DNA testing and HPV-16,18 vaccination. J Natl Cancer Inst 2008;100(5):308–20.
24. de Kok IM, van RJ, Dillner J, et al. Primary screening for human papillomavirus compared with cytology screening for cervical cancer in European settings: cost effectiveness analysis based on a Dutch microsimulation model. BMJ 2012;344:e670.
25. Solomon D, Schiffman M, Tarone R. Comparison of three management strategies for patients with atypical squamous cells of undetermined significance: baseline results from a randomized trial. J Natl Cancer Inst 2001;93(4):293–9.
26. Wright TC Jr, Cox JT, Massad LS, et al. 2001 Consensus Guidelines for the management of women with cervical cytological abnormalities. JAMA 2002; 287(16):2120–9.
27. Saslow D, Runowicz CD, Solomon D, et al. American Cancer Society guideline for the early detection of cervical neoplasia and cancer. CA Cancer J Clin 2002; 52(6):342–62.
28. ACOG Committee on Practice Bulletins–Gynecology. ACOG Practice Bulletin No. 109: cervical cytology screening. Obstet Gynecol 2009;114(6):1409–20.
29. Saslow D, Solomon D, Lawson HW, et al. American Cancer Society, American Society for Colposcopy and Cervical Pathology, and American Society for Clinical Pathology screening guidelines for the prevention and early detection of cervical cancer. CA Cancer J Clin 2012 Mar;14:10.
30. Saslow D, Solomon D, Lawson HW, et al. American Cancer Society, American Society for Colposcopy and Cervical Pathology, and American Society for Clinical Pathology screening guidelines for the prevention and early detection of cervical cancer. CA Cancer J Clin 2012;62(3):147–72.
31. Committee on Practice Bulletins–Gynecology. ACOG practice bulletin 131: screening for cervical cancer. Obstet Gynecol 2012;120(5):1222–38.
32. Saraiya M, Berkowitz Z, Yabroff KR, et al. Cervical cancer screening with HPV and the Pap test vs. the Pap test alone: what screening intervals are physicians recommending? Arch Intern Med 2010;170(11):977–85.
33. Lee JW, Berkowitz Z, Saraiya M. Low-risk human papillomavirus testing and other nonrecommended human papillomavirus testing practices among U.S. health care providers. Obstet Gynecol 2011;118(1):4–13.
34. Castle PE, Fetterman B, Thomas CJ, et al. The age-specific relationships of abnormal cytology and human papillomavirus DNA results to the risk of cervical precancer and cancer. Obstet Gynecol 2010;116(1):76–84.
35. Yabroff KR, Saraiya M, Meissner HI, et al. Specialty differences in primary care physician reports of Papanicolaou test screening practices: a national survey, 2006 to 2007. Ann Intern Med 2009;151(9):602–11.
36. Kyrgiou M, Koliopoulos G, Martin-Hirsch P, et al. Obstetric outcomes after conservative treatment for intraepithelial or early invasive cervical lesions: systematic review and meta-analysis. Lancet 2006;367(9509):489–98.
37. Siegel R, Naishadham D, Jemal A. Cancer statistics, 2012. CA Cancer J Clin 2012;62(1):10–29.
38. Freeman HP, Wingrove BK. Excess cervical cancer mortality: a marker for low access to health care in poor communities. Bethesda (MD): National Institutes of Health; 2007. Report No.: 05-5282.
39. Simard EP, Fedewa S, Ma J, et al. Widening socioeconomic disparities in cervical cancer mortality among women in 26 states, 1993-2007. Cancer 2012; 118(20):5110–6.

40. Scarinci IC, Garcia FA, Kobetz E, et al. Cervical cancer prevention: new tools and old barriers. Cancer 2010;116(11):2531–42.
41. Zhao FH, Lewkowitz AK, Chen F, et al. Pooled analysis of a self-sampling HPV DNA test as a cervical cancer primary screening method. J Natl Cancer Inst 2012;104(3):178–88.
42. Balasubramanian A, Kulasingam SL, Baer A, et al. Accuracy and cost-effectiveness of cervical cancer screening by high-risk human papillomavirus DNA testing of self-collected vaginal samples. J Low Genit Tract Dis 2010; 14(3):185–95.
43. Virtanen A, Nieminen P, Luostarinen T, et al. Self-sample HPV tests as an intervention for nonattendees of cervical cancer screening in Finland: a randomized trial. Cancer Epidemiol Biomarkers Prev 2011;20(9):1960–9.
44. Gok M, Heideman DA, van Kemenade FJ, et al. HPV testing on self collected cervicovaginal lavage specimens as screening method for women who do not attend cervical screening: cohort study. BMJ 2010;340:c1040.
45. Gok M, Heideman DA, van Kemenade FJ, et al. Offering self-sampling for human papillomavirus testing to non-attendees of the cervical screening programme: characteristics of the responders. Eur J Cancer 2012;48(12):1799–808.
46. Szarewski A, Cadman L, Mesher D, et al. HPV self-sampling as an alternative strategy in non-attenders for cervical screening–a randomised controlled trial. Br J Cancer 2011;104(6):915–20.
47. Lindell M, Sanner K, Wikstrom I, et al. Self-sampling of vaginal fluid and high-risk human papillomavirus testing in women aged 50 years or older not attending Papanicolaou smear screening. BJOG 2012;119(2):245–8.
48. Castle PE, Rausa A, Walls T, et al. Comparative community outreach to increase cervical cancer screening in the Mississippi Delta. Prev Med 2011;52(6):452–5.
49. Ferlay J, Shin HR, Bray F, et al. GLOBOCAN 2008 v2.0, Cancer incidence and mortality worldwide: IARC CancerBase No. 10. Lyon (France): International Agency for Research on Cancer; 2010.
50. Kitchener HC, Castle PE, Cox JT. Achievements and limitations of cervical cytology screening. Vaccine 2006;24(Suppl 3):S63–70.
51. Qiao YL, Sellors JW, Eder PS, et al. A new HPV-DNA test for cervical-cancer screening in developing regions: a cross-sectional study of clinical accuracy in rural China. Lancet Oncol 2008;9(10):929–36.
52. Schweizer J, Lu PS, Mahoney CW, et al. Feasibility study of a human papillomavirus e6 oncoprotein test for diagnosis of cervical precancer and cancer. J Clin Microbiol 2010;48(12):4646–8.
53. Belinson JL, Du H, Yang B, et al. Improved sensitivity of vaginal self-collection and high-risk human papillomavirus testing. Int J Cancer 2012;130(8):1855–60.
54. Gage JC, Castle PE. Preventing cervical cancer globally by acting locally: if not now, when? J Natl Cancer Inst 2010;102(20):1524–7.
55. Stoler MH, Castle PE, Solomon D, et al. The expanded use of HPV testing in gynecologic practice per ASCCP-guided management requires the use of well-validated assays. Am J Clin Pathol 2007;127(3):1–3.
56. Meijer CJ, Berkhof J, Castle PE, et al. Guidelines for human papillomavirus DNA test requirements for primary cervical cancer screening in women 30 years and older. Int J Cancer 2009;124(3):516–20.

Counseling the Patient with HPV Disease

Maria Lina Diaz, MD

KEYWORDS

- Human papillomavirus • Genital warts • Abnormal cytology
- High-risk HPV DNA test • Colposcopy • Loop electrosurgical excision procedure

KEY POINTS

- Human papillomavirus (HPV) genital infections are a common occurrence in human beings. Most infections are transient with potential oncogenic progression probably limited to cases of persistent high-risk strains.
- The diagnosis, evaluation, and treatment of HPV-related diseases can cause anxiety and distress, and have a negative psychosocial impact on patients.
- Clinicians should have expertise in the natural history of HPV diseases and implement counseling strategies to help patients throughout all stages of diagnosis, evaluation, and treatment.
- The presentation of a patient with HPV disease presents an opportunity for counseling regarding lifestyle modifications, transmission, and HPV vaccination in age-appropriate patients.

As health care providers and patients become more aware of the relationship between human papillomavirus (HPV) and abnormal cytology, as well as lower genital tract diseases (eg, premalignant and malignant anogenital tract conditions), it becomes critical to disclose accurate medical information and counsel the patient effectively and compassionately. It is of upmost importance that the provider not only stay abreast of the latest scientific information regarding HPV diseases but, in addition, develop a strategy for counseling that is educational and informative, as well as minimizing of potential psychological distress. Disclosing information regarding a sexually transmitted virus that is linked to lower genital tract cancers has the potential to instill fear, decreased self-esteem, provoke anxiety and depression, and negatively affect interpersonal relationships. It is, therefore, crucial to develop expertise and ease when disclosing abnormal results to patients. It may be equally important to train ancillary office support staff to do the same so that the patient receives the same message from all medical personnel interacting with them. Clear and concise discussions that

Section of Ambulatory Gynecology, Department of Gynecology, Cleveland Clinic Florida, 2950 Cleveland Clinic Boulevard, Weston, FL 33331, USA
E-mail address: marialinadiazmd@gmail.com

Obstet Gynecol Clin N Am 40 (2013) 391–402
http://dx.doi.org/10.1016/j.ogc.2013.02.003
0889-8545/13/$ – see front matter © 2013 Published by Elsevier Inc.

obgyn.theclinics.com

are appropriately targeted toward the patients' level of medical literacy, are appropriately timed, and include supportive undertones may minimize psychological damage and avoid adversely affecting patients and their partners. It is important to recognize that the presentation of a patient with HPV disease provides an opportunity to screen for other sexually transmitted diseases (STDs) and identify and modify high-risk sexual behaviors, as well as provide a means to increase awareness of HPV-related diseases. Finally, many of these clinical presentations represent an opportunity to encourage patients to accept HPV vaccination counseling and immunization.

INTRODUCTION

HPV acquisition is virtually ubiquitous among human beings. Many studies support the finding that HPV infections are common shortly after the sexual debut. A hallmark study that is often cited demonstrated that a significant portion of sexually naïve female college students became HPV-positive within several years of sexual debut.[1] HPV, a double-stranded DNA virus, is divided into two strains: nononcogenic or low-risk HPV (LR-HPV), and oncogenic or high-risk HPV (HR-HPV). It is recognized that genital warts are mainly caused by nononcogenic HPV strains, principally 6 and 11.[2] Recurrent laryngeal papillomatosis, benign growths of papillomas caused mainly from HPV 6 and 11 in the respiratory tree, can pose problems for children born of infected mothers[3] and for some adults who may acquire the infections from sexual activity.[4] HR-HPV strains, particularly 16 and 18, are implicated in abnormal cytology, cervical intraepithelial neoplasms, cervical cancer, and anal squamous cell carcinomas.[5] Additionally, HR-HPV is implicated in vaginal intraepithelial neoplasms and vaginal carcinomas,[6] as well as in vulvar intraepithelial neoplasms and vulvar carcinomas.[7] Finally, there is a growing body of evidence implicating HR-HPV in a significant portion of squamous cell carcinomas of the oropharynx.[8]

It is important to understand and to counsel patients that HPV infections are usually transient and do not represent risk for progression. Persistence of oncogenic HPV, however, is a prerequisite for cervical cancer. In the small segment of women with this type of infection, the process of oncogenesis can be lengthy, allowing ample opportunity for identifying and successfully treating premalignant cervical conditions. It may be useful to counsel patients that most cervical cancers occur in never-screened or underscreened women.[9] There are recognized factors and cofactors that may play a role in oncogenesis in the case of cervical cancer. Risk factors for cervical cancer include early age at onset of sexual activity, multiple sexual partners, having high-risk sexual partners, and high parity. Another risk factor for the development of cervical cancer is history of STDs, specifically Chlamydia trachomatis[10] and herpes simplex virus.[11] Other risk factors include cigarette smoking[12] and prolonged use of oral contraceptive pills,[13] particularly in adenocarcinoma of the cervix.[14] An incompetent immune system, such as in the cases of women with HIV,[15] and immunosuppressive drugs, such as in the cases of transplant recipients,[16] may also play a role in the body's ability to clear HPV infections, allowing for persistence of the viral infection that may facilitate oncogenesis. Patients can be made aware of prevention strategies such as delaying intercourse until age 21, limiting the number of sexual partners, avoiding high-risk sexual partners, and avoiding of tobacco products. Additionally, the consistent use of condoms has shown to decrease the incidence of cervical and vulvovaginal HPV infections in women.[17] There is a concern that condom use is limited because condoms do not entirely cover exposed sexual skin during intercourse and, therefore, leaves these areas vulnerable to skin-to skin transmission of HPV infections. Interestingly, in a review of the evidence comparing the HPV vaccines to condoms in the prevalence of HPV infections, the greatest degree of protection from specific types of HPV infection was provided by the vaccines. However, the investigator noted that the use of condoms in addition to the HPV vaccines provides the greatest protection from the untoward effects of HPV infection and may provide protection against HPV types and other STDs not in the vaccine.[18] Because other STDs are potential cofactors in the development of cervical cancer, the consistent use of condoms should be recommended to patients who are at risk for contracting these diseases.

The introduction of the HPV vaccines has provided a novel approach to the prevention of cervical cancer and other HPV-related diseases. The prophylactic HPV vaccines include the quadrivalent and the bivalent HPV vaccines. The quadrivalent HPV vaccine provides immunogenicity against HPV 6, 11, 16, and 18. The vaccine is indicated in women for the prevention of cervical, vulvar, vaginal, and anal cancers caused by HPV 16,18; cervical precancers (cervical intraepithelial neoplasia [CIN] 2/3) and adenocarcinoma in situ (AIS); CIN 1; vulvar intraepithelial neoplasia 2/3, vaginal intraepithelial neoplasia 2/3, and anal intraepithelial neoplasia 1/2/3; and genital warts and CIN caused by HPV types 6 and 11.[19] To date, the quadrivalent HPV vaccine is the only vaccine with indications for women and men and has been approved for the prevention of genital warts (caused by HPV 6 and 11), anal cancer (caused by HPV 16 and 18), and AIS 1/2/3 caused by HPV 6, 11, 16, or 18 in men. The bivalent vaccine, which provides immunogenicity against HPV 16 and 18, has indications for the prevention of cervical cancer and CIN 2, and, worse, AIS and CIN 1.[20] Both vaccines are especially effective in prevention of the respective HPV-related diseases studied when administered to sexually naïve individuals, but they also are effective in patients who have initiated sexual activity. The Advisory Committee on Immunization Practices, the Centers for Disease Control, and the American College of Obstetricians and Gynecologist recommend vaccine administration to girls and women aged 9 to 26 years.[21–23] It has been shown that, in the United States, the HPV vaccination capture rate lags behind many other countries and sadly represents a lost opportunity for prevention of HPV diseases. Clinicians caring for young women should not only emphasize the safety profile of the vaccines[24] but also the benefits of vaccination to nonvaccinated or incompletely vaccinated patients.

The role of the clinician in making an impact toward modifying high-risk behaviors is perhaps underestimated. A Cochrane review of behavioral interventions for young women to encourage safer sexual behaviors to prevent transmission of STDs, including HPV, showed that these interventions can be effective, primarily in encouraging condom use.[25] Women's health care providers are in a unique position to positively affect their patients' health by educating and counseling them regarding preventative measures, including healthy lifestyle practices and regular age-appropriate screenings and vaccinations that can reduce the burden of HPV disease. **Box 1** summarizes key points to discuss with all patients when counseling regarding modifiable lifestyle changes that are protective against HPV diseases.

External Genital Warts

Genital warts are a common sexually transmitted infection and, therefore, the cost of the evaluation and treatment of genital warts is staggering to our society. In the United States, it is estimated that there are more than 300,000 annual visits to health care providers for this.[26] Because of the obvious visibility of external genital lesions and because of the physical discomfort associated with treatment, the diagnosis of genital warts, despite their largely asymptomatic nature, proves to be quite distressing to most patients. The incubation period of genital warts ranges between 2 to 3 months

Box 1
Key points to discuss with all patients
Regular condom use
Limitation of number of sexual partners
Tobacco cessation or avoidance
Routine screening for sexually transmitted infections
Adherence to age-appropriate Papanicolaou (Pap) smear screening schedule
HPV vaccination in age-appropriate cases

and genital warts are quite infectious with an infectivity rate of 64%.[27] Although HPV 6 and 11 are responsible for 90% of genital warts, patients may have coinfection with oncogenic HPV types because higher risks of anogenital cancers are reported in patients with a history of genital warts.[28] Therefore, it is important to screen genital wart patients for multicentric HPV disease. Other considerations in the evaluation and treatment of patients with genital warts is screening for other STDS because some studies report a significant prevalence of chlamydia and gonorrhea in these patients.[29]

Treatment of external genital warts include medical and surgical methods. Medical methods include local application of chemodestructive therapies, which can be further subdivided into provider-applied versus patient-applied treatment. The provider-applied chemodestructive agents include bichloroacetic or trichloroacetic acid and podophyllin. The bichloroacetic or trichloroacetic acid therapies act by denaturing or precipitating proteins, thus destroying the genital wart and affected mucosa and skin.[30] Podophyllin therapy works by blocking cell division at metaphase and promoting cell death.[31] Both methods may cause pain and irritation to surrounding skin and measures can be taken, such as applying paraffin to surrounding skin before application or neutralizing excess acid with either bicarbonate or talc. Patient-applied therapies include podophyllin, imiquimod, and sinecatechins. The immune-modulating imiquimod,[32] as well as the botanic ointment sinecatechins,[33] can cause local skin irritation that can be managed by temporarily prolonging treatment intervals. Surgical management of genital warts includes excisional removal of condylomas through traditional excision with scalpel or electrosurgical procedures. Laser ablation of genital warts for extensive involvement is usually undertaken in the surgical suite with general anesthesia. An outpatient ablative technique is cryosurgery with nitrous oxide. Because these treatments have a significant failure rates, careful follow-up and surveillance is important. Immunocompromised patients may have more difficulty clearing genital warts and are at higher risk for recurrence.

Psychosexual vulnerability along with depression, anxiety, and anger have been reported by patients with genital warts.[34] In other studies, the negative psychological and social effect of the diagnosis and treatment of genital warts included anxiety about love and sexual life, stigma of the diagnosis of a venereal disease, distress about uncertain treatment times and success, and concerns regarding transmission to others, as well as anger, fear of HPV-related malignancies, depression, self-loathing, and worries about the future.[35] During the diagnosis and treatment of genital warts, the clinician should consider not only the patient's physical healing but also the emotional impact and implications of the diagnosis. During counseling following the diagnosis of genital warts, a brief description of the natural history of genital warts, method of acquisition, and transmissibility, as well as a discussion of treatment options, is essential. Patients should be counseled regarding the sometimes protracted course of treatment to establish a realistic and, therefore, not disappointing time frame for resolution. When counseling patients with genital warts, it has been recommended that shared decision making between patient and clinician may help a patient make more informed decisions, be compliant with the chosen treatment, and make lifestyle modifications that may help reduce the risk of HPV transmission, including informing current or new sexual partners.[36]

In a national survey that examined messages US clinicians practice when counseling patients with anogenital warts, most providers reported counseling patients regarding STD prevention, including condoms, limiting sexual partners, or practicing monogamy or abstinence.[37] Providers in this survey identified potential barriers to counseling, including definitive answers about to now the HPV infection was acquired, dealing with patients' psychological issues, and adequate reimbursement. Patients often focus on identifying a partner to blame and may try to engage the provider in this activity. Redirecting the conversation and focusing on the treatment needed to resolve the patient's genital warts and perhaps recommending that current partner or partners be evaluated may be a better approach. The accurate documentation of the time spent counseling the patient may overcome the concerns regarding reimbursement. Additionally, written information that reinforces the discussion seems to be appreciated and should be offered in a patient's preferred language, if available. However, it should never be substituted for face-to-face counseling. **Box 2** summarizes key points to discuss with patients with genital warts.

Abnormal Cytology and/or HR-HPV Testing

With the advent of HR-HPV DNA testing as part of cervical cancer screening, more and more women are recognizing and understanding that HR-HPV is the necessary agent for the development of abnormal Papanicolaou (Pap) smears and premalignant lesions of the cervix, as well as of cervical cancer. Before this development, it was not uncommon to inform women of abnormal cytology results without disclosing that the abnormality was due to the presence of a sexually acquired infectious viral agent. HR-HPV DNA testing became available in the United States in 2004. Current applications of this test include the triage of atypical squamous cells of undetermined significance from Pap smear results, cotesting of women 30 years and older as part of routine a cervical cancer screening program, and the posttreatment surveillance of CIN. Owing to the addition of the HR-HPV DNA test in these clinical settings, women are learning that they have tested positive for the HPV virus, many times in the setting of a normal Pap smear. It has been demonstrated that, irrespective of cytologic status, women who test positive for the HPV DNA test experience more anxiety and distress than women who test negative and, additionally, feel worse about their sexual

---

Box 2
Key points to discuss with genital wart patients

Natural history of genital warts

Treatment options and time frame for resolution

Recurrence rate and need for posttreatment surveillance

Modifiable risk factors (condom use, limiting numbers of sexual partners, smoking cessation)

Screening for other STDs

Quadrivalent HPV vaccination if age-appropriate

relationships.[38] Keeping in mind that it is distressing for patients to learn they are positive for HR-HPV, it becomes important to use the test appropriately. A concerning observation is that, despite the aforementioned approved indications of the HR-HPV DNA testing, surveys have demonstrated inappropriate use of this test,[39] which may subject many patients to undue and unnecessary psychological distress. Examples of inappropriate use of HPV DNA testing includes cotesting women less than 30 years of age and the use of LR-HPV DNA testing in any clinical setting.

When discussing abnormal cytologic and or HR-HPV DNA testing, the clinician should recognize that, for many patients, this is a distressing situation and patients may experience a host of unpleasant reactions. Some of these reactions may be due to lack of knowledge or familiarity with the HPV, which may lead a patient to feel vulnerable owing to fear, stigma, and confusion regarding her diagnosis. A patient may express anger at her partner for exposing her to the virus and fear that their partner has been unfaithful. Younger patients may misinterpret the results to indicate that they will not be able to have children. Older patients may be less concerned about perceived loss of fertility but more concerned regarding the possibility of infidelity or shortened lifespan due to cancer. The clinician should be aware of potential emotional reactions and ask open-ended question in a nonjudgmental and reassuring manner. It is crucial to explain the disease process in language the patient can understand. It may be equally inappropriate to simplify information to a highly educated patient as it is to speak in scientific terminology to a medically illiterate patient.

When reviewing the literature pertaining to the emotional reactions and feelings that patients experience on learning of an abnormal Pap smear or HR-HPV status, one can find several studies that were conducted as surveys to patients in these clinical scenarios. Much can be learned from reviewing these studies to formulate counseling strategies that support patients and minimize the psychological burden associated with abnormal results. Many times, patients express a desire to have their health care provider be the primary source of education regarding their disease process and secondarily defer to their close social contacts and the Internet.[40] A study of 10 demographically diverse women with a history of at least one abnormal pap smear demonstrated that the initial anxiety on learning of the diagnosis was followed by urgent need for information and that information obtained from health care providers was deemed supportive if facts were accompanied by reassurance. Using too much medical jargon, not enough time spent explaining the information, or perceived lack of interpersonal concerns was viewed as nonsupportive.[41] Many patients struggle with a negative influence on sexuality and report difficulties with relationships and may enlist the help of the clinician in trying to determine from whom they may have contracted HPV. It is usually best to explain to the patient that it may be impossible to determine this. It is important to impart to the patient that although HPV infections are common, particularly in younger women, the development of cervical cancer is actually rare in screened populations. Reassuring the patient and removing the stigma of the diagnosis of a sexually acquired viral disease process, helps redirect the conversation toward the necessary next steps for her evaluation.

A significant counseling dilemma can arise when a woman has negative cytology but positive HR-HPV on cotesting. In a recent study, this combination of results occurred 3.7% in women more than 30 years old.[42] Currently, there are two accepted management algorithms for the management of this combination. The first scenario is to repeat both the cytology and the HR-HPV test in 1 year. This is an accepted option because the probability of significant pathologic disease is very low in this group.[43] The second option is to pursue immediate HPV genotype-specific testing for HPV 16 or HPV 16/18. Women who test positive for HPV 16 or HPV 16/18 are then triaged to immediate colposcopy. Women who test negative are rescreened with cytology and HR-HPV testing in 1 year. For some women, being told they have an HPV infection but, because their pap is normal, they will be rescreened again in 1 year may be distressing. It is not uncommon for the clinician to be challenged on the perception they are "doing nothing" and "letting this go on unchecked". It is important to explain to the patient that most HPV infections are transient and that only in cases of persistence of the HR-HPV virus does the potential for cancer exist. Patients who seem anxious about potential HR-HPV results may be counseled regarding genotyping to reduce their anxiety of having to wait 1 year for additional testing. **Boxes 3–5** summarize key points to include when counseling patients with abnormal cytology and/or HR-HPV results, colposcopy candidates, and CIN patients.

COLPOSCOPY

For patients who are candidates for colposcopy, a thoughtful explanation of this diagnostic test is important to increase knowledge and satisfaction with the procedure and should be delivered by a provider or extender who is competent to discuss the topic in a reassuring manner. In a study of women attending a colposcopy clinic, women reported preferring to receive information about colposcopy at or before the time of receiving their abnormal results.[44] At minimum, a preliminary discussion of what the procedure involves and the rationale behind it should be offered to the patient with a more comprehensive counseling session scheduled with time for questions with the provider at time of the colposcopy. Although a study demonstrated that women scheduled for colposcopy have a similar level of mild anxiety and depression as women scheduled for a primary care appointment,[45] some patients are highly anxious and distressed in anticipation of the procedure. Patients express fear of experiencing pain during the procedure, and express fear and uncertainty about the results the procedure may reveal. It has been shown that isolated distribution of informational leaflets before colposcopy is not useful in reducing anxiety or psychosexual scores.[46] Studies also suggest that informational discussions before colposcopy, either on the telephone[47] or in sessions with colposcopy nurses,[48] do little to reduce patient anxiety but are important in improving knowledge scores and satisfaction. In a meta-analysis that reviewed mean differences of anxiety levels, knowledge scores, pain, patient satisfaction, and psychosexual dysfunction in women who underwent colposcopy it seemed that playing music during colposcopy reduced anxiety and pain experienced.[49] Other strategies to help reduce patient stress include the prescription of mild anxiolytics in extreme cases of anxiety, allowing supportive family members in the examination room, and offering the patient the opportunity to view their procedure (if the technology in the examination room allows). Even if the patient declines to view the procedure, having the choice may be beneficial because it restores a small portion control to the patient.

Box 3
Key points to discuss with abnormal cytology/HR-HPV patients
HPV genital infections are common and most are transient
Cervical cancer develops slowly, allowing ample opportunity for detection and treatment in premalignant states
Cervical cancer is rare in screened populations
Colposcopy is a diagnostic tool that helps determine degree of HPV effect on the cervix

> **Box 4**
> **Key points for colposcopy candidates**
>
> Colposcopy is a diagnostic tool that helps determine the degree of HPV effect on cervix
>
> Biopsies can be uncomfortable but most patients describe mild cramping that is not prolonged
>
> Playing music during procedure reduces anxiety
>
> Treatment plan is based on correlation between cytology, colposcopic impression, and biopsy results

Management and Treatment of Cervical Dysplasia

Once the colposcopic evaluation has been completed, patients are traditionally counseled on their results and offered a treatment plan. When possible, this session is best scheduled for a face-to-face discussion with the provider. Patients may have a lot of fears, anxieties, and questions that may not be optimally determined and addressed on the telephone. If a face-to-face session is not feasible and the provider uses clinical staff to discuss results and impart recommendations for treatment plans, it is important that the staff be knowledgeable and competent in discussing the many nuances that may come up on the telephone. This expertise and comfort in counseling patients usually comes from highly trained ancillary staff members who have either acquired this information during on-the-job training or have taken targeted courses on this topic.

Patients with mild cytologic intraepithelial lesions on colposcopic-directed biopsies may be counseled regarding the high rate of spontaneous regression of low-grade lesions and of the American Society for Colposcopy and Cervical Pathology 2006 consensus guidelines that allow for observation of these lesions.[50] The patient should be counseled to understand that, although observation is encouraged in these cases, it must be coupled with excellent compliance with surveillance visits. Various patient-level interventions are effective in increasing follow-up rates and include mail and telephone reminders, telephone counseling, and print educational interventions.[51]

In patients receiving recommendations for treatment of CIN due to abnormal cytology and histology, much of the distress experienced may attributable to the lack of easily understandable information about the significance of the abnormality and the misperception of a cancer diagnosis. Furthermore, it has been shown that face-to-face individualized education and support after colposcopy with informational booklets as a background for discussion can decrease a patients' distress at

> **Box 5**
> **Key points to discuss with CIN patients**
>
> CIN 1 lesions have a high degree of spontaneous resolution and can often be observed
>
> In cases of observation, compliance with follow-up visits is important
>
> CIN is not cervical cancer
>
> Treatments for CIN are very effective
>
> Loop electrosurgical excision procedure (LEEP) may be associated with the pregnancy complication of preterm delivery
>
> It is important to adhere to posttreatment surveillance appointments

subsequent treatment visits.[52] Counseling before the procedure should include the rationale for the treatment, details regarding logistics of the procedure, pain control strategies routinely used during the procedure, and the need for posttreatment surveillance. Women undergoing treatment of CIN who are interested in future childbearing, should be counseled that the procedure may place them at higher risk for pregnancy complications such as preterm delivery, premature rupture of membranes, and low-birthweight infants. Studies on pregnancy after loop electrosurgical excision procedure (LEEP) are limited by differing methodologies and lack of information on potential confounders, as well as lack of data on LEEP depth, volume of tissue excised, or the degree of neoplasia prompting the procedure itself.[53] There is some evidence that women undergoing conization with either cold knife technique or LEEP have an increased risk of preterm delivery before the 34th week,[54] although recently it has been observed that increasing the depth of cervical cone removed by LEEP is directly associated with preterm delivery.[55] Although the exact relationship between LEEP and pregnancy complications may be difficult to study, it is best to make patients aware of the potential issues should a pregnancy after LEEP be a consideration. In cases in which cryosurgery is recommended, patients should be counseled that pregnancy complications are not observed[56] but that the procedure can be uncomfortable due to cramps, hydrorrhea, and odor.[57] Regardless of treatment option, patients should be counseled regarding the importance of posttreatment surveillance and the clinician should have protocols in place for the recall of patients who have undergone treatment.

SUMMARY

The clinician plays an important role in counseling the patient with HPV disease. It is paramount that the clinician have an excellent understanding of the natural history of HPV disease and is able to relay this information to the patient in a manner that is educational, timely, and understandable. It is equally important to relay this information in a manner that is supportive and reassuring. The diagnosis, evaluation, and treatment of HPV diseases across the board are anxiety-provoking to patients and are capable of producing significant negative psychosocial and psychosexual disturbances. Having ancillary staff partner in the understanding of HPV disease and in appropriate counseling strategies is important to the patient because this facilitates the similar messages being voiced by all individuals involved in her care, eliminating confusion and further unnecessary anxiety. Finally, the clinical presentation of the patient with HPV disease presents a unique opportunity to counsel.

REFERENCES

1. Winer RL, Lee SK, Hughes JP, et al. Genital human papillomavirus infection: incidence and risk factors in a cohort of female university students. Am J Epidemiol 2003;157:218–26.
2. Brown DR, Schroeder JM, Bryan JY, et al. Detection of multiple human papillomavirus types in condyloma acuminata lesions from otherwise healthy and immuno-compromised patients. J Clin Microbiol 1999;37:3316–22.
3. Quick CA, Watts SL, Krzyzek RA, et al. Relationship between condyloma and laryngeal papillomata. Clinical and molecular evidence. Ann Otol Rhinol Laryngol 1980;89:467–71.
4. Kashima HK, Shah F, Lyles A, et al. A comparison of risk factors in juvenile-onset and adult-onset recurrent respiratory papillomatosis. Laryngoscope 1992;102: 9–13.

5. Koutsky LA, Galloway DA, Holmes KK. Epidemiology of genital human papilloma-virus infection. Epidemiol Rev 1988;10:122–63.
6. Wharton JT, Totolero-Luna G, Linares AC, et al. Vaginal intraepithelial neoplasia and vaginal cancer. Obstet Gynecol Clin North Am 1996;23:325–45.
7. Jones RW, Rowan DM. Vulvar intraepithelial neoplasia III: a clinical study of the outcome in 113 cases with relation to the later development of invasive vulvar carcinoma. Obstet Gynecol 1994;84:741–5.
8. Gillison ML, Koch WM, Copone RB, et al. Evidence for causal association between Human Papillomavirus and a subset of head and neck cancers. J Natl Cancer Inst 2000;92:709–20.
9. Sung HY, Keaerney KA, Miller M, et al. Papanicolaou smear history and the diag-nosis of invasive cervical cancer among members of a large prepaid health plan. Cancer 2000;88:2283–9.
10. Herrington CS. Human papilloma virus and cervical neoplasia II. Interaction of HPV with other factors. J Clin Pathol 1995;48:1.
11. Smith JS, Herrero R, Boseetti C, et al. Herpes simplex virus-2 as a human papil-lomavirus cofactor in the etiology of invasive cervical cancer. J Natl Cancer Inst 2002;94:1604–13.
12. Plummer M, Herrero R, Franceschi S, et al. Smoking and cervical cancer: pooled analysis of the IARC multicentric case-control study. Cancer Causes Control 2003;14:805–14.
13. Moreno V, Bosch FX, Munoz N, et al. International agency for research on cancer multicentric cervical cancer study group. Effect of oral contraceptives on risk of cervical cancer in women with human papillomavirus infection: the IARC multi-centric case-control study. Lancet 2002;359:1085–92.
14. Chilvers C, Mant D, Pike MC. Cervical adenocarcinoma and oral contraceptives. BMJ 1987;295:1446–7.
15. Levi JE, Kleter B, Quint WG, et al. High prevalence of human papillomavirus (HPV) infections and high risk frequency of multiple HPV genotypes in human immuno-deficiency virus-infected women in Brazil. J Clin Microbiol 2002;40:3341–5.
16. Penn I. Cancers of the anogenital region in renal transplant patients. Cancer 1986;58:611–6.
17. Winer RL, Hughes JP, Fen Q, et al. Condom use and the risk of genital human papillomavirus infection in young women. N Engl J Med 2006;354:2645–54.
18. Miksis S. A review of the evidence comparing the human papillomavirus vaccine versus condoms in the prevention of human papillomavirus infections. J Obstet Gynecol Neonatal Nurs 2008;37:329–37.
19. Gardasil [package insert]. Whitehouse Station, NJ: Merck and CO, Inc; 2010. Available at: http://www.fda.gov/downloads/BiologicsBloodVaccines/Vaccines/ApprovedProducts/UCM111263.pdf. Accessed December 8, 2012.
20. Cervarix [package insert]. Rixensart, Belgium: GlaxoSmithKline Biologists; 2011. Available at: http://www.fda.gov/downloads/BiologicsBloodVaccines/Vaccines/ApprovedProducts/UCM186981.pdf. Accessed December 8, 2012.
21. Centers for Disease Control and Prevention (CDC). FDA licensure of bivalent human papillomavirus vaccine (HPV2, Cervarix) for use in females and updated HPV vaccination recommendations from the Advisory Committee on Immuniza-tions Practices (ACIP) [Erratum appears in MMWR Morb Mortal Wkly Rep 2010;59:1184]. MMWR Morb Mortal Wkly Rep 2010;59:626–9.
22. Markowits LE, Dunne EF, Saraiya M, et al. Quadrivalent human papillomavirus vaccines: recommendations of the Advisory Committee of Immunization Prac-tices (ACIP). MMWR Recomm Rep 2007;56(RR–2):1–24.

23. Human papillomavirus vaccination. Committee Opinion No.467. American College of Obstetricians and Gynecologists. Obstet Gynecol 2010;116:800–3.
24. Velicer C. Post-licensure safety study of quadrivalent human papillomavirus vaccines among 189,629 females. Paper presented at: advisory committee on immunization practices meeting. Atlanta, October 25, 2011. Available at: http://www.cdc.gov/VACCINes/recs/acip/downloads/mtg-slides-oct11/03-HPV-CVelicer.pdf. Accessed November 27, 2012.
25. Shepherd JP, Fampton GK, Harris P. Interventions for encouraging sexual behaviours intended to prevent cervical cancer. Cochrane Database Syst Rev 2011;(12):CD001035.
26. Department of Health and Human Services and Centers for Disease Control and Prevention. STD surveillance. 2004.
27. Garland SM, Quinn MA. How to manage and communicate with patients about HPV? Int J Gynecol Obstet 2006;94(Suppl 1):S106–12.
28. Koutsky L. Epidemiology of genital human papillomavirus infection. Am J Med 1997;102:3–8.
29. Sturgiss EA, Jin F, Martin SJ, et al. Prevalence of other sexually transmissible infections in patients with newly diagnosed anogenital warts in a sexual health clinic. Sex Health 2010;7:55–9.
30. Wiley DJ, Douglas J, Beutner K, et al. External genital warts: diagnosis, treatment and prevention. Clin Infect Dis 2002;35:S210–24.
31. Helberg D, Svarrer T, Nilsson E, et al. Self treatment of female genital warts with 0.5% podophyllotoxin cream (Condyline) vs weekly applications of 20% podophyllin solution. Int J STD AIDS 1995;6:257–61.
32. Sauder DN, Skinner RB, Fox TL, et al. Topical imiquimod 5% cream as an effective treatment for external genital and perianal warts in different patient populations. Sex Transm Dis 2003;30:124–8.
33. Tatti S, Swinehart JM, Thielert C, et al. Sinecatechins, a defined green tree extract, in the treatment of external genital warts: a randomized controlled trial. Obstet Gynecol 2008;111:1371–9.
34. Graziottin A, Serafini A. HPV infection in women: psychosexual impact of genital warts and intraepithelial lesions. J Sex Med 2009;3:633–45.
35. Mortansen GL, Larsen HK. The quality of life of patients with genital warts: a qualitative study. BMC Public Health 2010;10:113.
36. Steben M, Labelle D. Genital warts: Canadians' perception, health-related behaviors and treatment preferences. J Low Genit Tract Dis 2012;4:409–15.
37. Henderson Z, Irwin KL, Montana DE, et al. Anogenital warts knowledge and counseling practices of US clinicians:results from a national survey. Sex Transm Dis 2007;34:644–52.
38. McCaffery K, Waller J, Forrest S, et al. Testing positive for human papillomavirus in routine cervical screening: examination of psychosocial impact. BJOG 2004;111:1437–43.
39. Irwin K, Monatano D, Kasprzyk D, et al. Cervical cancer screening, abnormal cytology management, and counseling practices in the United States. Obstet Gynecol 2006;108:397–409.
40. Monsonego J, Cortes J, da Silva DP, et al. Psychological impact, support and information needs for women with an abnormal Pap smear: comparative results of a questionnaire in three European countries. BMC Womens Health 2011;11:18.
41. Bertram CC, Magnussen L. Information needs and the experiences of women with abnormal Papanicolaou smears. J Am Acad Nurse Pract 2008;20:455–62.

42. Katki HA, Kinney WK, Fetterman B, et al. Cervical cancer risk for women undergoing concurrent testing for human papillomavirus and cervical cytology: a population based study in routine practice [Erratum appears in Lancet Oncol 2011;12:722]. Lancet Oncol 2011;12:663–72.
43. Saslow D, Solomon D, Lawson HW, et al. American Cancer Society, American Society for Colposcopy and Cervical Pathology, and American Society for Clinical Pathology screening guidelines for the prevention and early detection of cervical cancer. CA Cancer J Clin 2012;62:147–72.
44. Byrom J, Dunn PD, Hughes GM, et al. Colposcopy information leaflets: what women want to know and when they want to receive this information. J Med Screen 2003;10:143–7.
45. Ferris DG, Gilman PA, Leyva Lopez AG, et al. Psychological effects women experience before and after a colposcopic examination and primary care appointment. J Low Genit Tract Dis 2003;7:89–94.
46. Howells RE, Dunn PD, Isasi T, et al. Is the provision of information leaflets before colposcopy beneficial? A prospective randomized study. Br J Obstet Gynaecol 1999;106:528–34.
47. de Bie RP, Massuger LF, Lenselink CH, et al. The role of individually targeted information to reduce anxiety before colposcopy: a randomized control trial. BJOG 2011;118:945–50.
48. Byrom J, Clarke T, Neale J, et al. Can pre-colposcopy sessions reduce anxiety at the time of colposcopy? A prospective randomized study. J Obstet Gynaecol 2002;22:415–20.
49. Galaal K, Bryant A, Deane KH, et al. Interventions for reducing anxiety in women undergoing colposcopy. Cochrane Database Syst Rev 2011;(7):CD006013.
50. Wright TC, Massad LS, Dunton CJ, et al. 2006 consensus guidelines for the management of women with cervical intraepithelial neoplasia or adenocarcinoma in situ. J Low Genit Tract Dis 2007;11:223–39.
51. Bastani R, Yabroff KR, Myers RE, et al. Interventions to improve follow-up of abnormal findings in cancer screening. Cancer 2004;101:1188–200.
52. Le T, Hopkins L, Menard C, et al. Psychologic morbidities prior to loop electrosurgical excision procedure in the treatment of cervical intraepithelial neoplasia. Int J Gynecol Cancer 2006;16:1089–93.
53. Werner C, Lo JY, Heffernan T, et al. Loop electrosurgical excision procedure and risk of preterm birth. Obstet Gynecol 2010;115:605–8.
54. Armarnik S, Sheiner E, Piura B, et al. Obstetric outcome following conization. Arch Gynecol Obstet 2011;283:765–9.
55. Noehr B, Jensen A, Frederiksen K, et al. Depth of cervical cone removed by loop electrosurgical excision procedure and subsequent risk of spontaneous preterm delivery. Obstet Gynecol 2009;114:1232–8.
56. Hemmingsson E. Outcome of third-trimester pregnancies after cryotherapy of the uterine cervix. Br J Obstet Gynaecol 1982;82:675–7.
57. Harper DM, Mayeaux EJ, Daaleman TP, et al. Healing experiences after cervical cryosurgery. J Fam Pract 2000;49:701–6.

Index

Note: Page numbers of article titles are in **boldface** type.

Obstet Gynecol Clin N Am 40 (2013) 403–411
http://dx.doi.org/10.1016/S0889-8545(13)00046-6
0889-8545/13/$ – see front matter © 2013 Elsevier Inc. All rights reserved.

Printed and bound by CPI Group (UK) Ltd, Croydon, CR0 4YY

03/10/2024

01040436-0003